Nailfold Capillaroscopy in Rheumatological Diseases

Ariane L. Herrick • Andrea Murray
Chris Taylor • Vanessa Smith
Maurizio Cutolo
Editors

Nailfold Capillaroscopy in Rheumatological Diseases

Springer

Editors
Ariane L. Herrick
Centre for Musculoskeletal Research, Division of Musculoskeletal and Dermatological Sciences
The University of Manchester, Manchester Academic Health Science Centre
Manchester, UK

Northern Care Alliance NHS Foundation Trust
Salford, UK

National Institute for Health and Care Research (NIHR) Manchester Biomedical Research Centre
Manchester, UK

Department of Rheumatology
Aberdeen Royal Infirmary, NHS Grampian
Aberdeen, UK

Centre for Arthritis and Musculoskeletal Health, University of Aberdeen
Aberdeen, UK

Chris Taylor
School of Engineering and School of Health Sciences
University of Manchester
Manchester, UK

Maurizio Cutolo
Laboratory of Experimental Rheumatology, Division of Rheumatology, Department of Internal Medicine and Medical Specialties (DiMI)
University of Genova, IRCCS San Martino Polyclinic Hospital
Genova, Italy

Andrea Murray
Centre for Musculoskeletal Research, Division of Musculoskeletal and Dermatological Sciences
The University of Manchester, Manchester Academic Health Science Centre
Manchester, UK

Northern Care Alliance NHS Foundation Trust
Salford, UK

National Institute for Health and Care Research (NIHR) Manchester Biomedical Research Centre
Manchester, UK

Vanessa Smith
Department of Internal Medicine/(Rheumatology)
Ghent University (Hospital), and Unit for Molecular Immunology and Inflammation, VIB Inflammation Research Center (IRC)
Ghent, Belgium

ISBN 978-3-032-03969-9 ISBN 978-3-032-03970-5 (eBook)
https://doi.org/10.1007/978-3-032-03970-5

This Springer imprint is published by the registered company Springer Nature Switzerland AG
The registered company address is: Gewerbestrasse 11, 6330 Cham, Switzerland

Foreword

Examination of the microcirculation, and specifically the capillary bed in the nailfolds of the fingers, has emerged as an unlikely but extremely powerful approach to diagnosis, management and understanding of autoimmune rheumatic disease. This specialised field has evolved over past decades with advances in the methods for visualisation of the nailfold capillaries and much better practical training for clinicians. More recently there has been remarkable progress in standardisation and validation of assessment leading to inclusion of capillaroscopy as an endpoint in clinical trials. This has provided the foundations for capillaroscopy to move into mainstream clinical medicine and to realise its full potential. Specifically, modern nailfold capillaroscopy tools provide opportunity to directly observe, record and analyse changes in structure and appearance of the microcirculation and have elucidated important clinical correlates.

Incorporation of disease-specific nailfold capillaroscopy abnormalities into the validated classification criteria for systemic sclerosis, published in 2013, was a landmark for the field because it facilitated earlier and more precise detection and diagnosis of this challenging disease. It also fuelled interest in defining and studying early-stage systemic sclerosis, raising the potential for future early intervention strategies for connective tissue disease.

This book provides the reader with unparalleled and comprehensive insight into all aspects of nailfold capillaroscopy. It covers a remarkable history of individuals that had the foresight to see its potential, and reviews technical advances in assessment and the exciting opportunities for automation, centralisation of assessment and computerised image analysis, including by machine learning and artificial intelligence. For the clinician there is expert guidance and demonstration of patterns of abnormality that are seen in practice. In this way the book also serves as an atlas of wonderful illustrative images that can be used as a reference source for those already proficient in capillaroscopy. Case reports and clinical examples illustrate how capillaroscopy helps in diagnosis and management of important rheumatic diseases in adults and children.

The future is indeed bright for nailfold capillaroscopy and this textbook, written by leading international experts, is a wonderful addition to the field.

Christopher P. Denton
Division of Medicine
University College London (UCL)
London, UK

Preface

It has been recognised for over 300 years that small blood vessels, capillaries, can be visualised under magnification at the nailfold. This 'experiment of nature', whereby capillaries at the nailfold run parallel rather than perpendicular to the skin surface, provides the basis for the technique of nailfold capillaroscopy which provides a unique, non-invasive window into the microcirculation. Advances in our understanding of the microcirculation, alongside technological advances, have led to an explosion of interest in the technique over the last 30 years. In this book we aim to bring together these advances and to provide the reader with updates on methods and applications of nailfold capillaroscopy, and to give pointers as to how the technique is likely to develop further in the coming years, both in clinical practice and in the research setting.

The book begins with an account of the history of nailfold capillaroscopy, highlighting the seminal work of Hildegard Maricq, who in the 1970s laid the foundations for the role of nailfold capillaroscopy in rheumatological practice, describing the 'scleroderma type' of capillaroscopic pattern with dilated loops, areas of avascularity and haemorrhages. Her work was built upon by Maurizio Cutolo who in 2000 described 'early', 'active' and 'late' scleroderma patterns.

Nailfold capillaroscopic abnormalities occur not only in systemic sclerosis but also in related conditions especially dermatomyositis. We discuss current clinical indications for nailfold capillaroscopy: primarily the assessment of the patient presenting with Raynaud's phenomenon or other clinical features leading to suspicion of an underlying systemic sclerosis-spectrum disorder, and the monitoring of patients with dermatomyositis. Most patients with systemic sclerosis present with Raynaud's phenomenon and nailfold capillaroscopy gives a window of opportunity for early diagnosis. Conversely those with normal capillaries can often be reassured that their Raynaud's is primary and will not progress to serious disease. Inclusion of abnormal nailfold capillaries into the 2013 American College of Rheumatology (ACR)/European Alliance of Associations for Rheumatology (EULAR) criteria for the classification of systemic sclerosis was a key milestone for nailfold capillaroscopy in rheumatological practice; as a result, all rheumatologists responsible for diagnosing connective tissue disease should be familiar with (and have access to) the technique.

However, at present not all rheumatologists use nailfold capillaroscopy in their everyday clinical practice, although uptake is increasing evidenced by more and more rheumatologists attending training courses: over the last 20 years the EULAR live courses have been attended by thousands of rheumatologists from over 100 different countries. There are two challenges for the practising rheumatologist related to performing nailfold capillaroscopy: first, acquiring high-quality images, and second, interpreting these images. A separate chapter is devoted to each of these. Advances in methodologies mean that images can be acquired not only with the gold standard of nailfold videocapillaroscopy but also with lower-cost methods (including USB microscopy and dermoscopy) which may be more accessible to rheumatologists. Image interpretation can be both qualitative and quantitative: recent advances in standardising these are described, including a 'fast-track' algorithm for easy identification of patients with marked scleroderma pattern abnormalities. Recent advances in quantifying nailfold capillaroscopic change are then discussed, including the application of artificial intelligence (AI) to image analysis. AI methods hold promise not only for clinical research, potentially allowing rapid analysis of images from large datasets, but also for clinical practice, providing 'remote' interpretation of images for rheumatologists less experienced in the technique.

Four clinically focussed chapters describe applications of nailfold capillaroscopy in patients with systemic sclerosis, with idiopathic inflammatory myopathies, with other rheumatological diseases, and in children. All of these subject areas have seen increasing numbers of papers published over the last 10 to 20 years. These publications have increased our understanding of how nailfold capillaroscopy can provide insights into the pathogenesis of rheumatological diseases in which there is a microvascular component, and of how nailfold capillaroscopy can not only aid diagnosis but may have a role in monitoring disease and in predicting disease trajectory. Although nailfold capillaroscopy can pose challenges in children, especially young children, many children are interested to see their capillaries 'live' on screen, and this can help them to understand their disease.

Three chapters then focus on research applications. Although nailfold capillaroscopy is used mainly to assess capillary structure, different aspects of capillary function (permeability, blood flow and oxygenation) can also be assessed and hold promise in furthering our understanding of the pathophysiology of microvascular disease and how this might be monitored. Nailfold capillaroscopy, being non-invasive, has huge potential as a biomarker of microvascular disease (especially with recent advances in quantification), and although there are certain challenges to be overcome, including ensuring high reliability and assessing capillaries in darker skin tones, progress is being made. The third research chapter places nailfold capillaroscopy in the context of other microvascular imaging techniques which provide complementary information and which can be used in combination with nailfold capillaroscopy: laser-based methods, infrared thermography and several cutting-edge technologies, including optical coherence tomography, hyperspectral imaging and multispectral photoacoustic imaging, are all discussed.

Finally, to place things into context for the clinician, five cases are presented describing how nailfold capillaroscopy plays a role in the diagnosis and monitoring of rheumatological disease.

We recognise that in ensuring that each chapter is standalone, there is some duplication of information between chapters, but hope that the reader will see this as reinforcement of key points. In writing this book, we pay tribute to all those who have advanced nailfold capillaroscopy to where it is now—a technique which continues to gain momentum as a diagnostic tool for all rheumatologists, and which continues to expand its potential as a research tool for studying pathophysiology and for predicting and monitoring disease trajectory and treatment response.

Manchester, UK Ariane L. Herrick

Manchester, UK Andrea Murray

Manchester, UK Chris Taylor

Ghent, Belgium Vanessa Smith

Genova, Italy Maurizio Cutolo

Contents

History of Nailfold Capillaroscopy

Sarah Smith and Richard M. Silver

Key Points

- First observed in the seventeenth century, nailfold capillaroscopy evolved into a clinically relevant tool in the twentieth century thanks to methodological refinement and imaging advances
- The identification of characteristic "scleroderma patterns" has positioned nailfold capillaroscopy as a central tool in diagnosing systemic sclerosis and differentiating primary from secondary Raynaud phenomenon
- Videocapillaroscopy enables real-time assessment of microvascular abnormalities and is becoming increasingly useful for diagnosis and prognosis of patients with Raynaud phenomenon and connective tissue diseases

Introduction

Remarkably, the most effective technique for assessing microvasculature today remains one of the oldest: intravital capillary microscopy, or capillaroscopy. Since its early beginnings, nailfold capillaroscopy has evolved to be an essential tool for assessing microvascular abnormalities across a range of medical conditions. Its clinical significance stems from the unique anatomical orientation of capillary loops in the nailfold region—aligned parallel to the skin surface—allowing for direct, non-invasive visualization of their entire structure. Unlike capillaries in other areas

S. Smith
Medical University of South Carolina, Charleston, SC, USA
e-mail: ssmit470@jh.edu

R. M. Silver (✉)
Division of Rheumatology & Immunology, Department of Medicine, Medical University of South Carolina, Charleston, SC, USA
e-mail: silverr@musc.edu

A. L. Herrick et al. (eds.), *Nailfold Capillaroscopy in Rheumatological Diseases*,
https://doi.org/10.1007/978-3-032-03970-5_1

of the body, which are oriented perpendicularly, this distinctive feature enables rapid, easy, and cost-effective assessment of microcirculation.

First described in 1663, nailfold capillaroscopy gradually gained recognition for its diagnostic value, particularly in vascular and connective tissue diseases. Over time, it has transformed from a purely observational technique into a standardized diagnostic tool integral to categorizing various rheumatic disorders, including a crucial role in distinguishing primary Raynaud phenomenon from systemic sclerosis where characteristic capillaroscopic findings can be diagnostic. The technique's growing clinical relevance is underscored by its incorporation into classification guidelines and the increasing body of research dedicated to its methodologies and applications.

In this chapter we trace the evolution of nailfold capillaroscopy, highlighting key milestones in its history, from its early development as a research tool to its modern role as a clinically validated diagnostic method. By examining the advancements in imaging technology, standardization efforts, and clinical applications, this chapter will provide a comprehensive overview of nailfold capillaroscopy's historical significance and its expanding role in medical diagnostics.

Pre-twentieth Century: Early Observations and Techniques

The earliest recorded observation of nailfold capillaries dates to 1663, when Johan Christophorus Kolhaus used a rudimentary microscope to visualize the tiny blood vessels surrounding the nails. Over 100 years later, Italian physician Giovanni Rasori (1766–1837) expanded on these early observations by employing a magnifying glass to examine capillary abnormalities. He notably described an "inextricable knot of capillary loops" in cases of conjunctivitis, suggesting a link between capillary alterations and inflammation [1]. This marked one of the earliest documented attempts to correlate microvascular changes with pathological conditions.

The next significant milestone in the study of microvascular function came in 1862, when Maurice Raynaud (1834–1881), son of a professor at the University of Paris, qualified for his doctorate in medicine upon presentation of a thesis titled *De l'asphyxie locale et de la gangrène symétrique des extrémités* (*Local Asphyxia and Symmetrical Gangrene of the Extremities*) (Fig. 1). In his thesis, Raynaud described 25 patients, 20 of whom were female, who had a series of color changes in their hands and feet when exposed to the cold or when the patients were under stress [2]. The hand-drawn illustrations included in his work depict these vascular changes, ranging from initial discoloration of the fingers and toes to the progression of gangrene (Fig. 2). Raynaud's work, while focused on the clinical manifestations of vascular dysfunction rather than direct microvascular visualization, underscored the significance of capillary abnormalities in systemic disease. The condition described in his thesis would later become eponymous, *Raynaud phenomenon,* and ultimately would come to be recognized as both a primary condition as well as a crucial early clinical vascular sign of several autoimmune diseases.

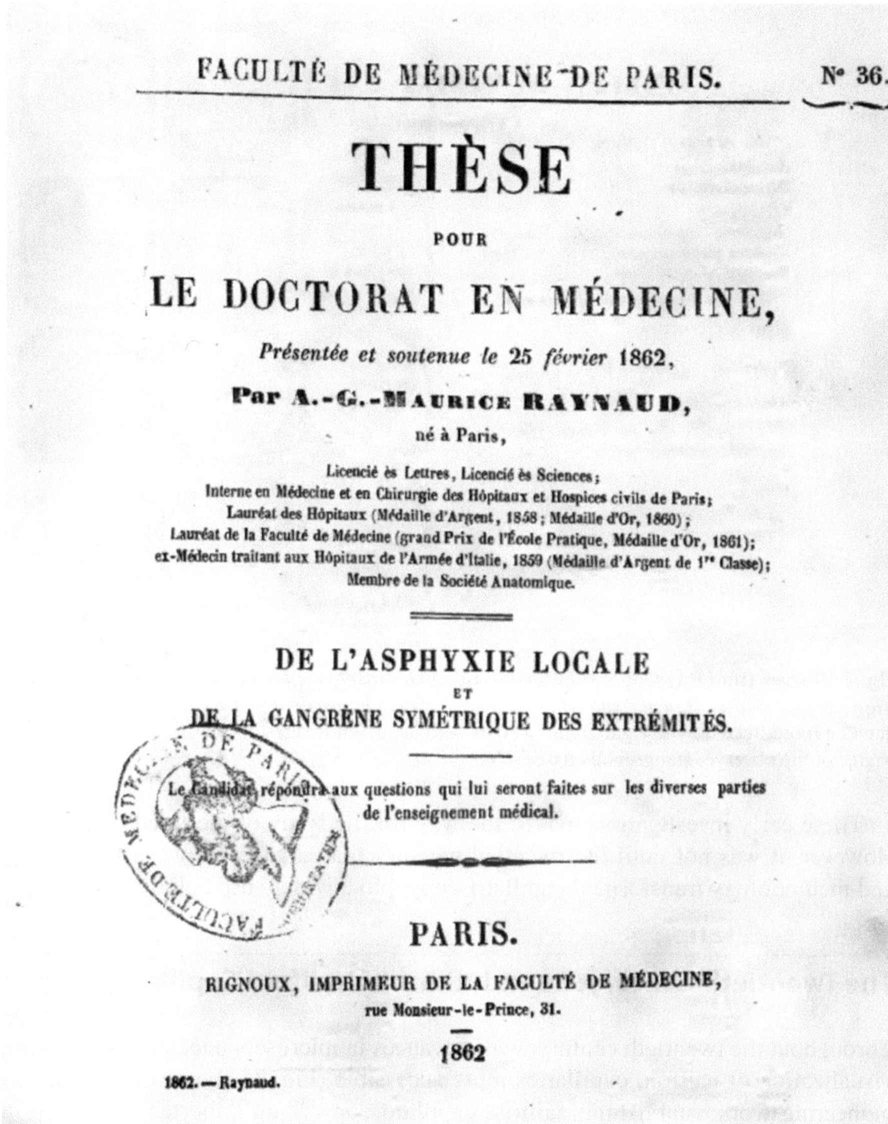

FACULTÉ DE MÉDECINE DE PARIS. N° 36.

THÈSE

POUR

LE DOCTORAT EN MÉDECINE,

Présentée et soutenue le 25 février 1862,

Par A.-G.-Maurice Raynaud,

né à Paris,

Licencié ès Lettres, Licencié ès Sciences;
Interne en Médecine et en Chirurgie des Hôpitaux et Hospices civils de Paris;
Lauréat des Hôpitaux (Médaille d'Argent, 1858; Médaille d'Or, 1860);
Lauréat de la Faculté de Médecine (grand Prix de l'École Pratique, Médaille d'Or, 1861);
ex-Médecin traitant aux Hôpitaux de l'Armée d'Italie, 1859 (Médaille d'Argent de 1re Classe);
Membre de la Société Anatomique.

DE L'ASPHYXIE LOCALE

ET

DE LA GANGRÈNE SYMÉTRIQUE DES EXTRÉMITÉS.

Le Candidat répondra aux questions qui lui seront faites sur les diverses parties de l'enseignement médical.

PARIS.

RIGNOUX, IMPRIMEUR DE LA FACULTÉ DE MÉDECINE,
rue Monsieur-le-Prince, 31.

1862

1862. — Raynaud.

Fig. 1 Image of the first page of Maurice Raynaud's 1862 thesis, titled *De l'asphyxie locale et de la gangrène symétrique des extrémités* (*Local Asphyxia and Symmetrical Gangrene of the Extremities*) [2]

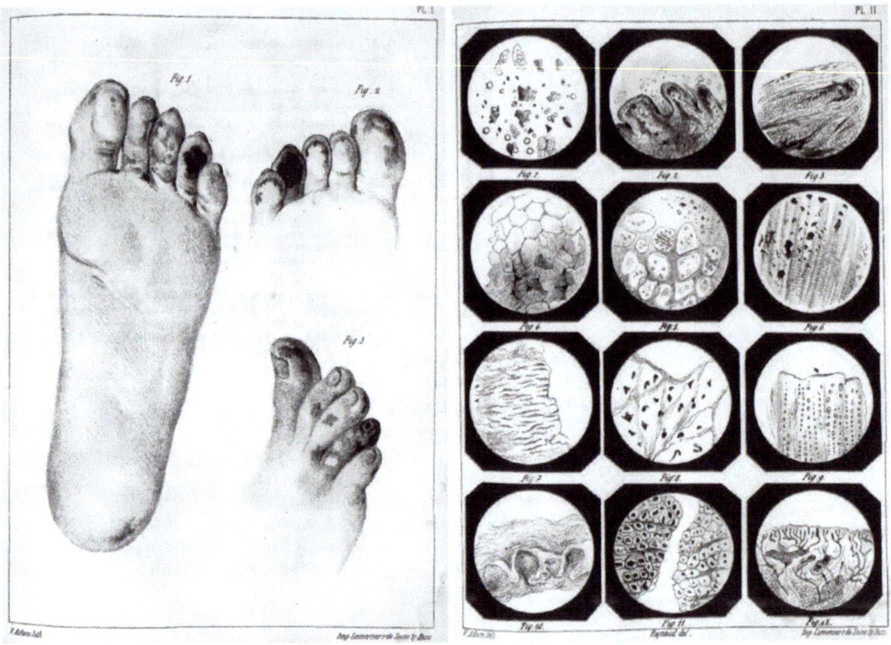

Fig. 2 Images from Raynaud's 1862 thesis, titled *De l'asphyxie locale et de la gangrène symétrique des extrémités* (*Local Asphyxia and Symmetrical Gangrene of the Extremities*) [2]. Images depict a foot affected by dry gangrene (left) as well as drawn images of microscopic examination (right) of the observed gangrenous tissue

These early investigations paved the way for the study of the microcirculation. However, it was not until the twentieth century that advancements in technology and methodology transformed capillaroscopy into a widely used clinical tool.

The Twentieth Century: Foundations of Nailfold Capillaroscopy

Throughout the twentieth century, with advances in microscope technology making visualization of nailfold capillaries more accessible (Fig. 3), there was substantial pioneering work establishing nailfold capillaroscopy as an important tool both in clinical diagnosis and in research. In particular, the adoption of microscopes with 100-300x magnification provided the ability to capture highly detailed images of capillary loops, further advancing the technique's diagnostic and investigative potential. Starting in 1901, Hutchinson was able to distinguish primary Raynaud phenomenon from Raynaud phenomenon secondary to systemic disease by detecting microvascular changes with capillaroscopy [4]. A decade later in 1911, Lombard discovered that a drop of immersion oil placed on periungual skin capillaries enabled easier visualization of the capillaries with a microscope [5]. This in turn influenced Weiss in 1916, who further standardized capillaroscopic techniques and

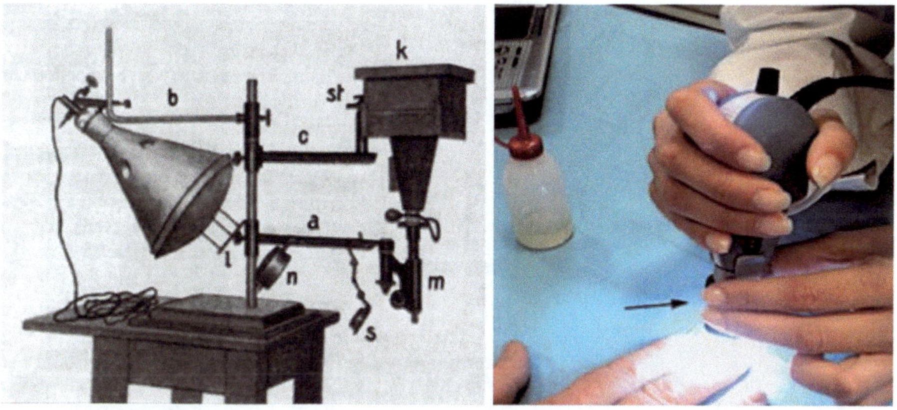

Fig. 3 Capillaroscope of the early twentieth century (left) compared with the new digitalized nailfold videocapillaroscope of the twenty-first century (right). (Image sourced from Cutolo and Smith's 2013 publication [3])

produced the first photographs of the capillaries using a primordial camera [6]. Following this, in 1925, nailfold capillaroscopy was linked with rheumatic diseases when Brown and O'Leary used capillaroscopic analysis to show some of the abnormalities characteristic of the microvasculature in secondary Raynaud phenomenon and particularly in systemic sclerosis. This was the first introduction of the concept of a 'scleroderma' pattern defined by capillaroscopy. Specifically, in their paper titled *Skin Capillaries in Scleroderma*, along with photographic images they detail the involvement of the microvasculature in Raynaud phenomenon and systemic sclerosis, describing normal capillaries in healthy individuals as having a predominant type of loop that is straight or hairpin patterned with small incidence of tortuosity, contrasted to the capillaroscopic changes in scleroderma as including giant capillary loops, elongated capillaries and low capillary number per millimeter. They also observed indistinct capillary borders with a feathery appearance in association with decreased visibility owing to increased collagen deposition in the skin of patients with scleroderma [7].

Following this work, Allen and Brown in 1932 [8] and Hunt in 1936 [9] refuted the microvascular theory that had first been proposed by Raynaud, and rather suggested that a macrovascular component was necessary to generate the profound damage of the acral tissues. Around that time, in 1939, Müller published a large collection of color capillaroscopic images that he had painted himself (Fig. 4) [10]. However, the considerable variability in capillary loop morphology, coupled with the lack of healthy control groups in many studies, made the narrow-field approach highly subjective. This led to inconsistent, non-reproducible results—factors that likely contributed to a period of stagnation in the field of nailfold capillaroscopy for the next three decades.

The study of nailfold capillaroscopy underwent a resurgence in the 1970s, driven in large part by the pioneering work of Hildegard Maricq (née Rand) (Fig. 5). During World War II she fled communism from her homeland Estonia to Germany

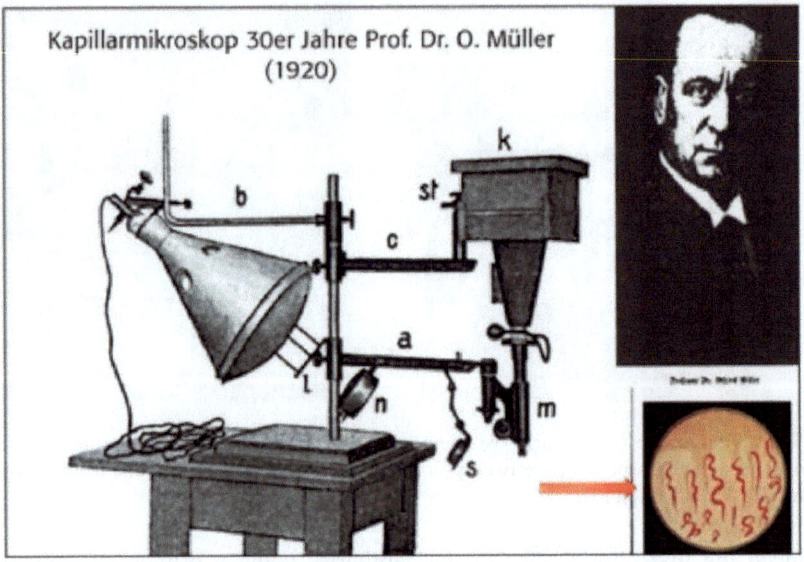

Fig. 4 Image from Cutolo's *Atlas of Capillaroscopy in Rheumatic Diseases* depicting a capillaroscope from the beginning of the twentieth century and the first depiction of capillaries by O Müller (red arrow) [1]

Fig. 5 Hildegard Rand Maricq (1925–2009), a twentieth century pioneer in the field of microcirculation and nailfold capillaroscopy

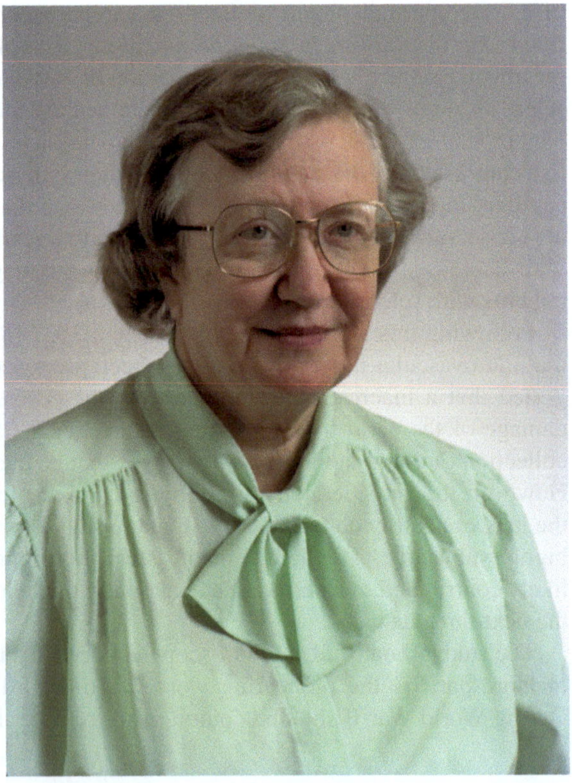

and from there to Belgium, where she met and married Jean (John) Maricq, who later would work side-by-side in her microcirculation laboratory. Hildegard graduated *cum laude* in medicine from the University Libre of Brussels in 1953. Soon thereafter she emigrated to the United States, where her first professional appointment was in Psychiatry, initiating studies of the microcirculation of patients with schizophrenia [11]. Her expertise in capillaroscopy attracted the attention of Dr. E. Carwile LeRoy, who recruited her to Columbia University's College of Physicians and Surgeons in New York City and later, in 1975, to the Medical University of South Carolina in Charleston. Maricq's research led to significant advances in the field, particularly when she established the advantages of utilizing panoramic "wide-field" capillaroscopy for the diagnosis of systemic sclerosis. Her work shifted from the subtle morphological variability in individual capillary loops, drawing attention toward the recognition of the importance of the microvascular landscape. In 1973, together with LeRoy she published the first study describing specific capillaroscopic patterns in systemic sclerosis (Fig. 6). They described the specific 'scleroderma type' capillaroscopic pattern as having hemorrhages and giant dilated, distorted capillaries alternating with areas of avascularity [12]. Maricq and colleagues later went on to suggest the presence of an 'active' and a 'slow' capillaroscopic pattern in systemic sclerosis, suggesting that the 'slow' pattern was associated with lower disease activity [13]. The 'slow' staging pattern described capillaroscopy findings of high numbers of giant capillary loops with mild capillary loss. The 'active' staging pattern described capillaroscopy findings of severe capillary loss with extensive avascular areas and new blood vessel formation. In 1976, Maricq and LeRoy further documented the continuous changes in capillary blood flow during cold exposure, observing that the capillary blood flow was at a complete standstill in systemic sclerosis and was intermittent in primary Raynaud phenomenon, whilst continuous in healthy individuals [14].

Shortly thereafter, in 1979, a new technique using fluorescent tracers for capillary videomicroscopy was introduced by A. Bollinger. In this method, a 20% sodium fluorescein solution is injected as a bolus into the antecubital vein, allowing the dye to circulate and reach the capillaries. This approach enabled visualization of the dye's movement through capillary walls and into the surrounding interstitial space. Bollinger demonstrated that in Raynaud phenomenon, one can identify increased transcapillary dye passage, indicating a compromised pericapillary diffusion barrier [15]. In 1991, Bollinger and colleagues then showed that conventional capillaroscopy and infrared fluorescence videomicroscopy with indocyanine green could be used as a new technique to allow for visualization of capillary aneurysms even when filled only by plasma (Fig. 7) [16]. While the use of dyes such as sodium fluorescein and indocyanine green in nailfold capillaroscopy provided valuable physiological insights into microvascular abnormalities and have advanced our understanding of capillary structure and function, they remain primarily research tools and are not routinely used in day-to-day clinical practice.

Around this time, Grassi and colleagues in 1993 utilized capillaroscopy at the nailfold as well as the lips. In addition to the typical 'scleroderma pattern' at the nailfold, labial capillaroscopy revealed a different morphological pattern of

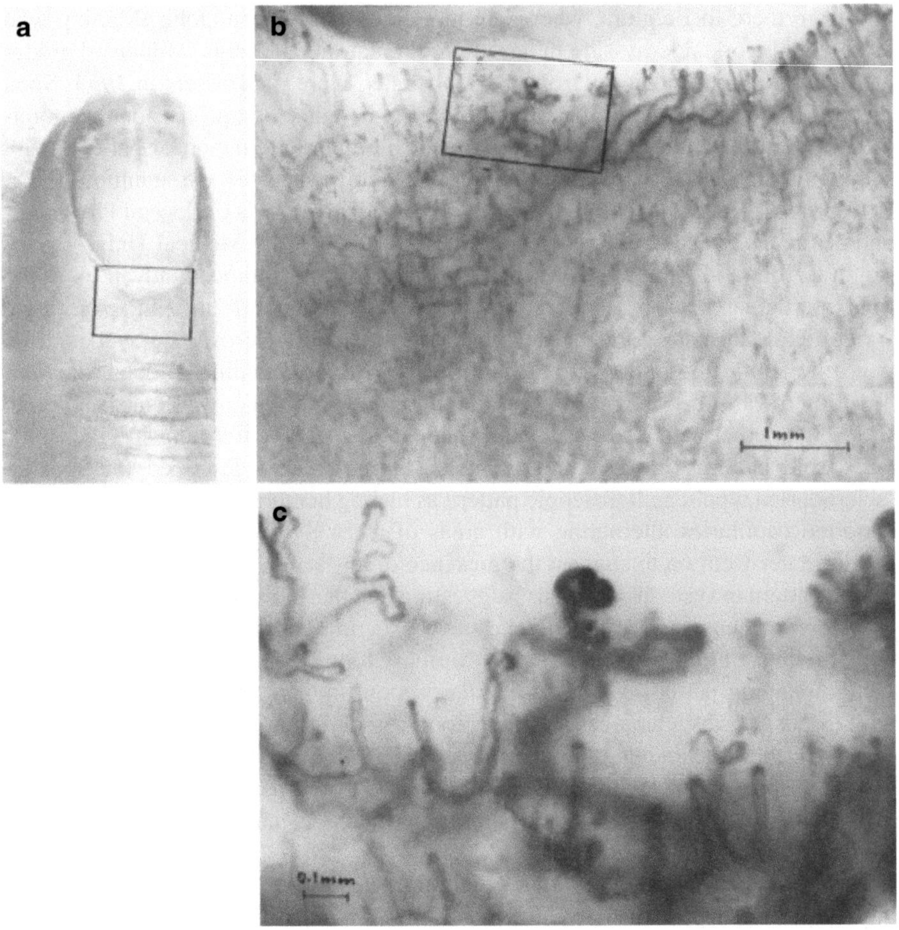

Fig. 6 Image from Maricq and Leroy's 1973 publication describing capillaroscopic patterns in systemic sclerosis.This image shows (**a**) photo of a finger of a patient with scleroderma; (**b**) nailfold vascular pattern with the wide-field technique; (**c**) a portion of the same nailfold at higher magnification [12]

microangiopathy in systemic sclerosis [17]. Ariane Herrick and colleagues from the University of Manchester, UK, in 1996 utilized video capillaroscopy to measure nailfold capillary dimensions in patients with primary Raynaud phenomenon, systemic sclerosis and controls. In this study, they utilized various measurements of nailfold capillaries and found that all dimensions other than distance between capillary limbs were significantly increased in primary Raynaud phenomenon and systemic sclerosis compared to controls [18]. A figure displaying capillary measurement in this study is shown in Fig. 8.

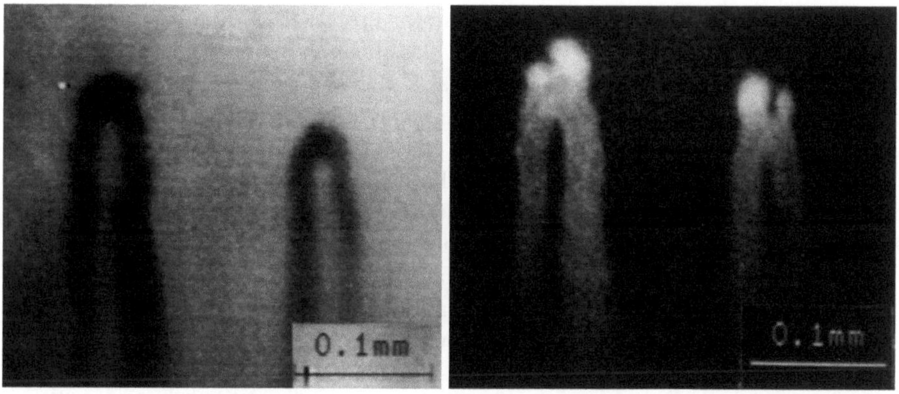

Fig. 7 Image from a 1991 publication by Bollinger et al. describing that conventional capillaroscopy and infrared fluorescence videomicroscopy with indocyanine green could be used as a new technique to allow for visualization of capillary aneurysms even when filled only by plasma. The images above were from a patient with mixed connective tissue disease. The left image shows conventional epi-illumination capillaroscopy. The right image shows infrared fluorescence videomicroscopy with indocyanine green revealing aneurysms at the apex of both loops [16]

Fig. 8 Image from a 1996 publication by Bukhari et al. on '*Increased nailfold capillary dimensions in primary Raynaud phenomenon and systemic sclerosis*'. In the image from their paper, the following were measured: (**a**) arterial diameter, (**b**) venous diameter, (**c**) loop diameter, (**d**) capillary width, (**e**) distance between limbs [18]

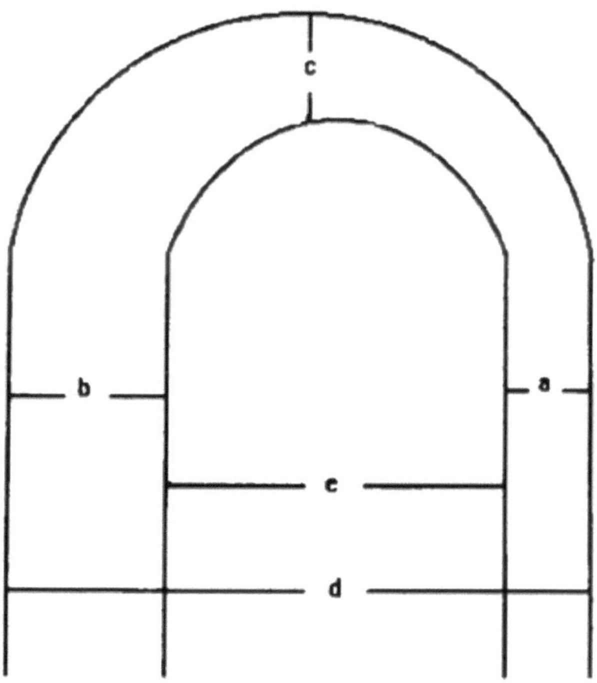

More recently, in 2000, Maurizio Cutolo, Professor of Rheumatology at the University of Genova, further refined the classification of 'scleroderma'-type nailfold capillaroscopic patterns used to assess the appearance and progression of microangiopathy in scleroderma [19]. These classifications are now widely utilized in clinical practice and include 3 distinct phases: early, active and late. The 'early' phase is characterized by few giant capillaries, microhemorrhages and preserved capillary distribution and density. The 'active' phase is characterized by a higher number of enlarged capillaries and microhemorrhage with moderate loss of capillaries and capillary derangement. The 'late' phase is characterized by advanced capillary derangement, extensive avasculature and the presence of ramified/bushy capillary loops [19]. In 2011, Cutolo published the *Atlas of Capillaroscopy in Rheumatic Diseases*, providing extensive insights into the history, techniques, and visual interpretation of capillaroscopy [1]. This work also offers practical guidance on troubleshooting and detailed findings across various rheumatic diseases, further advancing the application of capillaroscopy in clinical practice.

The twentieth century was a turning point in establishing nailfold capillaroscopy as a vital diagnostic tool in rheumatology, driven by advancements in microscopy, evolving techniques, and groundbreaking research. A timeline of the history of nailfold capillaroscopy leading up until present times is shown in Fig. 9. From Hutchinson's early differentiation of Raynaud phenomenon in 1901, to Maricq's development of wide-field capillaroscopy in the 1970s, the field evolved through a series of key discoveries that refined both methodology and clinical applications. The standardization of scleroderma pattern classification by Cutolo further cemented capillaroscopy's role in assessing microvascular changes in systemic sclerosis. These pivotal contributions paved the way for capillaroscopy to become an essential tool in modern rheumatology, shaping both clinical practice and research into microvascular pathology.

Fig. 9 Historical timeline of the history of nailfold capillaroscopy

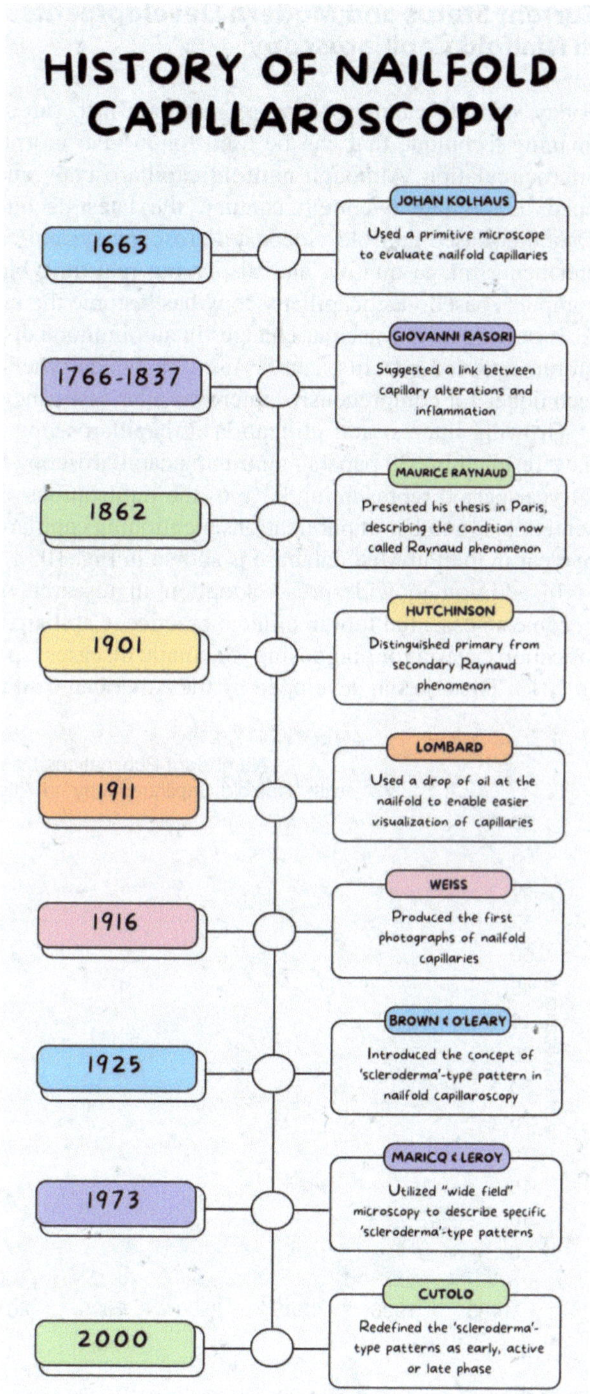

Current Status and Modern Developments in Nailfold Capillaroscopy

Today, nailfold capillaroscopy represents a fast, safe, and affordable noninvasive imaging technique that can be used for in vivo morphological assessment of the microcirculation. Although nailfold capillaroscopy analysis was primarily developed in the late twentieth century, the latest technological advancement is a computer-based nailfold videocapillaroscopy system capable of capturing images, enhancing image quality, and displaying real-time blood flow and velocity. The computer-based videocapillaroscopy has become the most commonly used method for assessing microvascular changes in autoimmune diseases and, in addition to the aforementioned benefits, can be used alongside other methods like laser Doppler techniques for comprehensive microvascular assessment [20–22].

Growing interest and utilization of capillaroscopy in research and diagnostics have resulted in 639 papers mentioning capillaroscopy from 2000 to 2024, with this 24-year period representing 93% of the publications since 1985. Graphical representation of number of publications mentioning capillaroscopy in the title or abstract by year in the PubMed database is shown in Fig. 10.

In addition to widespread adoption in research, nailfold capillaroscopy has become an essential tool in clinical practice. Capillaroscopy was added to the classification criteria for diagnosing rheumatic diseases, specifically systemic sclerosis, in 2013. The criteria, developed by the American College of Rheumatology (ACR)

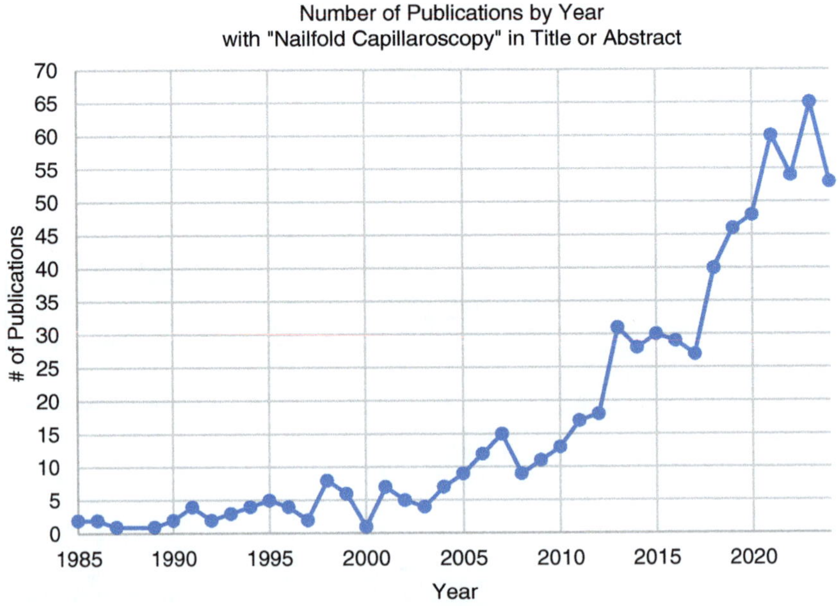

Fig. 10 Number of publications by year with "nailfold capillaroscopy" mentioned in the title or abstract in the PubMed database

and the European League Against Rheumatism (EULAR), now includes abnormal nailfold capillaries as one of the seven additive items used to classify individuals with systemic sclerosis, with varying weights assigned to each item [23]. This update significantly improved the sensitivity and specificity of the classification criteria compared to the previous 1980 preliminary criteria, allowing for better identification of patients with early or limited cutaneous systemic sclerosis. The update in the 2013 ACR/EULAR classification criteria for systemic sclerosis further reflects the clinical importance of microvascular changes in the early and accurate diagnosis of scleroderma. Additionally, since 2004, international courses on capillaroscopy offered by the EULAR and attended by participants from all over the world have been organized by leading experts including Maurizio Cutolo from Genova and Vanessa Smith from Ghent University Hospital, Belgium. These courses provide clinicians and researchers with essential training in this valuable technique.

In summary, nailfold capillaroscopy has evolved from an observational research tool to an essential component of both clinical practice and scientific investigation. Advancements in imaging technology have enhanced its diagnostic capabilities, enabling real-time visualization of microvascular changes, with an increasing number of publications and global educational initiatives further highlighting widespread recognition of its use. The inclusion of nailfold capillary abnormalities as a component in the 2013 ACR/EULAR classification criteria for systemic sclerosis underscores its clinical significance, improving early detection and diagnosis of systemic sclerosis. As research continues to refine its applications, capillaroscopy will remain a cornerstone in the assessment of microvascular pathology in autoimmune diseases.

References

1. Cutolo M. Atlas of capillaroscopy in rheumatic diseases. Elsevier; 2011.
2. Raynaud M. Thèse de Médecine: De l'asphyxie locale et de la gangrène des extrémités. Paris: Leclerc; 1862.
3. Cutolo M, Smith V. State of the art on nailfold capillaroscopy: a reliable diagnostic tool and putative biomarker in rheumatology? Rheumatology (Oxford). 2013;52(11):1933–40.
4. Hutchinson H. Raynaud's phenomenon. La Presse médicale. 1901;71:403–5.
5. Lombard W. The blood pressure in the arterioles, capillaries, and small veins of the human skin. Am J Phys. 1911;29:355–62.
6. Weiss W. Demonstration von Hautkapillarveraenderungen bei akuter Nephritis. Med Bl Landerver. 1916;LXXXVI:383.
7. Brown GE, O'Leary PA. Skin capillaries in scleroderma. Arch Intern Med. 1925;36(1):73–88.
8. Allen EV, Brown GE. Raynaud's disease: a critical review of minimal requisites for diagnosis. Am J Med Sci. 1932;183:187–200.
9. Hunt JH. The Raynaud phenomena: a critical review. QJM. 1936;5(3):399–444.
10. Müller O. Die feinsten blutgefäessen des menschen. Stuttgart: E Enke Verlag; 1939.
11. Maricq HR. Relationship between nailfold capillary patterns and finger blood flow in schizophrenic patients. Bibl Anat. 1975;13:246–7.
12. Maricq HR, LeRoy EC. Patterns of finger capillary abnormalities in connective tissue disease by "wide-field" microscopy. Arthritis Rheum. 1973;16(5):619–28.

13. Maricq HR, Harper FE, Khan MM, Tan EM, LeRoy EC. Microvascular abnormalities as possible predictors of disease subsets in Raynaud phenomenon and early connective tissue disease. Clin Exp Rheumatol. 1983;1(3):195–205.
14. Maricq HR, Downey JA, LeRoy EC. Standstill of nailfold capillary blood flow during cooling in scleroderma and Raynaud's syndrome. Blood Vessels. 1976;13(6):338–49.
15. Bollinger A, Jäger K, Roten A, Timeus C, Mahler F. Diffusion, pericapillary distribution and clearance of Na-fluorescein in the human nailfold. Pflugers Arch. 1979;382(2):137–43.
16. Bollinger A, Saesseli B, Hoffmann U, Franzeck UK. Intravital detection of skin capillary aneurysms by videomicroscopy with indocyanine green in patients with progressive systemic sclerosis and related disorders. Circulation. 1991;83(2):546–51.
17. Grassi W, Core P, Carlino G, Blasetti P, Cervini M. Labial capillary microscopy in systemic sclerosis. Ann Rheum Dis. 1993;52(8):564–9.
18. Bukhari M, Herrick AL, Moore T, Manning J, Jayson MI. Increased nailfold capillary dimensions in primary Raynaud's phenomenon and systemic sclerosis. Br J Rheumatol. 1996;35(11):1127–31.
19. Cutolo M, Sulli A, Pizzorni C, Accardo S. Nailfold videocapillaroscopy assessment of microvascular damage in systemic sclerosis. J Rheumatol. 2000;27(1):155–60.
20. Szabo N, Csiki Z, Szanto A, Danko K, Szodoray P, Zeher M. Functional and morphological evaluation of hand microcirculation with nailfold capillaroscopy and laser Doppler imaging in Raynaud's and Sjögren's syndrome and poly/dermatomyositis. Scand J Rheumatol. 2008;37(1):23–9.
21. Anderson ME, Allen PD, Moore T, Hillier V, Taylor CJ, Herrick AL. Computerized nailfold video capillaroscopy--a new tool for assessment of Raynaud's phenomenon. J Rheumatol. 2005;32(5):841–8.
22. Cutolo M, Smith V. Detection of microvascular changes in systemic sclerosis and other rheumatic diseases. Nat Rev Rheumatol. 2021;17(11):665–77.
23. van den Hoogen F, Khanna D, Fransen J, Johnson SR, Baron M, Tyndall A, et al. 2013 classification criteria for systemic sclerosis: an American college of rheumatology/European league against rheumatism collaborative initiative. Ann Rheum Dis. 2013;72(11):1747–55.

Clinical Indications

Ariane L. Herrick

Key Points

- The main clinical indication for nailfold capillaroscopy is the assessment of the patient with Raynaud's phenomenon (RP).
- In the patient presenting with RP, normal nailfold capillaries are reassuring (consistent with primary RP). Conversely, abnormal capillaries (especially capillary enlargement or capillary loss) are suggestive of an underlying systemic sclerosis (SSc)-spectrum disorder or that the patient is at risk of developing this.
- The second most important clinical indication is in the assessment of the patient with dermatomyositis. The degree of capillary abnormality can help in monitoring disease activity.
- Nailfold capillaroscopy is also indicated in patients without RP but in whom a SSc-spectrum disorder is nonetheless suspected.
- These clinical indications apply in children as well as in adults.
- In the future, it is likely that nailfold capillaroscopy will be used in predicting disease trajectory (e.g. the risk of digital ulceration) in patients with SSc-spectrum disorders.

A. L. Herrick (✉)
Centre for Musculoskeletal Research, Division of Musculoskeletal and Dermatological Sciences, The University of Manchester, Manchester Academic Health Science Centre, Manchester, UK

Northern Care Alliance NHS Foundation Trust, Salford, UK

National Institute for Health and Care Research (NIHR) Manchester Biomedical Research Centre, Manchester, UK

Department of Rheumatology, Aberdeen Royal Infirmary, NHS Grampian, Aberdeen, UK

Centre for Arthritis and Musculoskeletal Health, University of Aberdeen, Aberdeen, UK
e-mail: ariane.herrick@manchester.ac.uk

A. L. Herrick et al. (eds.), *Nailfold Capillaroscopy in Rheumatological Diseases*,
https://doi.org/10.1007/978-3-032-03970-5_2

Introduction

The technique of nailfold capillaroscopy is underpinned by the anatomy of the nailfold, because here capillaries run parallel rather than perpendicular to the skin surface (Fig. 1). This allows direct visualisation of the microcirculation. Sometimes the nailfold capillaries are so abnormal that they can be seen with the naked eye (Fig. 2) but usually magnification is required using one of the different systems described in chapter "Nailfold Capillaroscopy—Image Acquisition". Chapter "History of Nailfold Capillaroscopy" has described how the technique has evolved over the years. As technology advances, the possibilities of maximising the potential of this unique window into the microcirculation increase. Up until now, nailfold capillaroscopy has been used primarily to study microvascular structure, but there is now increasing interest in applying the technique to studying microvascular function, as will be described in chapter "Research Methods; Functional Measures of Nailfold Capillaroscopy Including Permeability, Perfusion and Oxygenation" (Research methods).

This chapter will describe main current clinical indications for nailfold capillaroscopy (Box 1), 'setting the scene' for the clinical applications described in later chapters. There will be a focus on nailfold capillaroscopy's main clinical indication which is in the assessment of the patient presenting with Raynaud's phenomenon (RP). Research applications will be discussed in later chapters.

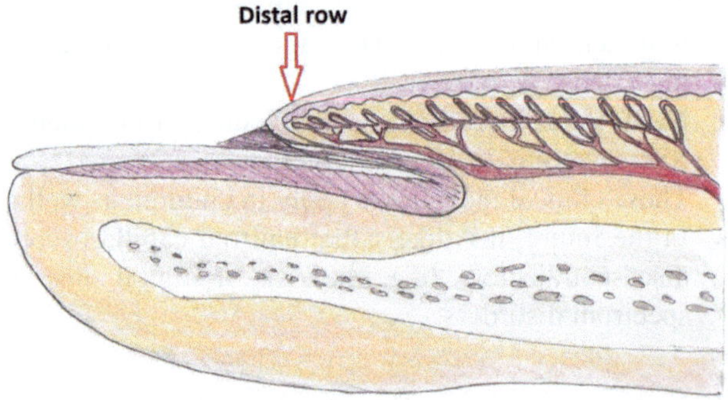

Fig. 1 Schematic of nailfold capillaries—at the nailfold the capillaries in the distal row run parallel to the skin surface. This is different from in other areas of skin, where they run perpendicular to the skin surface

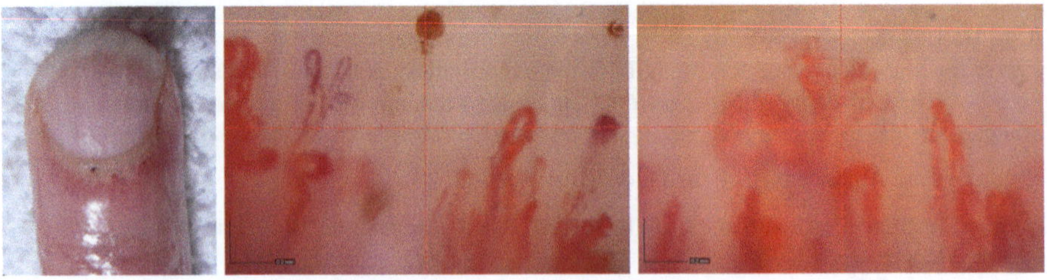

Fig. 2 Abnormal nailfold capillaries. Here these are so abnormal that they can be seen with the naked eye (left panel). However, usually magnification is required. The two panels to the right show sections of the same nailfold as visualised by videocapillaroscopy, demonstrating capillary enlargement, areas of avascularity, distortion of the normal nailfold architecture, and haemorrhages. (Figure courtesy of Hector Chinoy)

Box 1: Clinical Indications for Nailfold Capillaroscopy

Current

Investigation of the patient presenting with RP (this is the main clinical indication).

Investigation of the patient with other (non-RP) features suggestive of a SSc-spectrum disorder (i.e. of SSc, dermatomyositis, mixed connective tissue disease/other overlap syndromes, undifferentiated connective tissue disease).

Monitoring of disease/treatment response in the patient with dermatomyositis.

Future

Predicting disease trajectory in the patient with a SSc-spectrum disorder e.g. predicting risk of future digital ulceration.

Rationale for Nailfold Capillaroscopy in Patients with Rheumatological Diseases

Some rheumatological diseases have a significant microvascular component to their pathophysiology, especially systemic sclerosis (SSc), discussed in chapter "Nailfold Capillaroscopy in Systemic Sclerosis (Including Associations)", and dermatomyositis, discussed in chapter "Nailfold capillaroscopy in idiopathic inflammatory myopathies". These two diseases are both associated with (and probably driven by) microvascular changes, with structural as well as functional microvascular abnormalities. Non-invasive visualisation of nailfold capillaries provides a unique insight into disease status, often helping to make a diagnosis (particularly an early diagnosis of SSc as discussed in the next section) and (in the case of dermatomyositis) allowing monitoring of response to drug treatment. As already stated, at present the main indication for nailfold capillaroscopy for most rheumatologists is in the assessment of the patient with RP [1, 2] and this is true in paediatric as well as adult practice [3, 4]. However, increasing accessibility to equipment and advances in image interpretation make it likely that clinical indications may in the future extend to include prediction of disease trajectories. Therefore nailfold capillaroscopy could play an integral role in a personalised medicine approach to the care of patients with SSc and related disorders. The increasing accessibility to equipment includes low-cost methodologies as discussed in chapter "Nailfold Capillaroscopy—Image Acquisition", allowing increased uptake of the technique amongst rheumatologists in different countries [5–7]. Advances in image interpretation include standardisation of analysis [8–10], and automated analysis [11–16] as discussed in chapter "Quantitative Analysis".

Although rheumatological conditions other than SSc and dermatomyositis have been associated with nailfold capillaroscopic abnormality (discussed in chapter "Nailfold Capillaroscopy in Other Rheumatological Diseases"), at present nailfold capillaroscopy is not a key investigation in their diagnosis and management. However, if a patient with (for example) undifferentiated connective tissue disease or an overlap syndrome develops RP or experiences progression of RP, or develops any other new features suggestive that their disease is evolving into a SSc pattern, then nailfold capillaroscopy can be useful in determining the likelihood of a significant microvascular component to their disease and informing whether the diagnosis has changed. This could have implications for drug treatment, for example, the clinician may wish to intensify vasodilator therapy as exemplified in chapter "Practical Approaches to Nailfold Capillaroscopy—Case Studies" (Case 1).

Background to Raynaud's Phenomenon—The Main Clinicial Indication for Nailfold Capillaroscopy

RP is episodic discolouration of the extremities (mainly reported in the fingers) in response to cold exposure or emotional stress. Characteristically the fingers turn white (Fig. 3), then blue, then red although many patients do not experience all three colour changes [17]. RP is common, affecting approximately 5% of the general population [18]. In the vast majority of patients with RP, the RP is 'benign' primary (idiopathic) RP. Primary RP is essentially an exaggeration of the normal physiological response to cold, and by definition does not progress to tissue injury [19, 20]. However, in a minority of patients RP is secondary to an underlying cause (Table 1). Therefore RP is not a diagnosis, but is a symptom complex and the first step in management is to identify the cause of the RP, because this may require specific treatment. For example, if RP is secondary to a blood dyscrasia then its treatment is primarily that of the underlying disease.

The relevance of RP to rheumatologists is two-fold. First, RP can be secondary to connective tissue disease and may be its presenting feature. Hence patients with

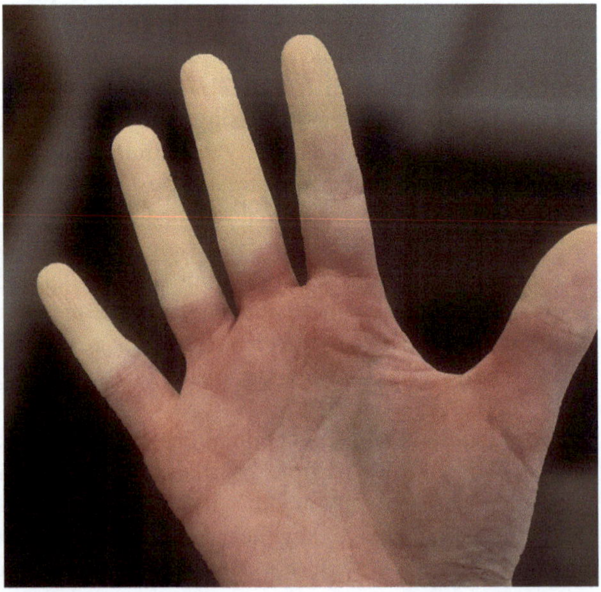

Fig. 3 The pallor phase of RP, photographed by a patient on her mobile phone (with background blurred and darkened)

Table 1 Main differential diagnosis of (and associations with) RP

Primary (idiopathic)
Secondary causes—Connective tissue diseases:
SSc and SSc-spectrum disorders (undifferentiated connective tissue disease, mixed connective tissue disease, other overlap syndromes)
Inflammatory muscle disease (including dermatomyositis)
Systemic lupus erythematosus
Sjogren's syndrome
Vasculitis
Secondary causes—Other:
Hand-arm-vibration syndrome ('vibration white finger')
Extrinsic vascular compression (including cervical rib)
Other causes of large vessel disease:
Atherosclerosis
Thromboangiitis obliterans (Buerger's disease)
'Intravascular' disease/conditions associated with increased viscosity, including:
Paraproteinaemia
Cryoglobulinaemia
Cryofibrinogenaemia
Malignancy
Certain drugs, chemicals, or other occupational exposures, including:
Beta-blockers
Chemotherapeutic agents
Clonidine
Ergotamine
Vinyl chloride
Other causes/associations, including:
Hypothyroidism
Carpal tunnel syndrome
Frostbite

RP are often referred to rheumatology for assessment. Second, when RP is secondary to connective tissue disease, especially to SSc, it can be very severe and difficult to treat. Nailfold capillaroscopy is a key investigation in diagnosis and potentially management, allowing separation between primary and SSc-related RP as discussed below and allowing identification of those patients with SSc-spectrum disorders at highest risk of disease progression. By 'SSc-spectrum disorders' are meant SSc, dermatomyositis, mixed connective tissue disease and other overlap syndromes, and a proportion of undifferentiated connective tissue disease.

The Role of Nailfold Capillaroscopy in Assessing the Patient with RP: Diagnosing Primary RP

Primary RP is a *functional* abnormality of the digital vasculature. Although its pathophysiology is incompletely understood, it is not associated with structural vascular change and the nailfold capillaries should therefore be normal. When defining primary RP, LeRoy and Medsger recognised the importance of normal nailfold capillaries [21] (Table 2), and this was reinforced in later international consensus criteria for the diagnosis of primary RP [22]. Conversely, if the nailfold capillaries are

Table 2 Proposed criteria for primary Raynaud's phenomenon [21]

Episodic attacks of acral pallor or cyanosis
Strong and symmetric peripheral pulses
No evidence of digital pitting, ulceration or gangrene
Normal nailfold capillaries
Negative antinuclear antibody (ANA) test (titre <1/100)
Normal erythrocyte sedimentation rate (ESR)

abnormal, then the patient cannot be diagnosed as having primary RP and an underlying connective tissue disease should be suspected.

That normal nailfold capillaries are reassuring was demonstrated in a study of 347 patients referred to a tertiary centre for nailfold capillaroscopy [23]: the absence of a 'scleroderma pattern' on capillaroscopy had a negative predictive value of 90% for identifying patients with definite or very early SSc. In another study also published in 2016 [24] it was suggested that a mean 'largest' capillary diameter of 30 μm or less had a high negative predictive value of 0.92, whereas the positive predictive value of a mean diameter greater than the cut-off was 0.44.

Although subtle nailfold changes have been reported in patients with primary RP [25, 26], these could be due to the case-mix of the patients who participated in these studies and who were seen in hospital practice. It is recognised that patients referred to hospital with what seems to be primary RP may be at higher risk of developing a SSc-spectrum disorder than patients who never seek medical advice, accounting for the high reported transition rates from 'isolated' RP to a connective tissue disease/SSc-spectrum disorder [27–29]. In the systematic review and meta-analysis reported by Ingegnoli et al. [29] which included 4051 patients with primary RP (mean follow-up duration 5.0 years) the mean incidence rate of transition from primary RP to a connective tissue disease was 2.65/100 patient years (95% confidence interval [CI] 0.44–5.73) and specifically to SSc 0.93/100 patient years (95% CI 0.27–2.13). This high transition rate probably lies in selection bias in reported hospital-based series. For example, the average age of the 4051 patients with primary RP reported by Ingegnoli et al. [29] and for whom age data were available was 34.1 years, whereas symptoms of primary RP generally begin in the teens and early twenties.

The conclusion therefore is that patients referred to a rheumatologist/secondary care with RP should be carefully assessed by history, examination, and investigations (Fig. 4). Nailfold capillaroscopy should form part of the investigative work up which should also include as a minimum a full blood count and testing for antinuclear antibody (ANA). Other testing will depend on the clinical scenario. Normal nailfold capillaries as shown in Fig. 5 (upper panel) are reassuring. In the absence of any other worrying features, such as puffy fingers or a positive ANA, then the patient can be safety discharged, sparing the patient unnecessary anxiety. However, if the RP is of recent onset, and especially if the patients is over 40 years old, then it may be prudent to reassess things, including repeating nailfold capillaroscopy, in around one year's time.

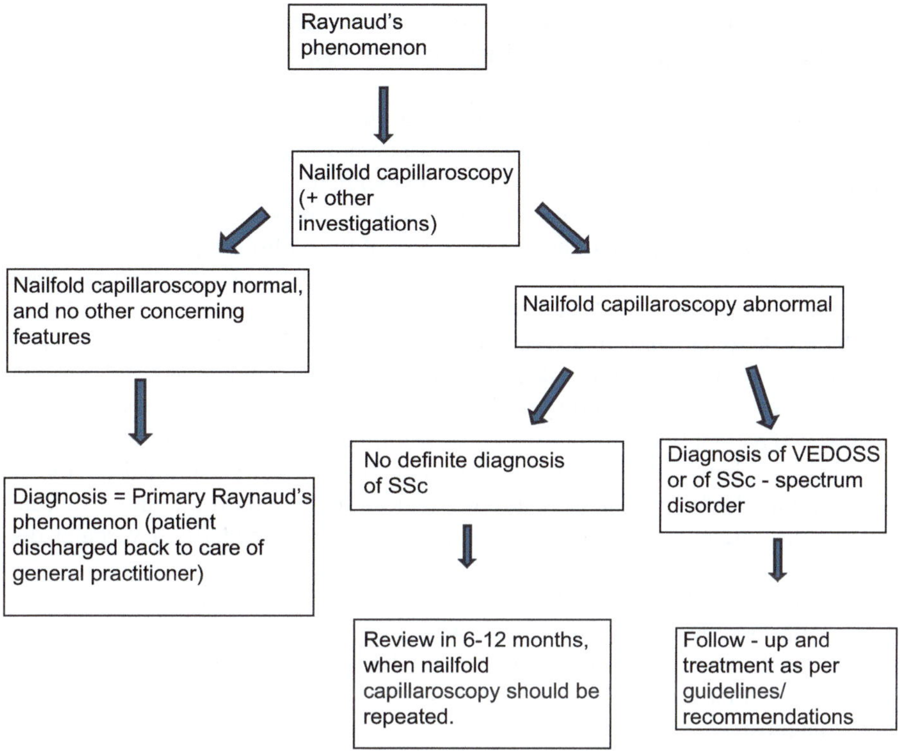

Fig. 4 Flow-chart describing the pivotal role of nailfold capillaroscopy in the assessment of the patient with RP. *SSc* = systemic sclerosis, *VEDOSS* = Very Early Diagnosis of SSc

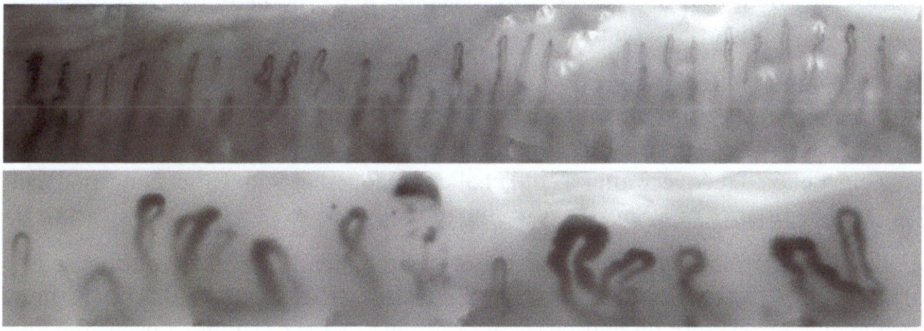

Fig. 5 Normal, evenly spaced nailfold capillaries (upper panel) compared to abnormal capillaries (lower panel) with dilated capillary loops (including giant capillaries), areas of avascularity (reduced capillary density), distortion of the normal nailfold architecture and haemorrhages

The Role of Nailfold Capillaroscopy in Assessing the Patient with RP—Making an Early Diagnosis of SSc

Identifying nailfold capillary abnormalities in the patient presenting with RP can either confirm a diagnosis of suspected SSc or demonstrate that the patient is at risk of progression to SSc. The seminal work by Maricq and colleagues in the early 1970s and 1980s [30, 31], already discussed in chapter "History of Nailfold Capillaroscopy", highlighted the abnormalities of the nailfold capillaries which are characteristic of the SSc disease process. These will be discussed in detail in chapters "Image Interpretation" and "Nailfold Capillaroscopy in Systemic Sclerosis (Including Associations)", but essentially comprise capillary enlargement, areas of avascularity (reduced capillary density), distortion of the normal nailfold architecture and (very often) haemorrhages [32], as demonstrated in Fig. 5 (lower panel). It is now well recognised that microvascular abnormality is a major contributor to SSc pathogenesis, but it remains unclear as to how microvascular abnormality, fibrosis and immune dysfunction inter-relate. It has been hypothesised that microvascular abnormality drives the disease process, and that SSc is primarily a vascular disease [33].

Irrespective of the exact pathogenesis of SSc, the key point with respect to nailfold capillaroscopy is that most patients with SSc have abnormal capillaries and that these abnormalities occur early on in disease. Because most patients with SSc have RP as their first symptom, this provides a unique window of opportunity for early diagnosis.

The Role of Nailfold Capillaries in the Diagnosis of SSc

LeRoy and Medger as far back as 2001 [34] proposed criteria for the early diagnosis and classification of SSc on the basis of either:

(i) Self-reported (i.e. 'subjective') RP together with abnormal nailfold capillaries and a SSc-specific autoantibody, or
(ii) 'Objective' evidence of RP (direct observation or abnormal response to cold e.g. delayed recovery after a cold challenge) together with either abnormal nailfold capillaries or a SSc-specific autoantibody.

Following on from this, criteria for very early diagnosis of SSc were proposed by the EULAR Scleroderma Trials and Research Group (EUSTAR) [35]. These criteria included a SSc pattern on nailfold capillaroscopy. A later Delphi Consensus Study in which physicians from 85 EUSTAR centres participated [36] provided further support for abnormal nailfold capillaroscopy (SSc pattern) being indicative of very early SSc. Specifically, RP, puffy fingers and ANA positivity were considered three red flags for very early diagnosis of SSc (VEDOSS) [37]. The finding of abnormal capillaroscopy and/or a SSc-specific autoantibody were considered indicative of very early SSc, but the authors were careful to point out that these proposed criteria needed to be validated in a prospective study, described in the next section. But already as a result of these expert opinion papers abnormal nailfold capillaries, defined as 'Enlarged capillaries and/or capillary loss with or without pericapillary haemorrhages' were included in the 2013 American College of Rheumatology (ACR)/EULAR criteria for the classification of SSc [38, 39], scoring 2 or the required 9 points.

Evidence for Abnormal Nailfold Capillaries Being Predictive of SSc in the Patient with RP

It is now well established that abnormal nailfold capillaries predict development of a SSc spectrum disorder [40–43]. Two large prospective studies have shown this. The first of these was a Canadian study in which 586 patients with RP were followed for 3197 person years [41]. Abnormal capillaroscopy and SSc-specifc autoantibodies were independent predictors of SSc: SSc developed in 8 patients (1.8%) with neither, in 8 (25.8%) with an abnormal capillary pattern, in 23 (35.4%) with a specific autoantibody and in 35 (79.5%) with both. The median duration of follow-up was 4 years. Koenig et al. reported that the earliest capillaroscopic abnormality was capillary enlargement [41]. The second study was the VEDOSS study [43], which sought to validate the criteria for very early diagnosis put forward by the Delphi exercise referred to in the previous section [36]. Of 553 patients meeting the VEDOSS criteria for study inclusion and who had at least one follow-up visit (median duration of follow-up 3.6 years), 254 (45.9%) completed the study (i.e. reached 5 years of follow-up or progressed to SSc) and of these 133/254 (52.4%) progressed to SSc. Abnormal nailfold capillaries helped to predict progression to SSc although not as strongly as puffy fingers or a SSc-specific autoantibody. Of the 35.2% of patients with abnormal nailfold capillaroscopy at baseline, 70.1% progressed to SSc, compared to 41.5% of the 64.8% in whom nailfold capillaroscopy was normal. The authors noted that the lack of standardisation of nailfold capillaroscopy (and the inclusion of 'non-specific abnormalities' when defining abnormality) might have influenced results (i.e. weakened the predictive value of capillaroscopy in this study). It would be interesting to see whether further longitudinal studies in which the approach to nailfold capillaroscopy image acquisition is standardised, and image analysis automated, can improve prediction.

An Italian study including 242 patients fulfilling VEDOSS criteria reported that 150 (64.1%) had a SSc capillaroscopic pattern [44] i.e. higher than reported by Bellando-Randone et al. [43].

The systematic review and meta-analysis already referred to by Ingegnoli et al. [29] in relation to predicting transition from primary RP to connective tissue disease, included 657 patients with 'suspected secondary RP' (defined by ANA positivity and/or capillary abnormalities). The mean follow-up duration was 3.6 years. These patients had much higher transition rates than those with primary RP: the mean incidence rate of transition to connective tissue disease was 11.01/100 patient years (95% CI 0.11–22.12) and to SSc 7.10/100 patient years (95% CI 1.02–13.19). Patients with both ANA positivity and abnormal nailfold capillaries were at particularly high risk, with a risk ratio for development of connective tissue disease of 16.96, and for SSc 40.45. Patients with negative ANA but abnormal nailfold capillaries had a risk ratio for development of connective tissue disease of 5.53, and for SSc 11.81.

In summary, the finding of abnormal nailfold capillaries increases the risk of the patient with RP progressing to SSc. It seems likely (as suggested in a study of 66 patients with VEDOSS [45]) that the degree of capillaroscopic change may help to stratify risk. However, this suggestion should be tested in prospective studies in which nailfold capillary images are acquired and interpreted in a standardised way. Improved risk stratification would be another step forward in optimising patient care.

In conclusion, nailfold capillaroscopy should always be performed in any patient with RP in whom there is any concern that there might be an underlying SSc-spectrum disorder. Essentially this means any patient referred to rheumatology with RP, and especially any patient with RP who is ANA positive, who has puffy fingers, or any other features of concern, for example late onset RP. As shown in Fig. 4, normal capillaries allow the patient to be reassured. Abnormal capillaries require actioning: at the very least the patient requires rheumatology follow-up: both patient and clinician need to be vigilant for development of any other features pointing to a connective tissue disease.

Assessment of the Patient Presenting with Other (Non-RP) Features Suggestive of a SSc-Spectrum Disorder

The reason why the main clinical indication for nailfold capillaroscopy is in the assessment of RP is that most patients with SSc present with RP which therefore (as already stated) provides a window of opportunity for early diagnosis. But SSc-spectrum disorders, including dermatomyositis discussed in chapter "Nailfold capillaroscopy in idiopathic inflammatory myopathies", can present with features other than RP and the clinician should always be alert to this possibility. For example, patients with early diffuse cutaneous SSc often develop RP only after development of skin thickening and so when investigating a patient with skin thickening, if there is any possibility that this could be SSc then the clinician should examine the nailfold capillaries.

Hong et al. [46]. examined the utility of nailfold capillaroscopy in patients without RP, and highlighted that this was particularly relevant in equatorial climates where RP is less prevalent in patients with SSc than in Western cohorts. In this study of 95 patients followed for a mean of 1.6 years [46], abnormal nailfold capillaries were associated with development of a SSc-spectrum disorder in the 49 patients without RP but with 'undifferentiated non-RP features' (for example interstitial lung disease). Another finding of the study was the high negative predictive of nailfold capillaroscopy in patients with SSc-associated antibodies (but without any other features of SSc), although numbers were small and this finding needs to be confirmed in larger studies.

In summary, if a diagnosis of a SSc-spectrum disorder is suspected, then nailfold capillaroscopy should be performed, irrespective of whether or not the patient has RP. Examples of scenarios in which nailfold capillaroscopy is indicated include:

1. A patient presenting with interstitial lung disease (ILD). Abnormal nailfold capillaroscopy may help to diagnose the presence of an underlying connective tissue disease [47], and this may have implications for management of the ILD.
2. A patient with known connective tissue disease (but no previous SSc features) who develops a sudden deterioration in renal function. While there is a broad differential diagnosis, abnormal nailfold capillaroscopy would suggest that this could represent a scleroderma renal crisis, and lead to a diagnosis of SSc [48].

Prediction of Digital Ulceration in the Patient with SSc

Results of several studies suggest that severity of nailfold capillary abnormality in patients with SSc helps to predict development of digital ulceration [49–54]. As an example, in 468 patients with SSc and with a history of digital ulceration followed over 6 months, the mean number of capillaries/mm in the middle finger of the dominant hand was one of the predictors of development of new digital ulceration [52]. This seems intuitive, because digital ulceration is thought to be driven by ischaemia and therefore patients with the most severe microvascular derangement are likely to be at highest risk.

Although many clinicians recognise that patients with severe nailfold capillaroscopic change are at high risk of progression from RP to digital ulceration, at present this has not as yet translated into a significant change in clinical practice. However, this could be relevant in the future, especially if new effective treatments to prevent digital ulcers are identified. Even now, it could be argued that patients with severe microvascular change should be especially closely monitored to ensure optimal treatment with vasoactive therapies. Conversely, a less intensive approach might be reasonable in patients with only minor capillary changes as these patients are at lower risk of irreversible tissue injury.

NFC as a Potential Biomarker of Microvascular Disease in Patients with SSc-Spectrum Disorders

Because nailfold capillaroscopy allows direct visualisation of the microcirculation, it has enormous potential as a tool to monitor disease activity/severity and/or treatment response, in both the clinical and the research setting. At present, the only clinical application as a biomarker is in the care of patients with dermatomyositis, a disease associated with marked nailfold changes. Following on from an early report of 9 children with dermatomyositis [55], it is recognised that the degree of nailfold capillary abnormality correlates with disease activity, and that appearances can normalise with effective treatment. This observation is now making its way into clinical practice as discussed in chapter "Nailfold capillaroscopy in idiopathic inflammatory myopathies". Dermatomyositis is an inflammatory disease with the potential for reversibility. Whether nailfold capillaroscopy will ever be used to monitor the non-inflammatory microangiopathy of SSc in the clinical setting is more contentious. More detailed discussion of capillaroscopy as a biomarker is given in chapter "Nailfold Capillaroscopy as a Biomarker for Monitoring Disease and Treatment Response".

Conclusions

The main clinical indication for nailfold capillaroscopy is in the assessment of the patient with RP, when the technique helps to differentiate between primary and SSc-related RP. Findings on nailfold capillaroscopy guide the clinician as to whether the patient can be reassured and discharged, or whether further follow-up and further investigation is required. A second important clinical indication is the follow-up of patients with dermatomyositis, when nailfold capillaroscopic findings help to gauge disease activity. As nailfold capillaroscopy becomes more widely used and as technologies (and treatments) advance, clinical indications may expand to include, for example, identification of patients with SSc-spectrum disorders most at risk of disease progression, as part of a personalised/stratified approach to treatment.

Acknowledgement I am grateful to Graham Dinsdale and to Sarah Groves for their help with the figures.

References

1. Herrick AL, Cutolo M. Clinical implications from capillaroscopic analysis in patients with Raynaud's phenomenon and systemic sclerosis-spectrum disorders. Arthritis Rheum. 2010;62:2595–604.
2. Smith V, Ickinger C, Hysa E, et al. Nailfold capillaroscopy. Best practice. Res Clin Rheumatol. 2023;37:101849.
3. Gerhold K, Becker MO. Nailfold capillaroscopy in juvenile rheumatic diseases: known measures, patterns and indications. Clin Exp Rheumatol. 2014;32(Suppl 86):S183–8.
4. Pain CE, Constantin T, Toplak N, et al. Paediatric Rheumatology European Society (PRES) Juvenile Scleroderma Working Group. Raynaud's syndrome in children: systematic review and development of recommendations for assessment and monitoring. Clin Exp Rheumatol. 2016;34(Suppl 100):200–6.
5. Snow MH, Saketkoo LA, Frech TM, et al. Results from an American pilot survey among scleroderma clinical trials consortium members on capillaroscopy use and how to best implement nailfold capillaroscopy training. Clin Exp Rheumatol. 2019;37(Suppl 119):151.
6. Eden M, Wilkinson S, Murray A, et al. Nailfold capillaroscopy: a survey of current UK practice and 'next steps' to facilitate generalised uptake. Rheumatology. 2022;62:335–40.
7. Jeelani S, Bali K, Hassan I, Bashir Y. Diagnostic utility of nailfold capillaroscopy using hand-held dermoscope in systemic sclerosis. Indian Dermatol Online J. 2023;14:200–6.
8. Kayser C, Bredemeier M, Caleiro MT, et al. Position article and guidelines 2018 recommendations of the Brazilian Society of Rheumatology for the indication, interpretation and performance of nailfold capillaroscopy. Adv Rheumatol. 2019;59:5.

9. Smith V, Herrick AL, Ingegnoli F, et al. Standardisation of nailfold capillaroscopy for the assessment of patients with Raynaud's phenomenon and systemic sclerosis. Autoimmun Rev. 2020;19:102458.
10. Ingegnoli F, Herrick A, Schioppo T, et al. Reporting items for capillaroscopy in clinical research on musculoskeletal diseases: a systematic review and international Delphi consensus. Rheumatology. 2021;60:1410–8.
11. Cutolo M, Trombetta AC, Melsens K, et al. Automated assessment of absolute nailfold capillary number on videocapillaroscopic images: proof of principle and validation in systemic sclerosis. Microcirculation. 2018;25:e12447.
12. Herrick AL, Berks M, Taylor C. Quantitative nailfold capillaroscopy—update and possible next steps. Rheumatology. 2021;60:2054–65.
13. Gurunath Bharathi P, Berks M, Dinsdale G, Murray A, Manning J, Wilkinson S, et al. A deep learning system for quantitative assessment of microvascular abnormalities in nailfold capillary images. Rheumatology. 2023;62:2325–9.
14. Garaiman A, Nooralahzadeh F, Mihai C, et al. Vision transformer assisting rheumatologists in screening for capillaroscopy changes in systemic sclerosis: an artificial intelligence model. Rheumatology. 2023;62:2492–500.
15. Gracia Tello B, Comet LS, Lledó G, et al. Capi-score: a quantitative algorithm for identifying disease patterns in nailfold videocapillaroscopy. Rheumatology. 2024;63:3315–21.
16. Ozturk L, Laclau C, Boulon C, et al. Analysis of nailfold capillaroscopy images with artificial intelligence: data from literature and performance of machine learning and deep learning from images acquired in the SCLEROCAP study. Microvasc Res. 2025;157:104753.
17. Wigley FM, Flavahan NA. Raynaud's phenomenon. N Engl J Med. 2016;375(6):556–65.
18. Kumar K, Maudrell A, Proudman SM. Epidemiology of Raynaud's phenomenon. In: Wigley FM, et al., editors. Raynaud's phenomenon: from pathogenesis to management. 2nd ed. Springer; 2024.
19. Herrick AL. Pathogenesis of Raynaud's phenomenon. Rheumatology. 2005;44:587–96.
20. Flavahan NA. A mechanistic approach to understanding and preventing the vasculopathy of Raynaud's phenomenon. In: Wigley FM, et al., editors. Raynaud's phenomenon: from pathogenesis to management. 2nd ed. Springer; 2024.
21. LeRoy EC, Medsger TA. Raynaud's phenomenon: a proposal for classification. Clin Exp Rheumatol. 1992;10:485–8.
22. Maverakis E, Patel F, Kronenberg DG, et al. International consensus criteria for the diagnosis of Raynaud's phenomenon. J Autoimmunity. 2014;48-49:60–5.
23. Bissell LA, Abignano G, Emery P, Del Galdo F, Buch MH. Absence of scleroderma pattern at nail fold capillaroscopy valuable in the exclusion of scleroderma in unselected patients with Raynaud's phenomenon. BMC Musculoskelet Disord. 2016;17:342.
24. Trombetta AC, Smith V, Pizzorni C, et al. Quantitative alterations of capillary diameter have a predictive value for development of the capillaroscopic systemic sclerosis pattern. J Rheumatol. 2016;43:599–606.
25. Bukhari M, Herrick AL, Moore T, Manning J, Jayson MIV. Increased nailfold capillary dimensions in primary Raynaud's phenomenon and systemic sclerosis. Br J Rheumatol. 1996;35:1127–31.
26. Bukhari M, Hollis S, Moore T, Jayson MIV, Herrick AL. Quantitation of microcirculatory abnormalities in patients with primary Raynaud's phenomenon and systemic sclerosis by video capillaroscopy. Rheumatology. 2000;39:506–12.
27. Spencer-Green G. Outcomes in primary Raynaud phenomenon: a meta-analysis of the frequency, rates and predictors of transition to secondary diseases. Arch Intern Med. 1998;158:595–600.
28. Hirschl M, Hirschl K, Lenz M, Katzenschlager R, Hutter H, Kundi M. Transition from primary Raynaud's phenomenon to secondary Raynaud's phenomenon identified by diagnosis of an associated disease. Arthritis Rheum. 2006;54:1974–81.
29. Ingegnoli F, Ughi N, Crotti C, Mosca M, Tani C. Outcomes, rates and predictors of transition of isolated Raynaud's phenomenon: a systematic review and meta-analysis. Swiss Med Wkly. 2017;147:w14506.

30. Maricq HR, LeRoy EC. Patterns of finger capillary abnormalities in connective tissue diseases by 'wide-field' microscopy. Arthritis Rheum. 1973;16:619–28.
31. Maricq HR. Widefield capillary microscopy. Technique and rating scale for abnormalities seen in scleroderma and related disorders. Arthritis Rheum. 1981;24:1159–65.
32. Cutolo M, Sulli A, Smith V. Assessing microvascular changes in systemic sclerosis diagnosis and management. Nat Rev Rheumatol. 2010;6:578–87.
33. Campbell PM, LeRoy EC. Pathogenesis of systemic sclerosis: a vascular hypothesis. Sem Arthritis Rheum. 1975;4:351–68.
34. LeRoy EC, Medsger TA. Criteria for the classification of early systemic sclerosis. J Rheumatol. 2001;28:1573–6.
35. Matucci-Cerinic M, Allanore Y, Czirják L, et al. The challenge of early systemic sclerosis for the EULAR Scleroderma Trial and Research group (EUSTAR) community. It is time to cut the Gordian knot and develop a prevention or rescue strategy. Ann Rheum Dis. 2009;68:1377–80.
36. Avouac J, Fransen J, Walker UA, et al. Preliminary criteria for the very early diagnosis of systemic sclerosis: results of a Delphi Consensus Study from EULAR Scleroderma Trials and Research Group. Ann Rheum Dis. 2011;70:476–81.
37. Bellando-Randone S, Matucci-Cerinic M. Very early systemic sclerosis. Best Pract Res Clin Rheumatol. 2019;33:101428.
38. Van den Hoogen F, Khanna D, Fransen J, et al. 2013 classification criteria for systemic sclerosis: an American College of Rheumatology/European League Against Rheumatism collaborative initiative. Ann Rheum Dis. 2013;72:1747–55.
39. Van den Hoogen F, Khanna D, Fransen J, et al. 2013 classification criteria for systemic sclerosis: an American College of Rheumatology/European league against rheumatism collaborative initiative. Arthritis Rheum. 2013;65:2737–47.
40. Ingegnoli F, Boracchi P, Gualtierotti R, et al. Prognostic model based on nailfold capillaroscopy for identifying Raynaud's phenomenon patients at high risk for the development of a scleroderma spectrum disorder. Arthritis Rheum. 2008;58:2174–82.
41. Koenig M, Joyal F, Fritzler MJ, et al. Autoantibodies and microvascular damage are independent predictive factors for the progression of Raynaud's phenomenon to systemic sclerosis. A twenty-year prospective study of 586 patients, with validation of proposed criteria for early systemic sclerosis. Arthritis Rheum. 2008;58:3902–12.
42. Ingegnoli F, Boracchi P, Gualtierotti R, et al. Improving outcome prediction of systemic sclerosis from isolated Raynaud's phenomenon: role of autoantibodies and nail-fold capillaroscopy. Rheumatology. 2010;49:797–805.
43. Bellando-Randone S, Del Galdo F, Lepri G, et al. Progression of patients with Raynaud's phenomenon to systemic sclerosis: a five-year analysis of the European scleroderma trial and research group multicentre, longitudinal registry study for very early diagnosis of systemic sclerosis (VEDOSS). Lancet Rheumatol. 2021;3:e834–43.
44. Ferri C, Giuggioli D, Guiducci S, et al. Systemic sclerosis progression INvestiGation (SPRING) Italian registry: demographic and clinico-serological features of the scleroderma spectrum. Clin Exp Rheumatol. 2020;38(Suppl 125):S40–7.
45. Vasile M, Avouac J, Sciarra I, et al. From VEDOSS to established systemic sclerosis diagnosis according to ACR/EULAR 2013 classification criteria: a French-Italian capillaroscopic survey. Clin Exp Rheumatol. 2018;26(Suppl 113):S82–7.
46. Hong C, Xiang L, Saffari SE, Low AH. Nailfold capillaroscopy for the early diagnosis of the scleroderma spectrum of diseases in patients without Raynaud's phenomenon. J Scleroderma Relat Disord. 2022;7:144–50.
47. Umashankar E, Abdel-Shaheed C, Plit M, Girgis L. Assessing the role for nailfold videocapillaroscopy in interstitial lung disease classfication: a systematic review and meta-analysis. Rheumatology. 2022;61:2221–34.
48. Abeygunaratne T, Herrick A, Chinoy H, Sowden E, Choudhury J, Sinha S. Simple tool in a complex case: use of the nailfold capillaroscopy. Kidney Int. 2016;89:1168.

49. Sebastiani M, Manfredi A, Colaci M, et al. Capillaroscopic skin ulcer risk index: a new prognostic tool for digital skin ulcer development in systemic sclerosis patients. Arthritis Rheum. 2009;61:688–94.
50. Smith V, De Keyser F, Pizzorni C, et al. Nailfold capillaroscopy for day-to-day clinical use: construction of a simple scoring modality as a clinical prognostic index for digital trophic lesions. Ann Rheum Dis. 2011;70:180–3.
51. Sebastiani M, Manfredi A, Vukatana G, Moscatelli S, Riato L, Bocci M, et al. Predictive role of capillaroscopic skin ulcer risk index in systemic sclerosis: a multicentre validation study. Ann Rheum Dis. 2012;71:67–70.
52. Cutolo M, Herrick AL, Distler O, et al. Nailfold videocapillaroscopic features and other clinical risk factors for digital ulcers in systemic sclerosis. A multicenter, prospective cohort study. Arthritis Rheumatol. 2016;68:2527–39.
53. Avouac J, Lepri G, Smith V, et al. Sequential nailfold videocapillaroscopy examinations have responsiveness to detect organ progression in systemic sclerosis. Sem Arthritis Rheum. 2017;47:86–94.
54. Friedrich S, Lüders S, Glimm AM, et al. Association between baseline clinical and imaging findings and the development of digital ulcers in patients with systemic sclerosis. Arthritis Res Ther. 2019;21:96.
55. Silver RM, Maricq HR. Childhood dermatomyositis: serial microvascular studies. Pediatrics. 1989;83:278.

Nailfold Capillaroscopy—Image Acquisition

Graham Dinsdale, Andrea Murray, and Tracy Frech

Key Points

- The usefulness of nailfold capillaroscopy in both clinical practice and research is dependent upon the acquisition of high quality images.
- Nailfold capillary images can be acquired using different imaging systems including nailfold videocapillaroscopy, USB microscope, stereomicroscope, dermatoscope, and ophthalmoscope.
- The different systems have their advantages and disadvantages including in terms of magnification, feasibility of making measurements, portability and cost.
- A non-toxic transparent oil should always be applied to the nailfold before imaging to facilitate visualisation of capillaries.
- Clinically, in order to identify (or rule out) abnormality, ideally all eight nailfolds (thumbs excluded) should be examined (over the whole nailfold), but if there are

G. Dinsdale
Department of Rheumatology, Salford Royal Hospital, Northern Care Alliance NHS Foundation Trust, Salford, UK
e-mail: graham.dinsdale@nca.nhs.uk

A. Murray (✉)
Centre for Musculoskeletal Research, Division of Musculoskeletal and Dermatological Sciences, The University of Manchester, Manchester Academic Health Science Centre, Manchester, UK

Northern Care Alliance NHS Foundation Trust, Salford, UK

National Institute for Health and Care Research (NIHR) Manchester Biomedical Research Centre, Manchester, UK
e-mail: andrea.murray@manchester.ac.uk

T. Frech
Division of Rheumatology and Immunology, Vanderbilt University Medical Center, Nashville, TN, USA
e-mail: tracy.frech@vumc.org

A. L. Herrick et al. (eds.), *Nailfold Capillaroscopy in Rheumatological Diseases*,
https://doi.org/10.1007/978-3-032-03970-5_3

constraints on time then a compromise is to examine the middle and ring fingers of each hand.

- When images are acquired for research purposes, to track change over time, it is important to ensure reliability of image acquisition.

Introduction

Nailfold capillaroscopy is a critical skill for rheumatologists to use in clinical as well as research settings for diagnosis, prognostication, and quantifying therapeutic response. There are several methods for nailfold capillaroscopy and these can be used for research studies as well as for clinical practice. The key point for both clinical practice and for research is that image clarity is imperative. From a clinical perspective, rheumatologists should assess the microcirculation of the nailfold in all patients presenting with Raynaud's phenomenon (RP) and/or concern for systemic sclerosis (SSc). This is underscored by the 2013 American College of Rheumatology (ACR)/ European League Against Rheumatism (EULAR) classification criteria for SSc [1], which allocate two points out of the nine required for classification to capillaroscopy. Practice will vary between countries, but even if a clinical provider is not certified in nailfold capillaroscopy, the importance of examining the nailfold and determining if an abnormality is present is a critical component of SSc assessment. The international community agrees that all patients experiencing RP and/or other criteria of SSc should be clinically screened for normal versus abnormal or nonspecific capillaroscopy.

Occasionally, nailfold capillaries are so abnormal as to be notable just by examining the fingers with the naked eye. Thus, every physical examination for a patient with RP and/or SSc should record whether the nailfolds appear normal or abnormal. However, since capillaries cannot usually be observed by eye, capillaroscopy systems all have optics to magnify. Most clinical practitioners have access to a portable ophthalmoscope, which can provide up to 15X magnification. However, these images cannot be recorded and systems with a higher magnification enable quantification of abnormalities. For research studies of SSc and/or RP, sufficient image clarity for quantification is mandatory. In this chapter, different nailfold capillaroscopy methods will be discussed in the context of benefits and limitations in both clinical and research settings.

The usefulness of nailfold capillaroscopy in either the clinical or research setting is dependent, first, on acquiring good quality images and, second, on interpretation of these images. In this chapter we discuss image acquisition; Chapter "Image Interpretation" discusses image interpretation. The particular challenges of image acquisition in children are discussed in chapter "Nailfold Capillaroscopy in Children".

Preparation for Nailfold Capillaroscopy and Some Practical Tips

Irrespective of the capillaroscopy device used, environmental conditions must be controlled and standardised as much as possible to minimise physiological variability [2]. A Delphi consensus on preparation and reporting standards highlighted several factors to be taken into account including acclimatisation, ensuring that the hands are clean, and ideally there should have been no recent manicure or trauma to the nailbeds: otherwise, this could influence capillary appearance [3].

Regardless of which nailfold capillaroscopy device is used transparent oil (e.g. immersion or olive oil) is placed on the nailfold surface (over the cuticle and adjacent skin) to enhance the translucency of the stratum corneum, facilitating imaging of the deeper capillary structures. In essence, the interface surface decreases light reflection and increases refraction, providing a clear view of the capillaries within the skin (Fig. 1). Oil on the surface can lead to glare on images in systems that have built-in LED/light sources concentric to the lens (specular reflections appearing as bright white spots on the image). These 'spots' can often be alleviated by varying the angle of the microscope to the finger. Some systems have built-in polarisers to remove these artifacts or use a diffuser to scatter light and even out the LED intensities, avoiding specular reflections.

Some capillaroscopy systems (including the stereomicroscope and some videocapillaroscopy systems) are non-contact although contact microscopes have gained popularity. Contact systems require less focusing, and as they are immersed in the oil, they do not tend to suffer from glare but they need to be used with caution as too much pressure will blanch capillaries and create what appears to be a lower capillary density or areas of avascularity. Gentle release of the probe pressure allows reperfusion of the capillaries enabling them to be observed.

Fixed versus handheld probes each have their advantages and disadvantages; a fixed probe may be easier to focus and minimise movement artifacts, facilitating imaging and image quality. A handheld microscope is often preferable for the patient with finger contractures (and a proportion of patients with SSc have flexion contractures of their fingers), offering flexible positioning on the finger and better comfort for the patient.

Imaging one nailfold takes between approximately a minute to 5 min, depending on the system used and whether the finger is viewed briefly in widefield view for screening or if multiple adjacent images are being saved. As discussed further below, fingers can be imaged in low optical magnification but widefield view to

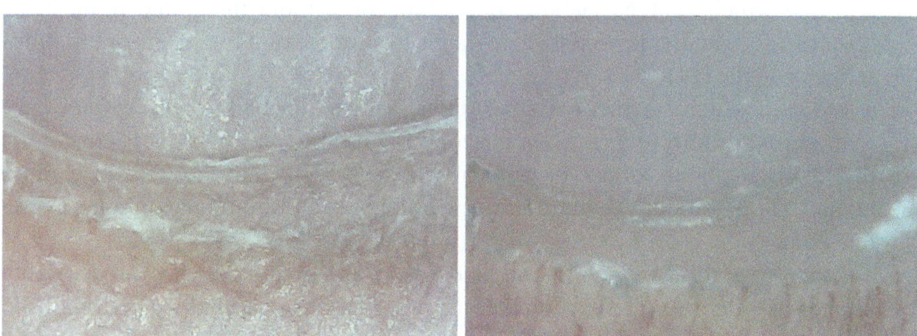

Fig. 1 Nailfold capillaroscopy without (left) and with (right) oil applied. The capillaries are much more clearly visualised after application of oil to the nailfold

observe/capture the whole or most of the nailfold. This is relatively quick and easy, possibly requiring only a single image view or capture but perhaps missing resolution and therefore detail. Conversely, images can be taken with higher optical/digital magnification systems, but this results in a smaller field of view with greater detail. With high magnification, the imaging system needs to be scanned across the nailfold, and several images viewed/taken in order to observe the whole nailfold field; this obviously takes longer than viewing/capturing a single field.

Consideration of how many fingers to image and whether to repeat imaging is discussed later in the chapter; however, from a clinical perspective once any specific abnormality has been observed (e.g. a giant capillary or an area of definite avascularity) it may be possible to make a diagnosis. Images can be acquired using high- or low-resolution imaging in one or more fingers and, although it is preferable to capture one or more images for the patient's clinical record, this may not be possible depending on the system used. When image capture is not possible then the capillaroscopy findings should be described/recorded by the clinician, for example in the clinical correspondence (including which fingers/number of fingers imaged).

In addition, it is worth noting that even an experienced operator may find that in some people (including 'healthy controls') imaging of capillaries is difficult, with poor visualisation. Whilst not fully understood, in some people capillary view is obscured, perhaps by damaged skin, oedema or fibrosis. Skin of colour may also be difficult to image since the melanin in the skin lies above the capillary layer and absorbs the light. This can lead to poor visualisation of the capillaries, and an underestimate of density or overestimate of avascular areas. This is discussed in detail in chapter "Nailfold Capillaroscopy as a Biomarker for Monitoring Disease and Treatment Response".

Points to Consider When Choosing a Nailfold Capillaroscopy System

Nailfold images may be acquired using 3 types of devices:

(a) a device which enables viewing only (with or without integrated light, these devices are usually low-cost, low magnification options, e.g. an ophthalmoscope or loupe) [4]
(b) a device to which a camera or smartphone can be attached to allow image capture and recording (e.g. a dermatoscope [4] or stereomicroscope). Of note is that a smart phone alone (or with an attached lens) may be able to capture images [5, 6] but as yet there are few studies examining smart phone use in this context
(c) a device that allows viewing and also has an integrated camera for recording images or videos (e.g USB microscope or digital videocapillaroscopy [Nailfold Video Capillaroscopy, NVC]).

Those with an integrated camera tend to have a better resolution (e.g. digital USB microscopy, or NVC) (Fig. 2).

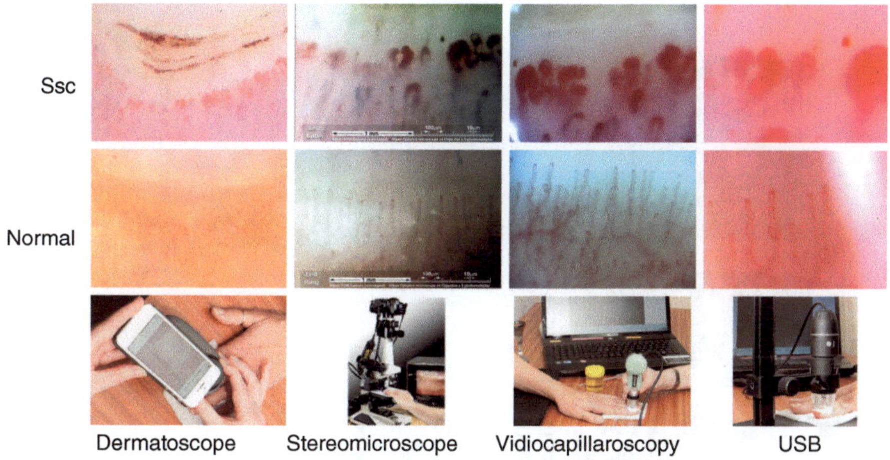

Fig. 2 Capillaroscopy techniques (lower row) and example images. The upper row shows images from a patient with SSc acquired using the different techniques, the middle row shows images from a healthy control subject. The images demonstrate the wide field of view captured with the dermatoscope and (to a lesser degree in this example) with the stereomicroscope. The individual capillaries are seen in more detail with the USB microscope and with videocapillaroscopy

It is worth a brief note at this point on resolution and magnification. Resolution refers to the ability of the device to capture detail, the pixel resolution (smallest unit of the image) defines the accuracy e.g. in terms of how precisely the inner and outer edges of the capillary can be identified for width measurement. In devices that have both optical (e.g. lenses) and electronic components (e.g. digital camera chips) the magnification (or increased size of viewing), depends on the combination of the initial optical magnification provided by the lens and then a further magnification of the captured image by the recording camera (digital zoom). The magnification can also be increased further by viewing images on a monitor/screen. Thus, when measures are to be made it is important to calibrate systems to be confident of values measured.

When deciding which device to choose/use it is critical to understand the components and properties of the device, including resolution and magnification. With digital devices the field of view and pixel resolution are the main points to take into account. For both clinical and research purposes, image storage (on-device, or via PC/laptop/smart device), and compatibility with software assisted image analysis systems also need to be considered: these are useful for later review and/or pattern categorisation or quantitative measurement. Table 1 summarises the properties of the different nailfold capillaroscopy systems, and Table 2 their advantages and disadvantages. It is to be noted that for clinical purposes direct image upload to the patient medical record may facilitate clinical communications between healthcare providers. If images are later to be extracted for research purposes, written consent should be considered when images are taken with purposes defined for the patient in terms of teaching, research and publication.

Table 1 Properties of different capillaroscopic methods

	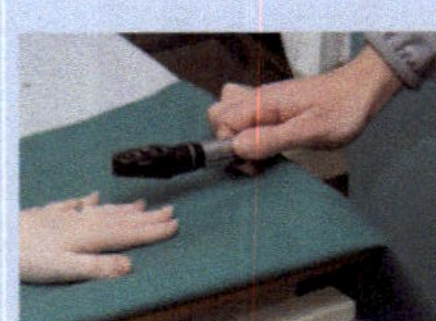	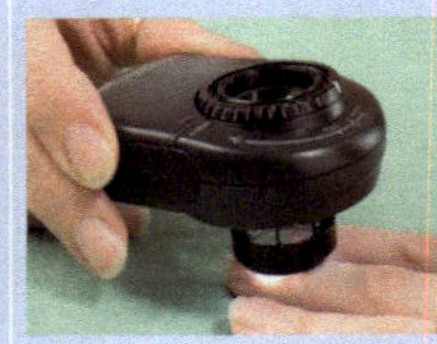	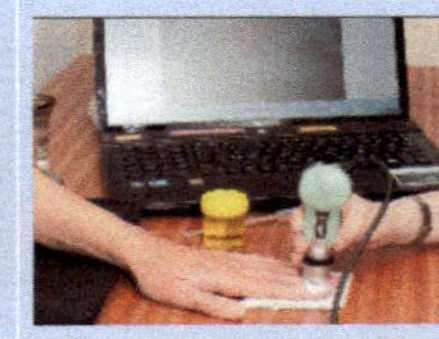	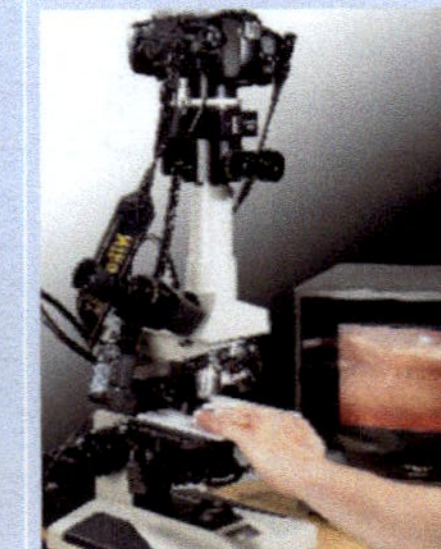	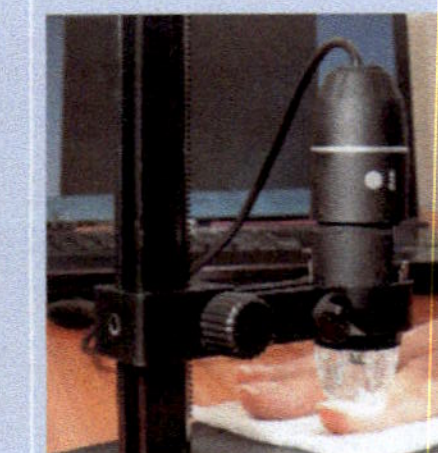
	Ophthalmoscope	Dermatoscope	NVC	Stereomicroscope	USB
Cost	$700	$2000	$5–12,000	$7000	$35
Easily portable	Yes	Yes	Depends on system	No	Yes
Image capture	No	With attached camera	Yes	Yes	Yes
Magnification	Low	Low	High	Variable	Variable
Resolution	Low	Medium	High	High	Medium
Whole field of view	No	Yes	No[a]	Yes	Yes
Measurement of density and capillary dimensions	No	No	Yes	Maybe	Maybe

NVC Nailfold videocapillaroscopy
[a]But possible via image mosaic

Table 2 Advantages and disadvantages of different capillaroscopic techniques

Technique	Advantages	Disadvantages
Nailfold videocapillaroscopy (NVC)	High magnification (×200 to ×600) Either hand-held probe or fixed microscope Measurements possible (of capillary density and dimensions) Image capture (for documentation in patient record) Can be used in both clinical and research practice	Small field of view at any one time with commercially available systems Not all systems portable Relatively high cost
Stereomicroscopy	Variable magnification Wide field of view Images rapidly acquired Image capture (for documentation in patient record)	Fixed microscope (can be problematic in patients with contractures) Measurements more complex then with NVC Not portable Relatively high cost
Dermoscopy	Easily portable, hand-held Wide field of view Relatively low cost	Low magnification Measurements not currently possible Image capture (for documentation in patient record) possible only if camera attached
USB microscopy	Portable, hand-held Variable field of view Measurements may be possible Image capture possible via attached computer Very low cost	Not specifically designed for capillaroscopy Lower resolution than videocapillaroscopy Can cause more glare than other techniques
Ophthalmoscopy	Readily available in the clinic Low cost	Narrow field of view Only obvious abnormalities can be easily seen (e.g. giant capillaries) Image capture (for documentation in patient record) not possible
Smartphone (with or without attached lens)	Portable, hand-held Variable field of view Relatively low cost	Not specifically designed for capillaroscopy Lower resolution than videocapillaroscopy

Images acquired using any of these systems can then be interpreted and abnormalities noted/scored or other analyses performed.

The main different capillaroscopy systems will now be considered in turn, beginning with low magnification systems and 'working up' to the current gold standard of nailfold videocapillaroscopy (NVC).

Ophthalmoscopy

As discussed above an ophthalmoscope or other standalone magnifying device can be used to observe but not record capillary shape and pattern, allowing a narrow field of view of the nailfold at low (×10–15) magnification. This device tends to be readily available in clinic and is low-cost. The ophthalmoscope can be used to identify very obvious changes e.g. giant capillaries, but more subtle changes will not be seen.

Dermoscopy

Portable dermatoscope devices contain lenses with LED illumination and are used by dermatologists to observe skin lesions. They can be used without a camera (generally ×10 optical magnification). Addition of a camera, or more recently a smartphone (camera) enables recording of the images and additional digital magnification. Due to the variation in magnification with automated focus, if an image is acquired with smartphone and dermatoscope in combination documentation of both the area of focus and a widefield view is required (or the use of a graticule captured at the same focus; some devices come with a scale bar on the surface that sits against the skin, automatically capturing the calibration data alongside the capillaries). Dermoscopy is often considered as a capillaroscopy screening procedure [7], and if marked abnormality is detected, for example obvious capillary enlargement or avascularity, then this would suffice for clinical diagnosis. However, it is more difficult to exclude abnormality with a smartphone or with dermoscopy than with NVC: this is because it is well recognised that dermoscopy is less sensitive (but more specific) in detecting abnormality than NVC [8, 9]. An advantage of dermoscopy for the clinician is that an image of the nailfold is acquired very quickly 'at a glance' which means that dermoscopy can be very easily applied in a busy out-patient clinic.

Optical magnification and suitable illumination are crucial for dermatoscope image interpretation [10]. For the dermatoscope and smartphone, a lack of uniform illumination can result in inconsistent image color, poor capillary contrast and make comparisons with future images difficult. It should also be noted that if the image is blurry, it is 'non-interpretable' and if changes are 'non-specific' further investigation with NVC is warranted [11]. Thus, it is important that if smartphone and dermoscopy screening procedures detect non-specific abnormalities there is a subsequent referral for further assessment to a SSc Clinical Center with NVC capabilities. If NVC is not available, then continued clinical follow-up with repeat nailfold assessment is indicated in 6–12 months.

Low-Cost USB Microscopy

Some of the devices discussed below are technically also "USB microscopes", in that they connect to a PC/tablet via USB. The difference is that the devices described in the next section are specifically designed with capillaroscopy in mind, while here, we refer to USB devices as general purpose and (almost always) much cheaper. These devices are widely available online for typically tens of pounds/Euros/US Dollars. They are not made by any recognisable brand-name companies. They are mostly plastic construction, including most of the optical components. They are designed to be used handheld but sometimes include a (low-cost plastic) stand for static imaging. They have standard USB connectors for PCs, but some now come with adaptors to micro-USB or USB-C for plugging directly into a smartphone or tablet. They usually include some very basic software for PCs and usually a suggested app for use with smartphones/tablets. The software, whether on a PC or other device, usually allows only live image viewing and image/video capture, so there are no measurement or annotation features. The devices are sold as having magnifications of 40×–1000×. The device placed on the finger and focused to observe capillaries. The devices operate with a "zoom-to-focus" mechanism, which results in varying field-of-view and pixel size, depending on focal distance. The optical mechanism used means there are usually two usable focal points: (1) a low magnification, wide field-of-view point, and (2) a high magnification, small field-of-view point. In practice this translates to a pixel resolution of around 2 μm at highest magnification, which is ample for viewing capillaries and detecting abnormalities. The lower magnifications offer a view similar to that given by a typical dermatoscope. Illumination is by some integrated LEDs around the lens which can result in artefacts/halos appearing in the image due to the poor-quality (plastic) optical components used. The advantages of these devices are that they provide reasonable resolution and work with most devices out of the box. Disadvantages include image artefacts due to low-cost optics, only basic software and non-durable construction. Images acquired with a low-cost USB system have been shown to be able to discriminate between patients with SSc and healthy controls [12].

Clinical Grade USB Microscopes

There are companies that specialise in clinically certified, USB microscopes (e.g. https://www.dinolite-uk.com/) whose price point is more in the range of high 100s of Pounds/Euros/US Dollars. Their specific devices, designed for nailfold capillaroscopy, include wireless and ultra-high magnification models. The devices tend to be a mixture of durable plastic and metal construction, with high-quality optical components used throughout. Connection is usually via standard USB to a PC (or wirelessly for specific models). Some have concavely shaped tips to fit the curvature of the fingers, facilitating the focusing of the device. The tips are removable for cleaning. Many systems come with their own software included which allows live image viewing, image/video capture, and measurement of different capillary parameters (e.g. capillary density, apical width) and annotation. Software often also includes a calibration routine which can enable a scale bar to be added to images. Focus/zoom is the same as for the low-cost devices, with two usable focal points as described above. Pixel resolution is around 1.5 μm at highest magnification. Devices sometimes incorporate a polariser or diffuser within the optical system to remove image artefacts such as glare/direct reflection caused by the LED illumination. This is controlled by a second wheel on the device body. Advantages of these USB microscopes include: relatively low-cost for a medical device, good resolution/image quality, robust design with easily cleaned parts. Full-featured software is included. Their disadvantages include that a variable field-of-view/magnifications for different zoom settings means careful calibration is required if image measurements are to be meaningfully compared with each other.

Stereomicroscopy

The widefield 'fixed' microscope or stereomicroscope (the technique used by Maricq in her early papers on nailfold capillaroscopy in rheumatological diseases [13, 14]), uses a 'traditional' microscope, often with a camera attachment to capture images. This can be used with different microscope lenses and thus magnifications. The finger is placed below the lens at the focal plane of the lens to capture images. The lens can be translated in three-dimensions to focus and move across the nailbed as required.

Nailfold Videocapillaroscopy (NVC)

NVC devices are also designed and made specifically for nailfold capillaroscopy. Features are similar to higher cost USB microscopes but with a fixed field-of-view which does not change while the focus adjusts. There is only one focal point available to the operator. The devices can have interchangeable lenses for different magnifications—the standard system is described as x200, but x500x and x20 lenses are also available (or may be supplied as part of a kit). Some companies supply hand held devices, others fixed stand microscopes as well as handheld (e.g. https://optilia.eu/, https://www.inspect-is.com/ and http://www.kktechnology.com). These clinical devices tend to have a full-featured software system, allowing imaging and annotation and patient demographic data storage. The optics are high-quality, and the illumination is dimmable to adjust for maximum contrast and to avoid glare. Pixel resolution is approximately 1 μm. Prices for systems are in the medium thousands of Pounds/Euros/US Dollars, including a laptop or pc. Devices are placed on the finger to capture images. Advantages of NVC include high image quality and full-featured software, and video capture is possible. Disadvantages include high cost.

Viewing Images on High Magnification Systems

As a general point, the magnification of a stereomicroscope, digital USB and NVC device can be set to a predetermined value (usually ×200–300) facilitating standardisation. It is again worth noting that autofocus of devices may change the exact magnification for USB and NVC devices, however, those with bespoke software often provide easy access to this information and sometimes record the magnification and a calibration bar on the image. Software may also enable display of a grid (with squares of a set size, e.g. 1 mm in length) overlaid on images to make capillary counting or estimation of capillary size easier. Examples of these grids/squares are included in chapter "Image Interpretation". Including as many frames as possible from each nailfold is likely to improve diagnostic accuracy [15].

Clinical Nailfold Capillary Reporting

Whilst this chapter covers image acquisition, we briefly consider clinical reporting here (whereas interpretation of images is covered in chapter "Image Interpretation"). Standard components of a nailfold capillaroscopy report may include reporting of capillary pattern as 'normal', 'early', 'active' or 'late', more quantitative measures such as capillary density and capillary dimension (apical diameter enlargement), and presence or absence of micro-haemorrahages or of abnormal capillary shapes. These are discussed in the next chapter (chapter "Image Interpretation"). The recognition of these abnormalities aid in the diagnosis of SSc-spectrum disease. The fast-track algorithm was developed to aid a practitioner in differentiating a scleroderma from a non-scleroderma pattern and has improved and standardised the training for image interpretation and highlights the importance of image clarity and storage [16, 17]. The purpose of mentioning this here is that although the fast-track algorithm can be applied with most capillaroscopy systems, more detailed analysis is unlikely to be possible with lower magnification techniques. Ingegnoli et al. [3] highlight the importance of describing the device used in their systemic review and international Delphi consensus of reporting items for capillaroscopy. This will help the person reviewing the report to understand any limitations. It is worth highlighting here nailfold capillaroscopy recognises only micro-circulation abnormalities, contrasting with macro-angiopathy assessments [18, 19].

Special Considerations When Acquiring Nailfold Capillaroscopy Images for Research Purposes

If nailfold capillaroscopy images are being recorded as part of a research project, nailfold capillaroscopy protocols should be clarified at the planning stage to optimise image interpretation, with relevant training if there are multiple users. This is especially important if there are multiple centres. It is common practice to collect clinically relevant digital vascular damage and severity variables in a nailfold capillaroscopy dataset at the outset of the project: these may include presence of digital ulcers, calcinosis, pitting, telangiectasia and/or amputation, duration of Raynaud's and non-Raynaud's disease features as well as other clinical features.

When capillaroscopy images are to be analysed for research purposes, then a greater level of detail may be necessary than for a clinical report and this may influence how the capillary images are acquired, and the capillaroscopy system used. For example, as discussed in later chapters, there is increasing interest in automating analysis, including machine learning, deep learning and other artificial intelligence (AI) techniques. If automated analysis is to be included in a research project, then the protocol needs to be ensure that sufficient numbers of images are collected from across each nailfold, and that image resolution/magnification is sufficient for the automation to be applied. The data generated will only be as good as the images used to generate them and quality assurance of results is always required to ensure data meet expectations and are interpreted correctly. This may influence choice of equipment and the imaging protocol.

Deep learning-based software can detect micro-hemorrhage, capillary enlargement, and abnormal shapes. Deep learning [20–24] can be applied to NVC and USB capillaroscopy images and aims to facilitate precision medicine in patients with SSc. However, at the present time it is unclear whether deep learning software is applicable to dermoscopy due to the lower resolution and variable image quality.

As automation of nailfold capillaroscopic analysis becomes more widely adopted, this will have implications for clinical practice as well as for research and clinical practice. This is because ease of automation of nailfold capillaroscopy reports may facilitate more widespread use in rheumatology clinical practice and facilitate early patient referrals to SSc Centers [24]. AI techniques are discussed further in chapter "Quantitative Analysis".

The increasing interest in research applications of nailfold capillaroscopy underscores the need for acquisition of high-quality images. Current knowledge about the nailfold microvascular changes in SSc supports both associations with disease activity and disease duration [25]. Cross-sectional data on capillaroscopy in an international multicentre cohort of SSc highlights the value of standardised protocols using NVC [26]. Relevant to multicentre research, and its challenges, a multicentre observational study—the Prospective Registry of Early Systemic Sclerosis (PRESS, an incident cohort of patients with early diffuse SSc with an aim to advance the understanding of disease pathogenesis and identify novel biomarkers) was unable to collect quality nailfold capillaroscopy images with a stereomicroscope platform despite a standardised protocol and training [27]. Difficulties in using the capillaroscopy system was the reason cited for missing capillaroscopy data in the PRESS cohort. It is noted that the stereomicroscope cannot provide quality images for patients with fixed contractures. Nonetheless, United States investigators at expert SSc Centers desire more training and are using an ophthalmoscope or dermatoscope in clinical practice [28], highlighting the importance of international collaborative efforts to standardise procedures and training [7, 11, 29]. It is clear that clinical registries and trials both benefit from standardised protocols for training in image acquisition and interpretation [7].

Relevant to this, there are several examples of formal capillaroscopy training facilitating image acquisition and interpretation [16, 17].

It is worth noting that the use of nailfold capillaroscopy systems varies between countries. Survey results suggest that in mainland Europe, NVC is the favoured technique [30] as opposed to lower cost techniques in the United States and the United Kingdom [28, 31, 32].

When to Consider Repeating Nailfold Capillaroscopic Images Over Time, Including—Longitudinal Measures in Research Studies

In clinical practice longitudinal measures are often not necessary: once abnormality has been identified then a diagnosis can usually be made. There are, however, exceptions to this, including borderline capillary changes when the clinician is not confident to make a firm diagnosis but prefers to follow up in a short period of time (e.g. 6 months). In addition, if a patient has clinical features of concern (for example late onset Raynaud's phenomenon) but no capillary changes then the clinician may again arrange longitudinal follow-up. If capillaroscopy is to be repeated, then it is prudent to record the finger with any abnormalities and from where the images were taken. Ideally images should be captured from across the whole nailfold to ensure that the same capillaries can be assessed at the follow-up visit to assess change.

From a research perspective, capillaroscopy has been used as an outcome measure in longitudinal studies to assess change in disease status with time or in response to therapeutics. Here, it is important to consider the frequency of data collection and reproducibility of taking images [33]. The requirements of capillaroscopy as a biomarker, including reliability of image acquisition are discussed in chapter "Nailfold Capillaroscopy as a Biomarker for Monitoring Disease and Treatment Response".

Number of Fingers to Be Imaged

Time constraints may impact nailfold capillaroscopy data collection in the clinical setting. In the United States, the critical importance of ease of nailfold image data collection and interpretation is underscored by billing-based practices [34]. During routine capillaroscopic examination, ideally all eight nailbeds (excluding thumbs) should be examined, otherwise some abnormalities will be missed. Single finger examination provides too low sensitivity to be recommended, but examination of a four-finger combination of both ring and both middle fingers gave a sensitivity of 66.7% for detection of SSc in a study of 2994 assessments of 1600 capillaroscopy images of 173 participants [35]. In addition, it should be noted that there can be significant heterogeneity both within and between fingers (Fig. 3). For these reasons

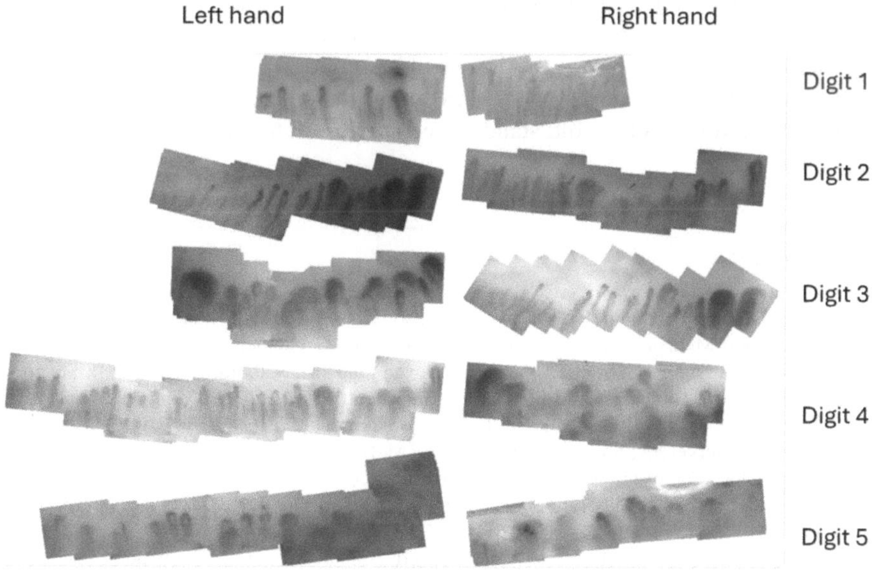

Fig. 3 Nailfold videocapillaroscopy images from 10 nailfolds (right and left thumb, index, middle, ring and little fingers). These images demonstrate the heterogeneity of capillary appearances both within and between nailfolds

it is imperative to image all eight fingers such that abnormalities that may be present in only one part of one digit are not missed.

Conclusions

Acquisition of high-quality images is essential for nailfold capillaroscopy to be useful in both clinical practice and research and is usually (although not always) achievable. Nailfold image acquisition is possible using a variety of devices, some standalone and some requiring a camera or smartphone to connect to record images. Whether the images are to be taken for clinical diagnostic or for research purposes may influence the choice of device to be used and the protocol followed. Image clarity is the most critical aspect to allow interpretation and quantification of capillary density, capillary dimensions (e.g. apical diameter enlargement), abnormal shape, and presence of micro-haemorrhages. Clarity depends upon magnification, resolution and good focus. Regardless of which nailfold capillaroscopy technique is used, application of oil to the nailfold and subject preparation is essential. If repeat capillaroscopic assessment is required, for example to confirm a diagnosis, to assess disease progression, or as an outcome measure in longitudinal research (for example to assess response to therapeutics), then the frequency of data collection should be carefully considered. Collection of digital vascular damage and severity variables in a nailfold capillaroscopy dataset should be included at the outset of research projects and may include presence of digital ulcers, calcinosis, pitting, telangiectasia and/or amputation or other clinical factors. While time constraints may impact nailfold capillaroscopy data collection obtained in the clinical setting, eight finger data acquisition is recommended. Application of data science to well-phenotyped patients with rheumatological conditions offers promise for more extensive use of nailfold capillaroscopy and underscores the need for acquisition of high-quality images. NVC remains the gold standard technique and training in this technique is imperative.

References

1. van den Hoogen F, Khanna D, Fransen J, Johnson SR, Baron M, Tyndall A, Matucci-Cerinic M, Naden RP, Medsger TA Jr, Carreira PE, Riemekasten G, Clements PJ, Denton CP, Distler O, Allanore Y, Furst DE, Gabrielli A, Mayes MD, van Laar JM, Seibold JR, Czirjak L, Steen VD, Inanc M, Kowal-Bielecka O, Müller-Ladner U, Valentini G, Veale DJ, Vonk MC, Walker UA, Chung L, Collier DH, Ellen Csuka M, Fessler BJ, Guiducci S, Herrick A, Hsu VM, Jimenez S, Kahaleh B, Merkel PA, Sierakowski S, Silver RM, Simms RW, Varga J, Pope JE. 2013 classification criteria for systemic sclerosis: an American college of rheumatology/European league against rheumatism collaborative initiative. Ann Rheum Dis. 2013;72(11):1747–55. https://doi.org/10.1136/annrheumdis-2013-204424. PMID: 24092682.
2. Herrick AL, Dinsdale G, Murray A. New perspectives in the imaging of Raynaud's phenomenon. Eur J Rheumatol. 2020;7(Suppl 3):S212–21. https://doi.org/10.5152/eurjrheum.2020.19124. Epub 2020 Jul 6. PMID: 33164735; PMCID: PMC7647685.

3. Ingegnoli F, Herrick AL, Schioppo T, Bartoli F, Ughi N, Pauling JD, Sulli A, Cutolo M, Smith V, European League against Rheumatism (EULAR) study group on microcirculation in rheumatic diseases and the Scleroderma Clinical Trials Consortium. Reporting items for capillaroscopy in clinical research on musculoskeletal diseases: a systematic review and international Delphi consensus. Rheumatology (Oxford). 2021;60(3):1410–8. https://doi.org/10.1093/rheumatology/keaa457. PMID: 32984894.
4. Ramani LT, Pullman-Mooar S, Meltzer M. Screening nailfold capillaroscopy using a jeweler's loupe. J Am Acad Dermatol. 2020;83:e1–e2. https://doi.org/10.1016/j.jaad.2019.09.006.
5. Parker MJS, Oliffe MT, McGill NW. An evaluation of two novel capillaroscopy techniques in suspected scleroderma-spectrum disorders: A single-centre cross-sectional study. Mod Rheumatol. 2018;28(4):676–80.
6. Ma Z, Mulder DJ, Gniadecki R, Cohen Tervaert JW, Osman M. Methods of assessing nailfold capillaroscopy compared to video capillaroscopy in patients with systemic sclerosis-a critical review of the literature. Diagnostics (Basel). 2023;13(13):2204.
7. Smith V, Herrick AL, Ingegnoli F, Damjanov N, De Angelis R, Denton CP, Distler O, Espejo K, Foeldvari I, Frech T, Garro B, Gutierrez M, Gyger G, Hachulla E, Hesselstrand R, Iagnocco A, Kayser C, Melsens K, Müller-Ladner U, Paolino S, Pizzorni C, Radic M, Riccieri V, Snow M, Stevens W, Sulli A, van Laar JM, Vonk MC, Vanhaecke A, Cutolo M, EULAR Study Group on Microcirculation in Rheumatic Diseases and the Scleroderma Clinical Trials Consortium Group on Capillaroscopy. Standardisation of nailfold capillaroscopy for the assessment of patients with Raynaud's phenomenon and systemic sclerosis. Autoimmun Rev. 2020;19(3):102458. https://doi.org/10.1016/j.autrev.2020.102458. Epub 2020 Jan 10. PMID: 31927087.
8. Hughes M, Moore T, O'Leary N, Tracey A, Ennis H, Dinsdale G, Murray A, Roberts C, Herrick AL. A study comparing videocapillaroscopy and dermoscopy in the assessment of nailfold capillaries in patients with systemic sclerosis-spectrum disorders. Rheumatology (Oxford). 2015;54(8):1435–42. https://doi.org/10.1093/rheumatology/keu533. Epub 2015 Mar 6. PMID: 25749623.
9. Dinsdale G, Peytrignet S, Moore T, Berks M, Roberts C, Manning J, Allen J, Anderson M, Cutolo M, Hesselstrand R, Howell K, Pizzorni C, Smith V, Sulli A, Wildt M, Taylor C, Murray A, Herrick AL. The assessment of nailfold capillaries: comparison of dermoscopy and nailfold videocapillaroscopy. Rheumatology (Oxford). 2018;57(6):1115–6. https://doi.org/10.1093/rheumatology/key018. PMID: 29447411.
10. Hanlon KL, Wei G, Correa-Selm L, Grichnik JM. Dermoscopy and skin imaging light sources: a comparison and review of spectral power distribution and color consistency. J Biomed Opt. 2022;27(8):080902. https://doi.org/10.1117/1.JBO.27.8.080902. Epub 2022 Aug 8. PMID: 36452032; PMCID: PMC9360608.
11. Radic M, Snow M, Frech TM, Saketkoo LA, Cutolo M, Smith V. Consensus-based evaluation of dermatoscopy versus nailfold videocapillaroscopy in Raynaud's phenomenon linking USA and Europe: a European League against Rheumatism study group on microcirculation in rheumatic diseases project. Clin Exp Rheumatol. 2020;125(3):132–6. Epub 2020 Aug 26. PMID: 32865167.
12. Berks M, Dinsdale G, Marjanovic E, Murray A, Taylor C, Herrick AL. Comparison between low cost USB nailfold capillaroscopy and videocapillaroscopy: a pilot study. Rheumatology (Oxford). 2021;60(8):3862–7. https://doi.org/10.1093/rheumatology/keaa723. PMID: 33232464; PMCID: PMC8328506.
13. Maricq HR, LeRoy EC. Patterns of finger capillary abnormalities in connective tissue diseases by 'wide-field' microscopy. Arthritis Rheum. 1973;16:619–28.
14. Maricq HR. Widefield capillary microscopy. Technique and rating scale for abnormalities seen in scleroderma and related disorders. Arthritis Rheum. 1981;24:1159–65.
15. Gracia Tello BDC, Sáez-Comet L, Lledó G, et al. POS0907 the significance of analysed millimeters in interpreting nailfold capillaroscopy images. Ann Rheum Dis. 2024;83:1146–7.
16. Smith V, Vanhaecke A, Herrick AL, Distler O, Guerra MG, Denton CP, Deschepper E, Foeldvari I, Gutierrez M, Hachulla E, Ingegnoli F, Kubo S, Müller-Ladner U, Riccieri V, Sulli A, van

Laar JM, Vonk MC, Walker UA, Cutolo M, EULAR Study Group on Microcirculation in Rheumatic Diseases. Fast track algorithm: How to differentiate a “scleroderma pattern” from a “non-scleroderma pattern”. Autoimmun Rev. 2019;18(11):102394. https://doi.org/10.1016/j.autrev.2019.102394. Epub 2019 Sep 11. PMID: 31520797.

17. Ng SA, Tan WH, Saffari SE, Low AHL. Evaluation of nailfold capillaroscopy online training using the fast track algorithm. J Rheumatol. 2023;50(3):368–72. https://doi.org/10.3899/jrheum.220794. Epub 2022 Dec 1. PMID: 36455942.
18. Schioppo T, Orenti A, Boracchi P, De Lucia O, Murgo A, Ingegnoli F. Evidence of macro- and micro-angiopathy in scleroderma: An integrated approach combining 22-MHz power Doppler ultrasonography and video-capillaroscopy. Microvasc Res. 2019;122:125–30. https://doi.org/10.1016/j.mvr.2018.07.001. Epub 2018 Jul 6. PMID: 29981761.
19. Frech TM. Imaging techniques for assessment of vascular involvement in systemic sclerosis. Curr Opin Rheumatol. 2022;34(6):311–8. https://doi.org/10.1097/BOR.0000000000000901. Epub 2022 Aug 24. PMID: 36001341; PMCID: PMC9936597.
20. Gracia Tello B, Ramos Ibañez E, Fanlo Mateo P, Sáez Cómet L, Martínez Robles E, Ríos Blanco JJ, Marí Alfonso B, Espinosa Garriga G, Todolí Parra J, Ortego Centeno N, Callejas Rubio JL, Freire Dapena M, Marín Ballvé A, Selva-O'Callaghan A, Guillén Del Castillo A, Simeón Aznar CP, Fonollosa PV. The challenge of comprehensive nailfold videocapillaroscopy practice: a further contribution. Clin Exp Rheumatol. 2022;40(10):1926–32. https://doi.org/10.55563/clinexprheumatol/6usce8. Epub 2021 Dec 16. PMID: 34936544.
21. Gracia Tello BC, Ramos Ibañez E, Saez Comet L, Guillén Del Castillo A, Simeón Aznar CP, Selva-O'Callaghan A, Espinosa G, Lledó G, Freire Dapena M, Martinez Robles E, Ríos JJ, Todolí Parra JA, Marí Alfonso B, Ortego Centeno N, Marín Ballvé A, Callejas Rubio JL, Fonollosa Plá V, Fanlo P. External clinical validation of automated software to identify structural abnormalities and microhaemorrhages in nailfold videocapillaroscopy images. Clin Exp Rheumatol. 2023;41(8):1605–11. https://doi.org/10.55563/clinexprheumatol/m6obl3. Epub 2023 May 4. PMID: 37140670.
22. Bharathi PG, Berks M, Dinsdale G, Murray A, Manning J, Wilkinson S, Cutolo M, Smith V, Herrick AL, Taylor CJ. A deep learning system for quantitative assessment of microvascular abnormalities in nailfold capillary images. Rheumatology (Oxford). 2023;62(6):2325–9. https://doi.org/10.1093/rheumatology/kead026. PMID: 36651676; PMCID: PMC10234192.
23. Ozturk L, Laclau C, Boulon C, Mangin M, Braz-Ma E, Constans J, Dari L, Le Hello C. Analysis of nailfold capillaroscopy images with artificial intelligence: Data from literature and performance of machine learning and deep learning from images acquired in the SCLEROCAP study. Microvasc Res. 2025;157:104753. https://doi.org/10.1016/j.mvr.2024.104753. Epub 2024 Oct 9. PMID: 39389419.
24. Gracia Tello BDC, Sáez Comet L, Lledó G, Freire Dapena M, Mesa MA, Martín-Cascón M, Guillén Del Castillo A, Martínez Robles E, Simeón-Aznar CP, Todolí Parra JA, Varela DC, Maldonado Vélez G, Marín Ballvé A, Aramburu Llorente J, Pérez Abad L, Ramos IE. Capiscore: a quantitative algorithm for identifying disease patterns in nailfold videocapillaroscopy. Rheumatology (Oxford). 2024;63(12):3315–21. https://doi.org/10.1093/rheumatology/keae197. PMID: 38530791; PMCID: PMC11637479.
25. Lambova SN, Müller-Ladner U. Nailfold capillaroscopy in systemic sclerosis—state of the art: the evolving knowledge about capillaroscopic abnormalities in systemic sclerosis. J Scleroderma Relat Disord. 2019;4(3):200–11. https://doi.org/10.1177/2397198319833486. Epub 2019 Apr 15. PMID: 35382505; PMCID: PMC8922564.
26. Ingegnoli F, Ardoino I, Boracchi P, Cutolo M, EUSTAR co-authors. Nailfold capillaroscopy in systemic sclerosis: data from the EULAR scleroderma trials and research (EUSTAR) database. Microvasc Res. 2013;89:122–8. https://doi.org/10.1016/j.mvr.2013.06.003. Epub 2013 Jun 17. PMID: 23792167.
27. Frech TM, Shanmugam VK, Shah AA, Assassi S, Gordon JK, Hant FN, Hinchcliff ME, Steen V, Khanna D, Kayser C, Domsic RT. Treatment of early diffuse systemic sclerosis skin disease. Clin Exp Rheumatol. 2013;31(2 Suppl 76):166–71. Epub 2013 Jul 23. PMID: 23910619; PMCID: PMC3889109.

28. Snow MH, Saketkoo LA, Frech TM, Stever JR, Lebedoff N, Herrick AL, Cutolo M, Smith V. Results from an American pilot survey among Scleroderma Clinical Trials Consortium members on capillaroscopy use and how to best implement nailfold capillaroscopy training. Clin Exp Rheumatol. 2019;119(4):151. Epub 2019 Apr 5. PMID: 31025929.
29. Smith V, Ickinger C, Hysa E, Snow M, Frech T, Sulli A, Cutolo M. Nailfold capillaroscopy. Best Pract Res Clin Rheumatol. 2023;37(1):101849. https://doi.org/10.1016/j.berh.2023.101849. Epub 2023 Jul 6. PMID: 37419757.
30. Ingegnoli F, Ughi N, Dinsdale G, Orenti A, Boracchi P, Allanore Y, Foeldvari I, Sulli A, Cutolo M, Smith V, Herrick AL, EULAR Study Group on Microcirculation in RheumaticDiseases. An international SUrvey on non-iNvaSive tecHniques to assess the mIcrocirculation in patients with RayNaud's phEnomenon (SUNSHINE survey). Rheumatol Int. 2017;37(11):1879–90. https://doi.org/10.1007/s00296-017-3808-0. Epub 2017 Sep 11. PMID: 28894946.
31. Eden M, Wilkinson S, Murray A, Bharathi PG, Vail A, Taylor CJ, Payne K, Herrick AL. Nailfold capillaroscopy: a survey of current UK practice and 'next steps' to increase uptake among rheumatologists. Rheumatology (Oxford). 2022;62(1):335–40. https://doi.org/10.1093/rheumatology/keac320. PMID: 35640131; PMCID: PMC9788809.
32. Anderson C, Leone V, Pain C. Comment on: Nailfold capillaroscopy: a survey of current UK practice and 'next steps' to increase uptake among rheumatologists. Rheumatology (Oxford). 2023;62(10):e303–4. https://doi.org/10.1093/rheumatology/kead386. PMID: 37527027.
33. Dinsdale G, Moore T, O'Leary N, Berks M, Roberts C, Manning J, Allen J, Anderson M, Cutolo M, Hesselstrand R, Howell K, Pizzorni C, Smith V, Sulli A, Wildt M, Taylor C, Murray A, Herrick AL. Quantitative outcome measures for systemic sclerosis-related Microangiopathy—reliability of image acquisition in Nailfold Capillaroscopy. Microvasc Res. 2017;113:56–9. https://doi.org/10.1016/j.mvr.2017.05.003. Epub 2017 May 8. PMID: 28495471.
34. Overbury R, Murtaugh MA, Fischer A, Frech TM. Primary care assessment of capillaroscopy abnormalities in patients with Raynaud's phenomenon. Clin Rheumatol. 2015;34(12):2135–40. https://doi.org/10.1007/s10067-015-3062-3. Epub 2015 Sep 23. PMID: 26400642.
35. Dinsdale G, Roberts C, Moore T, Manning J, Berks M, Allen J, Anderson ME, Cutolo M, Hesselstrand R, Howell K, Pizzorni C, Smith V, Sulli A, Wildt M, Taylor C, Murray A, Herrick AL. Nailfold capillaroscopy-how many fingers should be examined to detect abnormality? Rheumatology (Oxford). 2019;58(2):284–8. https://doi.org/10.1093/rheumatology/key293. PMID: 30247696.

Image Interpretation

Vanessa Smith and Maurizio Cutolo

Abbreviations

CTD	Connective Tissue Disease
EULAR	European Alliance of Associations for Rheumatology
EUSTAR	European Scleroderma Trials and Research group
mm	millimeter
µm	micrometer
NVC	Nailfold Videocapillaroscopy
RP	Raynaud's Phenomenon
SCTC	Scleroderma Clinical Trials Consortium
SDS	Scleroderma Spectrum Diseases
SSc	Systemic Sclerosis
VEDOSS	Very Early Diagnosis of Systemic Sclerosis

Key Points

- There is wide variability in capillaroscopic characteristics in healthy controls. Consequently 34% of healthy controls may have abnormalities in their capillaroscopy.

V. Smith (✉)
Department of Internal Medicine/(Rheumatology), Ghent University (Hospital), and Unit for Molecular Immunology and Inflammation, VIB Inflammation Research Center (IRC), Ghent, Belgium
e-mail: vanessa.smith@ugent.be

M. Cutolo
Laboratory of Experimental Rheumatology, Division of Rheumatology, Department of Internal Medicine and Medical Specialties (DiMI), University of Genova, IRCCS San Martino Polyclinic Hospital, Genova, Italy
e-mail: mcutolo@unige.it

A. L. Herrick et al. (eds.), *Nailfold Capillaroscopy in Rheumatological Diseases*,
https://doi.org/10.1007/978-3-032-03970-5_4

- Variation in capillaries may more easily be appreciated with a 200× magnification (nailfold videocapillaroscope [NVC]) than with a 20× magnification (dermatoscope).
- The EULAR/SCTC consensus concerning standardised reporting of capillaroscopy describes the following capillaroscopic characteristics per linear millimeter (mm): density, dimension, abnormal shapes and presence/absence of microhaemorrhages (quantitative scoring). Based on how these capillaroscopic characteristics are combined an image may be categorised as a scleroderma, or a non-scleroderma pattern.
- The fast track algorithm is a simple algorithm to categorize capillaroscopic images reliably into a scleroderma pattern or not.
- The following quantitative individual capillaroscopic characteristics, as per EULAR/SCTC consensus have been shown to have a high interrater reliability: density, giants and abnormal shapes.
- Qualitative interpretation allows classification as scleroderma patterns, normal patterns or as images with non-specific abnormalities.

Introduction

Capillaroscopy is the safest and fastest diagnostic system to detect structural alterations of the microcirculation [1, 2]. Since capillaroscopy may detect even minimal changes of the microvessel structure, its use is mandatory in presence of clinical symptoms of microangiopathy, i.e. in presence of RP, which affects 5% of the population [3] (see chapter "Clinical Indications").

Diverse terminology had been described for RP, until in 1992 LeRoy and Medsger proposed criteria for the strict definition of primary RP and of secondary RP [4]. A patient was defined as having primary RP when having, in addition to other criteria, 'normal nailfold capillaries'. In 2001, LeRoy and Medsger proposed criteria for the 'early' diagnosis of SSc, which included RP, SSc-specific autoantibodies and 'scleroderma-type' changes on nailfold capillaroscopy [5]. Scleroderma patterns are also incorporated in the Very Early clinical Diagnosis of SSc (VEDOSS) criteria (see chapter "Clinical Indications"). Both sets of criteria have been validated [6, 7]. Recent international efforts (SCTC and EULAR) have produced a consensus document to standardise description of capillaroscopic characteristics (see below) and to classify capillaroscopic images as 'normal', 'non-specific abnormalities' or 'scleroderma patterns' (see below): "EULAR/SCTC consensus on standardised interpretation of capillaroscopic images" [8, 9]. Standardized image interpretation is an aid for the clinician in daily practice as well as in research setting.

Normal, Scleroderma and Non-specific Patterns

Normal

Figure 1 depicts a normal capillary pattern taken with NVC with a 200× magnification. The capillaries are spaced at regular intervals, like the teeth of a hair comb.

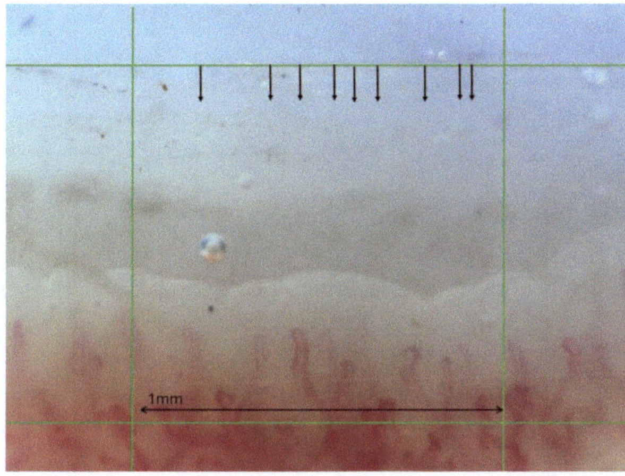

Fig. 1 A normal capillaroscopic pattern on NVC
A capillaroscopic image taken in a 12-year-old with RP with NVC with a 200× magnification. The capillaries of the distal row (black arrows) have a hairpin shape and lie at equal distances to each other. The capillaries are counted per linear mm

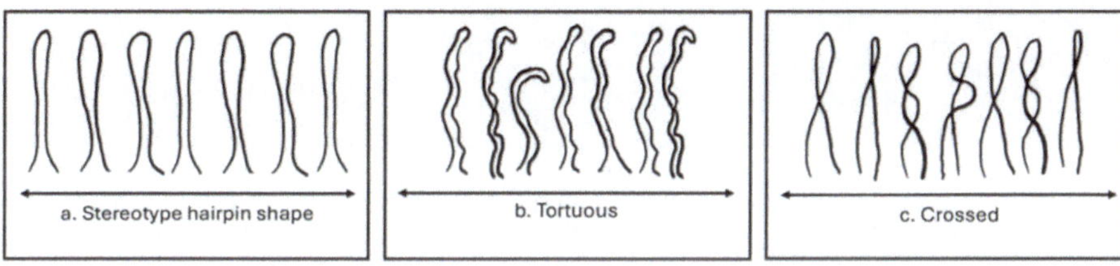

Fig. 2 Normal and non-specific variations of nailfold capillary morphology
Drawings representing the most frequent patterns Andrade and colleagues described in healthy controls with low magnification technique [11]. (**a**) Stereotype hairpin shape: the limbs are straight and do not cross each other (**b**) Tortuous type: the limbs are curled but do not cross each other (**c**) Crossed type: the limbs cross each other once or twice

This can be perceived visually (qualitative interpretation, see below). In a stereotype normal image the capillaries of the distal row of the nailfold have an open hairpin shape, a homogenous size, are regularly arranged in a parallel fashion and their number ranges between 7 and 12 capillaries per linear mm [8, 10]. The pattern of the nailfold capillaries is remarkably constant in healthy individuals. However, across the population there exists a wide variation in the ranges of the normal capillaroscopic characteristics, which has most extensively been reported by Andrade *et al.* He described with a 10×–16× magnification widefield technique, capillaroscopic findings in the largest described healthy persons study population (800 healthy individuals). Besides the stereotypical open loop ('hairpin shaped' capillary), subtle variations of the morphology of the distal row capillaries were noted. According to the most prevalent morphology, morphological dominant patterns were defined, such as open patterns (Fig. 2a), tortuous patterns (the limbs are curled but do not cross each other) (Fig. 2b), crossed patterns (the limbs cross each other once or twice) (Fig. 2c), undefined patterns and mixed patterns. Also, capillary 'abnormalities' (unusual distinctive capillary alterations), were quantified in the entire sample of healthy individuals: 'meandering' loops (limbs cross upon themselves or with another several times) (Fig. 3a) in 25%, 'ectatic' loops (dimension of

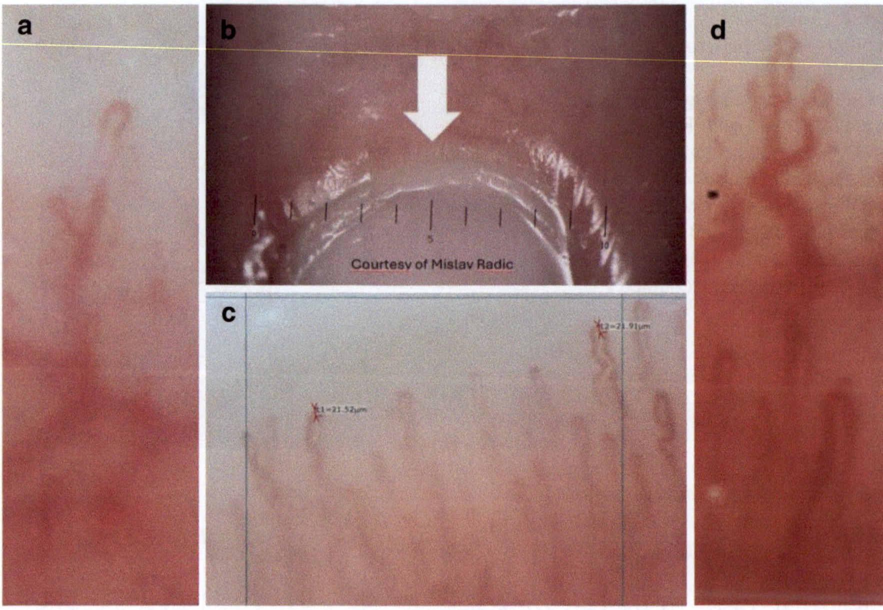

Fig. 3 Non-specific abnormalities in capillary morphology on NVC
Non-specific abnormalities that were described by Andrade et al. in 800 healthy controls [11]. (**a**) Meandering loop: non-specific abnormality of morphology in a 200× magnification capillaroscopic image. (**b**) Ectasia (increased dimension) taken with a 20× magnification (dermatoscopic image). (**c**) Ectasia taken with a 200× magnification (NVC image): apical diameter of 21.5 and 21.9 micrometer (μm). (**d**) Bushy capillary (non-specific abnormality of morphology) in a 200× magnification capillaroscopic image. Notably, certain abnormalities are barely visible with low magnification, whilst clearly visible with a 200× magnification

afferent, apical and efferent limbs is moderately enlarged) (Fig. 3b and c) in 12%, 'bushy' loops (Fig. 3d) in 7% and 'bizarre' loops ("striking atypical morphology, but not classifiable in the previous categories") in 2%.

These capillaroscopic anomalies were seen in 34% of the entire population of healthy individuals, but few in each individual. Haemorrhages (Fig. 4a and b) and avascular areas (Fig. 4c and d) may also exist [11]. In recent consensus literature between the SCTC and the EULAR study group on microcirculation in rheumatic diseases (EULAR SG MC/RD) on how to describe capillaroscopic images in a standardised way these anomalies have been classified as 'non-specific' abnormalities (see below: "EULAR/SCTC consensus on standardised interpretation of capillaroscopic images"). Ectasia (Fig. 3b and c), i.e. dilation of the apical limb >20μm and <50 μm is a 'non-specific' abnormality in dimension. Any shape that does not have a convex tip or that has more than two crossings of the limbs is called a 'non-specific' abnormal morphology (=shape) (Fig. 3a, d and also see below) [8, 12, 13]. In short, the landmark study of Andrade taught us that in a normal population not only stereotype 'normal' but also 'non-specific' abnormalities may occur.

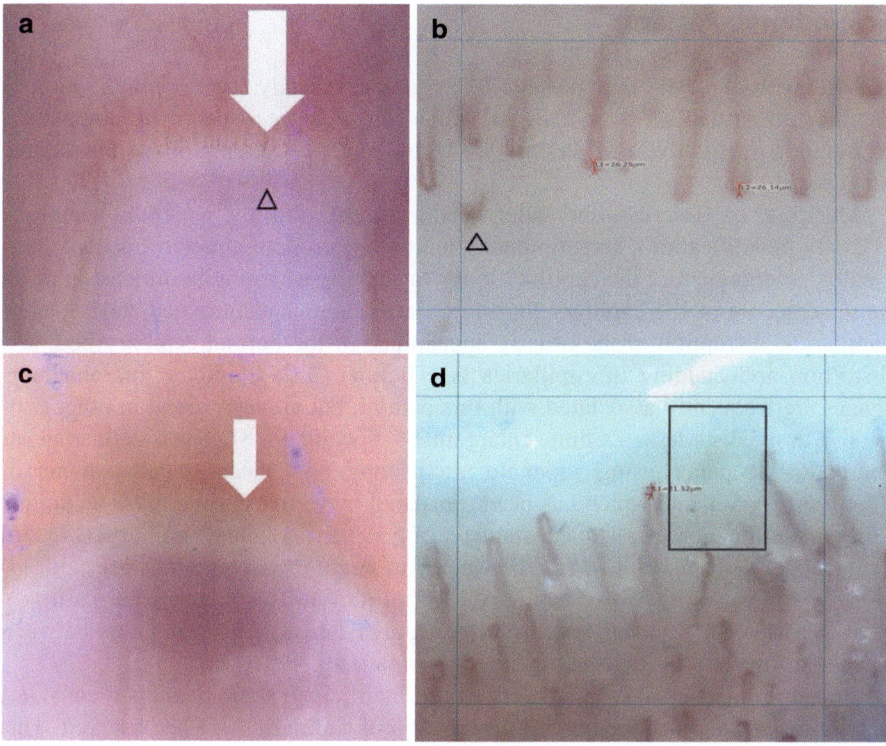

Fig. 4 Haemorrhages and avascular areas on NVC
Haemorrhages and avascular areas in healthy controls both with low magnification (20×) and high magnification (200×). **4(a).** Notably this haemorrhage (brown deposit Δ) is almost invisible with the low magnification, as it only looks like a brown punctation. The white arrow shows the area that is displayed in Fig. 4b with the NVC technique with a 200× magnification. (**b**) The haemorrhage is clearly visible as a brown deposit on the left lower quadrant of the 200× magnification capillaroscopic image (Δ). (**c**) Low magnification (20×) capillaroscopic image of a healthy control. The white arrow shows the area that is displayed in (**d**) with the NVC technique with a 200× magnification. (**d**) High magnification (200×) capillaroscopic image of a healthy control where the rectangular area depicts an area with a deletion of a capillary (= avascular area). Note that this avascular area can almost not be perceived with the low magnification (**c**)

However, certain features, such as giant capillaries (see below: section "Scleroderma patterns") or extensive avascularity (an extreme low density) do not seem to be present in a normal population. In fact, in recent consensus literature, giant capillaries and the combination of extreme loss of capillaries combined with abnormal shapes are 'specific' abnormalities indicative of scleroderma spectrum diseases (SDS) [9].

Scleroderma Patterns

Patients with clinically recognisable SSc characteristically show a combination of capillary abnormalities in the nailfold, which can easily be assessed through pattern recognition (qualitative assessment) (see below section: "Scoring of capillaroscopic images").

Maricq *et al.* described the 'scleroderma pattern' with the widefield technique (12–14× magnification), and stipulated that the 'scleroderma pattern' is characterised by enlargement of the capillary loops (a striking widening in dimension of all three segments of the capillary loop [arterial, venous and intermediate]), loss of capillaries, disruption of the orderly appearance of the normal capillary bed, and distortion and budding of capillaries (see below) [14]. Capillary microhaemorrhages are frequently associated with this pattern, but are also found in other connective tissue disorders. 'Definite enlargement', specific for SDS, was defined in her seminal 1986 paper, using widefield microscopy, as a mean apical diameter of 47.7μm (Fig. 5a), and which has been translated by Cutolo for the NVC technique (200× magnification) as an apical diameter of ≥50μm (i.e. 'giant' capillary) (Fig. 5b) [15]. Moderate capillary loss (i.e. between 2 to 4mm^2 avascular zones per nailfold) (Fig. 5c and d) and extensive capillary loss (>4 mm^2 avascular zones per nailfold), later on adopted by Lonzetti *et al.* and Koenig *et al.*, are also discriminatory between 'scleroderma patterns' and 'non-scleroderma patterns' [6, 16–18].

In addition to the above-mentioned abnormalities, in some patients a considerable disorganisation of the normal distribution of capillaries can be observed. This occurs mainly in combination with a marked loss of capillaries and is accompanied in some cases by many branched, 'bushy' capillaries (nowadays by consensus called 'abnormal morphology') (Fig. 5d) suggesting an attempt of budding capillary neoformation, wrote Maricq [19]. This description is the basis for the third step of the fast track algorithm to discern 'scleroderma patterns' from 'non-scleroderma patterns' [9], see below. Of note, scleroderma-type changes are also seen in diseases 'other than' clinically recognisable SSc such as patients with RP without a definite diagnosis of an associated disease, dermatomyositis, mixed connective tissue disease and undifferentiated connective tissue disease [9]. Maricq *et al.* suggested that all these diseases may share some common pathogenetic factors and referred to these diseases as the family of SDS [20].

In 2000, Cutolo *et al.* qualitatively assessed the nailfolds of an SSc cohort with patients fulfilling the 1980 American College of Rheumatology criteria for SSc with a newer technique, the NVC (200× magnification). The advantage of this NVC technique is that it consists of a handheld probe that can be moved along the nailfold and allows images to be taken of SSc patients with severe flexion contractures. Cutolo *et al.* classified the 200× magnification nailfold videocapillaroscopic patterns of the SSc patients in 'early', 'active' and 'late' scleroderma patterns (Fig. 6a–c). Each 'scleroderma pattern' is characterised by different proportions of the following scleroderma-type hallmark parameters: giants, ramifications (nowadays per consensus called 'abnormal morphology') and capillary loss. Optionally, to refer to the patterns of SDS with SSc specific characteristics, but not in the

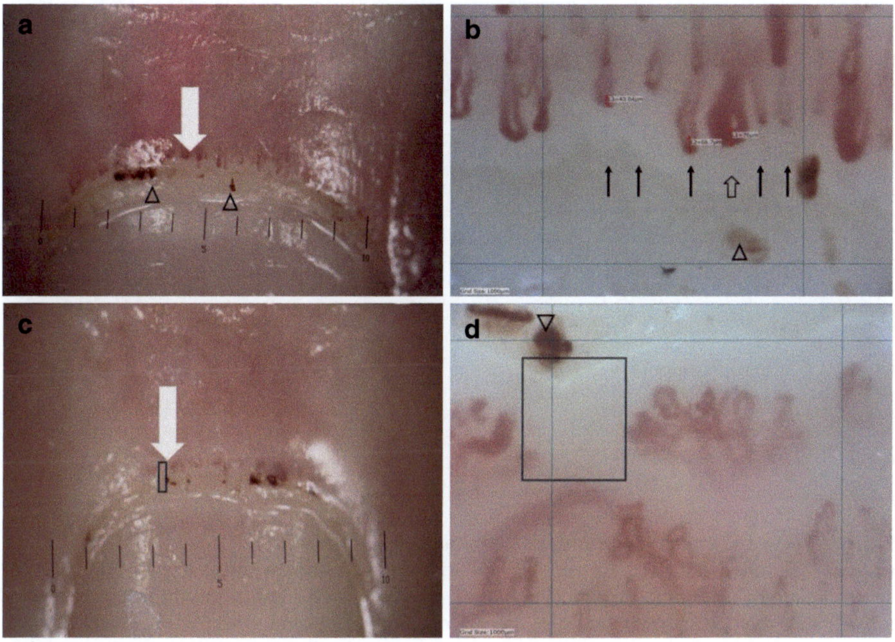

Fig. 5 Scleroderma pattern as seen on low and high magnification
(**a**) Scleroderma pattern with low magnification (20×). 'Definite enlargement' of the capillary loops (a striking widening in dimension of all three segments of the capillary loop, loss of capillaries, haemorrhages [brown deposits Δ]). The white arrow shows the area that is displayed in (**b**) with the NVC technique with a 200× magnification. (**b**) Scleroderma pattern on NVC with 200× magnification. Density: 6 capillaries per linear mm (5 black arrows plus one wide transparent arrow pointing at a giant capillary); dimension: presence of a giant; microhaemorrhages (brown deposits Δ). (**c**) Scleroderma pattern with low magnification (20×). The rectangle denoting an avascular area. The white arrow shows the area that is displayed in (**d**) with the NVC technique with a 200× magnification. (**d**) Avascular area is denoted with the rectangle. Within the one linear mm only one capillary is seen that has the shape of a tree (also called in former literature 'arborised', 'ramified' or 'neoangiogenic' capillary). For reasons of reliability this capillary is called an 'abnormal shape' according to the EULAR/SCTC consensus (see below). Of note, the combination of an extremely lowered density with neoangiogenesis (abnormal shape) is called a 'late' scleroderma pattern

proportions expected in the 'early', 'active', or 'late' scleroderma pattern this group uses the terminology: 'scleroderma-like' [17, 21](Fig. 6e, f). A two centre reliability study between two expert centres showed a high inter-rater reliability in distinguishing the whole group of 'scleroderma patterns' from 'normal' (positive agreement of 90%), whilst the inter-rater agreement within the scleroderma patterns ('early', 'active', 'late' and 'scleroderma-like') themselves was only 62% [21]. Hence further efforts in training of capillaroscopy, such as the fast track algorithm, has placed emphasis on learning to reliably categorise a capillaroscopic image as either a scleroderma pattern or a non-scleroderma pattern, and this with success (see below).

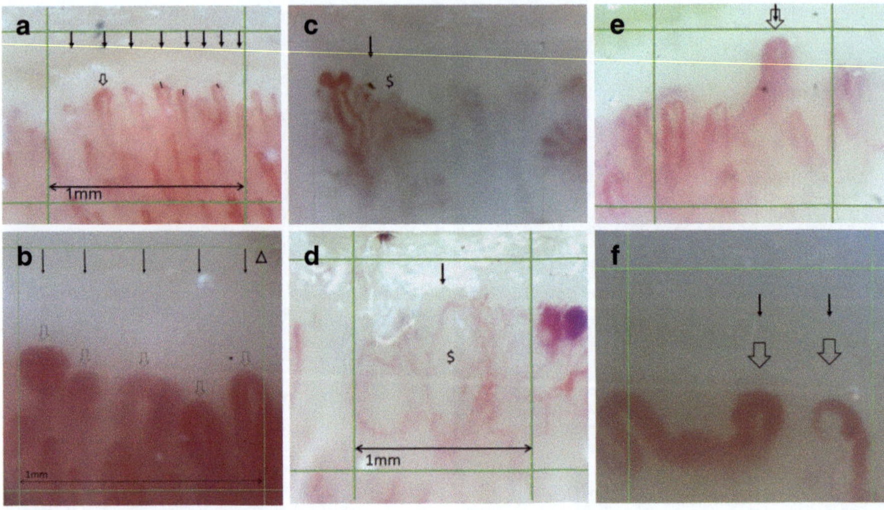

Fig. 6 Types of scleroderma patterns on 200× magnification NVC
(**a**) Early scleroderma pattern. Density: 8 capillaries/mm in distal row (black arrows); dimensions: several dilations (>20 µm, <50 µm, see line on image: -), one giant (>50 µm, transparent wide arrow); morphology: normal (hairpin) shapes of capillaries; hemorrhages: absent. (**b**) Active scleroderma pattern. 5 giants (transparent wide arrows) in the distal row (which is a lowered density) and one haemorrhage (Δ) in the extreme right upper corner (brown deposit, which is, in this image less evident to see). (**c**) and (**d**) Late scleroderma patterns. Density: 1 capillary in the distal row (black arrow); dimension: no dilation; morphology: grossly abnormal shape = neoangiogenesis ($); haemorrhages: absent. (**e**) and (**f**) Sclerodermalike patterns. One (**e**) and two (**f**) giants in the distal row. Giants are usually seen in the 'early' and 'active' scleroderma patterns where, per definition, the density is higher than the one giant capillary per linear mm, which is seen in image (**e**) In this way one expects a density >6 in the 'early' pattern and a density not lower than 4 in the 'active' pattern. Because these images have markers of the scleroderma pattern (in this case a giant) but not in the proportions of the definitions of 'early', 'active', or 'late' scleroderma pattern, we call it 'scleroderma-like'

Non-specific Patterns

In contrast to the SDS, the other connective tissue diseases (CTD), such as systemic lupus erythematosus, Sjögren's Syndrome etc. do not have 'unique' capillary patterns (chapter "Nailfold Capillaroscopy in Other Rheumatological Diseases"). Normal patterns as well as a variety of abnormalities in capillaroscopic characteristics have been observed, such as a lowered capillary density (Fig. 7a), changes in dimension (Fig. 7b), presence of abnormal morphology (i.e. bushy capillaries or bizarre capillaries, nowadays per consensus called 'abnormal' shapes etc.) (Fig. 7c) and presence of microhaemorrhages [22, 23](Fig. 7d and e). These abnormalities are not in themselves predictive of a defined condition, and hence are referred to as

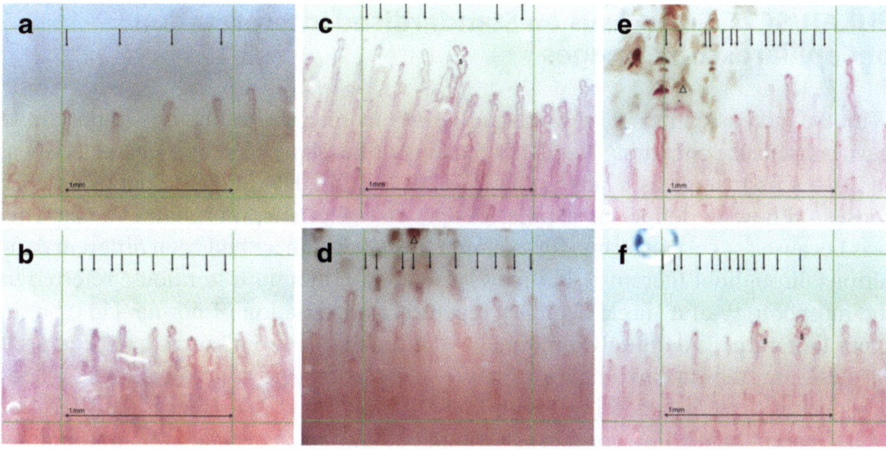

Fig. 7 Non-specific abnormalities on NVC. (**a**) Capillary image with non-specific abnormalities of the capillaroscopic characteristic density. Density: 4 capillaries/mm in distal row (black arrows). Dimensions: within normal limits (<20 μm). Morphology: normal shapes of capillaries .Haemorrhages: absent (**b**) Capillary image with non-specific abnormalities of the capillaroscopic characteristic dimension. Density: 10 capillaries/mm in distal row (black arrows). Dimensions: within normal limits, dilation (>20 μm, <50 μm, –). Morphology: normal shapes of capillaries. Haemorrhages: absent. (**c**) Capillary image with non-specific abnormality of the capillaroscopic characteristic morphology. Density: 7 capillaries/mm in distal row (black arrows). Dimensions: within normal limits, dilation (>20 μm, <50 μm, –). Morphology: abnormal shapes of capillaries ($). Haemorrhages: absent. (**d**) Capillary image with non-specific abnormalities due to the presence of haemorrhages. Density: 10 capillaries/mm in distal row (black arrows). Dimensions: within normal limits, dilation (>20 μm, <50 μm, –). Morphology: normal shapes of capillaries. Haemorrhages: present (Δ). (**e**) Capillary image with non-specific abnormalities due to the presence of haemorrhages. Density: 9 capillaries/mm in distal row (black arrows). Dimensions: within normal limits, dilation (>20 μm, <50 μm, –). Morphology: normal shapes of capillaries. Haemorrhages: present (Δ). (**f**) Capillary image with non-specific abnormalities in two capillaroscopic characteristics, dimension as well as morphology. Density: 14 capillaries/mm in distal row (black arrows). Dimensions: within normal limits, dilation (>20 μm, <50 μm, –). Morphology: abnormal shapes of capillaries ($). Haemorrhages: absent

'non-specific abnormalities' in recent consensus literature (see below). The fact that non-specific changes may occur in primary RP may sometimes cause difficulties in distinguishing between extreme variations of normal (in primary RP) or secondary RP. In general, the elaborative evaluation of healthy controls by Andrade taught us that when anomalies are isolated or uncommon, they may represent variation of normal. When the anomalies are numerous or when several anomalies occur in one individual, they are indicative of an underlying CTD. In this way, Andrade *et al.* registered a single anomaly in 25% of healthy individuals, while 8% showed two types and 1% showed three types of anomalies [11] (Fig. 7).

EULAR/SCTC Consensus on Standardised Interpretation of Capillaroscopic Images

With the increasing use of nailfold capillaroscopy internationally, it is important to have consensus concerning standard reporting of the capillaroscopic characteristics. In 2016 a first step was taken by the EULAR SG MC RD/SCTC to publish a consensus on how to define the capillaroscopic characteristic, morphology [12]. This was because for certain terms, for example 'tortuosity' there had been different definitions throughout literature. In this way, in certain literature 'tortuous' referred to the morphology of a single capillary regarded as a variation of normal [11], but in other literature, as definitely abnormal. Additionally, different terms had been used to describe the morphology of single capillaries (i.e. 'ramifications', 'neoangiogenesis' or 'meandering') with low reliability [11, 21]. Hence, the EULAR/SCTC had published by consensus a simple definition to evaluate the morphology of a single capillary as 'normal' or 'abnormal', adoptable to all rheumatic diseases and capillaroscopic evaluations for a standardized interpretation in 2016. In summary, capillaries with a 'hairpin' shape, a (once or twice) crossing shape or tortuous shape (the afferent and efferent limb bend [=undulate] but do not cross) are defined as being 'normal'. To optimize reliability of this definition, in 2018, an extra criterion had been added. In this way a capillary is called normal only if the tip of the capillary is convex [13](Fig. 2). This simple evaluation of single shapes of capillaries as 'normal' or 'abnormal' has attested excellent in a multicentre international study [13]. In this way a mean Cohen's kappa between the gold standard and experienced attendees was 0.83, between the gold standard and moderately experienced attendees was 0.81 and between the gold standard and novices was 0.80. This definition of 'normal' or 'abnormal' morphology of a single capillary was incorporated later on into the EULAR/SCTC consensus on standardized reporting of capillaroscopic images (see below).

To align interpretation of capillaroscopic images both in daily practice and research the EULAR SG MC RD/SCTC recently published a consensus framework to report capillaroscopic characteristics in a standard way [8]. The following capillary characteristics should be evaluated when assessing an image: capillary density (number of capillaries per linear mm), capillary morphology (shape of individual capillaries), capillary dimension (calibre of the apical limb of the capillary [Fig. 8]) and presence or absence of microhaemorrhages. Fig. 9 describes the stereotypic normality, the non-specific abnormalities (non-scleroderma patterns) and the SSc-specific abnormalities (scleroderma patterns) for each of these capillaroscopic characteristics according to international consensus [8].Based on the combination of these capillaroscopic characteristics a capillaroscopic image can be classified as a scleroderma pattern or a non-scleroderma pattern (stereotype normal and non-specific abnormalities) (see Figs. 6 and 7).

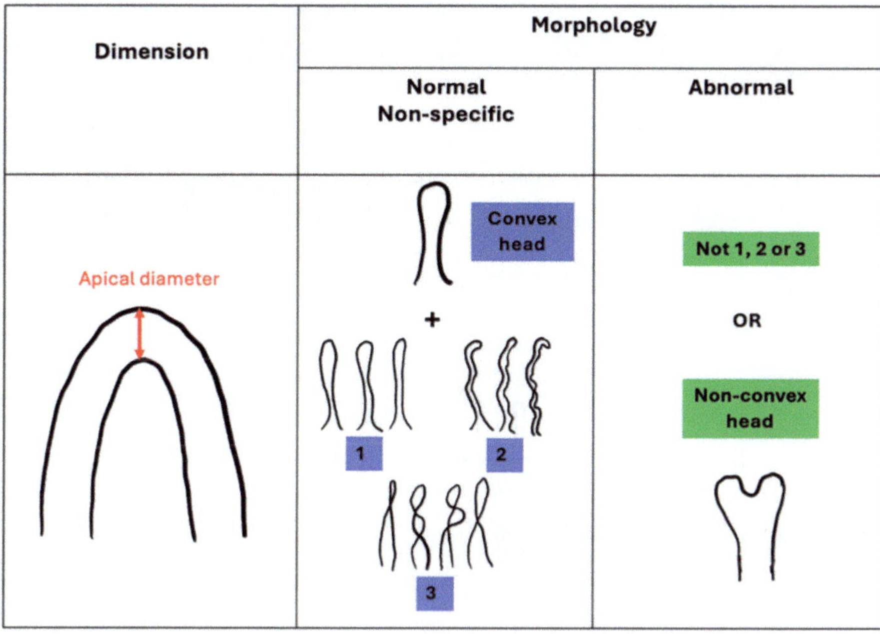

Fig. 8 Evaluation of capillary dimension and morphology
Capillary dimension as measured at the apex of the capillary loop **(left panel)**. **Capillary morphologies** are described according to consensus definitions as normal or abnormal shapes. Normal shapes must have a convex head and 'hairpin' shape **(1)** or non-specific variations of morphology, tortuous **(2)** and once or twice crossed **(3)** **(middle panel)**. Abnormal shapes are defined as either having a non-convex head or any shape that does not fall under 1, 2 or 3 **(right panel)**

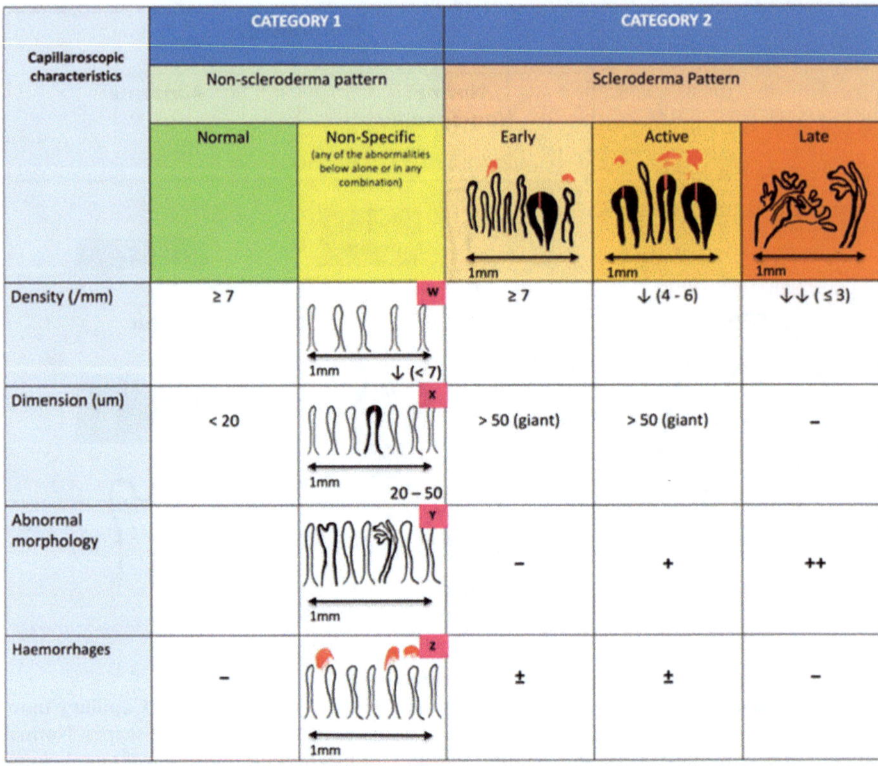

Fig. 9 EULAR/SCTC study group on microcirculation in rheumatic diseases standardized capillaroscopy evaluation chart. (Adapted from Smith V et al. [8])
This chart represents a consensus framework to standardize reporting of capillaroscopic characteristics when using NVC with a 200× magnification. Each NVC image is evaluated for capillary density (number of capillaries per linear mm), capillary dimension (measurement of the apical limb), capillary morphology (shape of individual capillaries) and the presence or absence of microhaemorrhages. **Non-scleroderma pattern** can be stereotype normal (capillary density ≥ 7capillaries per linear mm in the distal row [row lying closest to the nailfold], a normal apical diameter ≤ 20 μm and no abnormal shapes or haemorrhages) or non-specific abnormality (if any of the 4 capillary characteristics are abnormal alone or in combination, such as a lowered capillary density [**panel W**], the presences of enlarged capillaries [**panel X**], the presence of abnormal shapes [**panel Y**], the presence of haemorrhages [**panel Z**]). **Scleroderma pattern** is made up of 'early', 'active' and 'late' patterns. The 'early' pattern is characterized by the presence of giants (normal shaped, with symmetrical widening of the three limbs, apical limb diameter ≥ 50 μm) and a normal density (≥ 7 capillaries/mm) and haemorrhage may be present. In the 'active' pattern there are giants combined with a lowered density (4–6 capillaries/mm). The late pattern is characterized by an extremely lowered density (≤3 capillaries/mm) and abnormal shapes. No giants are present in the late pattern

The Fast Track Algorithm

The vast majority of 'non-specific abnormalities' that might be present in a healthy population may render it difficult for the non-experienced capillaroscopist to classify an image as a 'scleroderma pattern' or a 'non-scleroderma pattern'. To address this, the EULAR study group has produced a 'fast track' algorithm which has been shown to have a high reliability to classify in a fast and simple way an image as a 'scleroderma pattern' or a 'non-scleroderma pattern', even by novices in the field of capillaroscopy [9]. In this way Mean Cohen's kappa was 1/0.96 versus the gold standard for the 6 experts/135 attendees of the 8th EULAR capillaroscopy course and 1/0.94 for the 3 experts/85 attendees of the 8th European Scleroderma Trials and Research group (EUSTAR) SSc course. Light's kappa was 1/0.92 at the 8th EULAR capillaroscopy course, and 1/0.87 at the 8th EUSTAR SSc course. The 'fast track' algorithm comprises three easy rules. First the rater evaluates if the image to be assessed complies with rule number one which states that a normal capillary density ($\geq$7 capillaries per linear mm) and the absence of giant capillaries permits the rater to classify the capillaroscopic image as a 'non-scleroderma pattern'. If the image to be evaluated does not comply with the criteria for rule number one then the rater checks if it complies with the criteria of rule number two. Rule number two states that an extremely lowered capillary density ($\leq$3 capillaries per linear mm) together with abnormal shapes (i.e., 'late scleroderma pattern') or the presence of giant capillaries permits the rater to grade the capillaroscopic image as a 'scleroderma pattern'. If the image in front of the rater doesn't comply with the criteria of rule number one or rule number two then the rater automatically grades the image in front of him/her as a 'non-scleroderma pattern' (= rule number three).

This binary classification as scleroderma pattern or non-scleroderma pattern of 200× magnification capillaroscopic images through the fast track algorithm is particularly valuable in clinical setting, such as in the outpatients RP evaluation clinic.

Scoring of Capillaroscopic Images

Qualitative

Discrimination between scleroderma pattern and non-scleroderma pattern may be executed 'by eye' (= qualitative assessment). This lies in line with the way a style of a painting is appreciated on sight and classified into a style: e.g. impressionism, expressionism. The scleroderma patterns can be further classified into 'early', 'active' and 'late' scleroderma pattern (see chapter "Nailfold Capillaroscopy in Systemic Sclerosis (Including Associations)").

(Semi-)Quantitative

Quantitation can be executed per linear mm, such as in the EULAR/SCTC consensus (see above). This consensus facilitates comparison of results from capillaroscopic studies conducted anywhere around the globe. In this way, non-exhaustively, capillaroscopic findings in healthy children, as well in as children with connective tissue diseases have been described in a worldwide study [24]. In this way also within CTD capillaroscopy has been evaluated to assess associations with development of organ involvement [25].

Also, semi-quantitative scoring exists. In this way, for example in 2008, the group of Cutolo proposed a semi-quantitative assessment of the hallmark parameters of the 'scleroderma pattern': capillary loss, giant capillaries, microhaemorrhages and abnormal shapes (i.e. ramifications). In this semi-quantitative evaluation of capillaroscopic images capillaroscopic characteristics are given a score between 0 and 3 in relation to the number of capillaries counted in 1 linear mm (0 = no changes, 1 = ≤33% of capillary alterations/reduction, 2 = 33–66% of capillary alterations/reduction, and 3 = ≥ 66% of capillary alterations/reduction, per linear mm) [26]. In 2011 the inter- and intra-rater agreement (reliability) of this semi-quantitative scoring was demonstrated [21]. Three capillaroscopic characteristics had a high inter rater reliability as expressed by an intra class correlation coefficient of >0.8. In this way the intra class correlation coefficient of capillary loss was 0.96, of giants was 0.84 and of microhaemorrhages was 0.83. As mentioned above the characteristic 'ramifications' had a lower reliability with an intra class correlation coefficient of 0.64, which led to further standardisation efforts of interpretation of morphology of individual capillaries as 'abnormal' shapes in 2016 and 2018 which subsequently led to reliable definition for the capillaroscopic characteristic evaluating morphology of a single capillary.

Research Agenda

- Whilst healthy controls have been described with low magnification, standardised capillaroscopic descriptions of large observational cohorts are missing with nailfold videocapillaroscopy (200× magnification).
- Whilst the EULAR/SCTC consensus allows consistent interpretation of the capillaroscopic image taken with a 200× magnification capillaroscopic technique, its role in interpretation of low magnification technique capillaroscopic images has not been evaluated.
- Automated fully reliable, inexpensive, fast systems generating accurate reports are needed to execute randomised clinical trials.

Conclusions

As of 2025, the field of capillaroscopy has undergone significant advancements, particularly in the realm of image interpretation. The SCTC and the EULAR published a consensus framework that standardized terminology and definitions used in capillaroscopic image interpretation with the 200× magnification technique. This framework enables consistent interpretation of nailfold capillaroscopy across clinicians, researchers and international studies. In addition, the fast track algorithm was introduced, a fast and reliable binary classification into scleroderma pattern or non-scleroderma pattern, which may be a support in the work up of patients with RP. It is considered a valid aid in screening, and has been shown to have high inter rater reliability, even in people who are new in the field of capillaroscopy. Eyes are geared towards development of fully automated systems adoptable to any magnification technique to reliably assist the capillaroscopist in research and or daily practice.

Acknowledgement Our deep gratitude to Mislav Radic for providing the dermatoscopic images as well as the nailfold videocapillaroscopic images in the same area of nailfold for teaching purposes (which he collected as part of an EULAR study group on microcirculation in rheumatic diseases/SCTC project). Our deep gratitude equally goes to Dr. Ramona Govender for her contribution in the further adaptation of the EULAR/SCTC consensus table into an educative figure. Prof. V. Smith and Prof. M. Cutolo are surrecting members of the EULAR study group on microcirculation in Rheumatic diseases and of the European Reference network on Rare Connective Tissue diseases.

References

1. Volkmann ER, Andreasson K, Smith V. Systemic sclerosis. Lancet. 2023;401(10373):304–18.
2. Cutolo M, Smith V. Detection of microvascular changes in systemic sclerosis and other rheumatic diseases. Nat Rev Rheumatol. 2021;17(11):665–77.
3. Herrick AL, Wigley FM. Raynaud's phenomenon. Best Pract Res Clin Rheumatol. 2020;34(1):101474.
4. LeRoy EC, Medsger TA Jr. Raynaud's phenomenon: a proposal for classification. Clin Exp Rheumatol. 1992;10(5):485–8.
5. LeRoy EC, Medsger TA Jr. Criteria for the classification of early systemic sclerosis. J Rheumatol. 2001;28(7):1573–6.
6. Koenig M, Joyal F, Fritzler MJ, Roussin A, Abrahamowicz M, Boire G, et al. Autoantibodies and microvascular damage are independent predictive factors for the progression of Raynaud's phenomenon to systemic sclerosis: a twenty-year prospective study of 586 patients, with validation of proposed criteria for early systemic sclerosis. Arthritis Rheum. 2008;58(12):3902–12.
7. Bellando-Randone S, Del Galdo F, Lepri G, Minier T, Huscher D, Furst DE, et al. Progression of patients with Raynaud's phenomenon to systemic sclerosis: a five-year analysis of the European scleroderma trial and research group multicentre, longitudinal registry study for very early diagnosis of systemic sclerosis (VEDOSS). Lancet Rheumatol. 2021;3(12):e834–43.
8. Smith V, Herrick AL, Ingegnoli F, Damjanov N, De Angelis R, Denton CP, et al. Standardisation of nailfold capillaroscopy for the assessment of patients with Raynaud's phenomenon and systemic sclerosis. Autoimmun Rev. 2020;19(3):102458.
9. Smith V, Vanhaecke A, Herrick AL, Distler O, Guerra MG, Denton CP, et al. Fast track algorithm: how to differentiate a "scleroderma pattern" from a "non-scleroderma pattern". Autoimmun Rev. 2019;18(11):102394.

10. Ingegnoli F, Ardoino I, Boracchi P, Cutolo M, Airò P, Ananieva LP, et al. Nailfold capillaroscopy in systemic sclerosis: data from the EULAR scleroderma trials and research (EUSTAR) database. Microvasc Res. 2013;89:122–8.
11. Andrade LE, Gabriel Junior A, Assad RL, Ferrari AJ, Atra E. Panoramic nailfold capillaroscopy: a new reading method and normal range. Semin Arthritis Rheum. 1990;20(1):21–31.
12. Smith V, Beeckman S, Herrick AL, Decuman S, Deschepper E, De Keyser F, et al. An EULAR study group pilot study on reliability of simple capillaroscopic definitions to describe capillary morphology in rheumatic diseases. Rheumatology. 2016;55(5):883–90.
13. Cutolo M, Melsens K, Herrick AL, Foeldvari I, Deschepper E, De Keyser F, et al. Reliability of simple capillaroscopic definitions in describing capillary morphology in rheumatic diseases. Rheumatology. 2018;57(4):757–9.
14. Maricq HR, LeRoy EC. Patterns of finger capillary abnormalities in connective tissue disease by "wide-field" microscopy. Arthritis Rheum. 1973;16(5):619–28.
15. Maricq HR. Comparison of quantitative and semiquantitative estimates of nailfold capillary abnormalities in scleroderma spectrum disorders. Microvasc Res. 1986;32(2):271–6.
16. Maricq HR, Maize JC. Nailfold capillary abnormalities. Clin Rheum Dis. 1982;8(2):455–78.
17. Cutolo M, Sulli A, Pizzorni C, Accardo S. Nailfold videocapillaroscopy assessment of microvascular damage in systemic sclerosis. J Rheumatol. 2000;27(1):155–60.
18. Lonzetti LS, Joyal F, Raynauld JP, Roussin A, Goulet JR, Rich E, et al. Updating the American College of Rheumatology preliminary classification criteria for systemic sclerosis: addition of severe nailfold capillaroscopy abnormalities markedly increases the sensitivity for limited scleroderma. Arthritis Rheum. 2001;44(3):735–6.
19. Maricq HR. Wide-field capillary microscopy. Arthritis Rheum. 1981;24(9):1159–65.
20. Maricq HR, Weinberger AB, LeRoy EC. Early detection of scleroderma-spectrum disorders by in vivo capillary microscopy: a prospective study of patients with Raynaud's phenomenon. J Rheumatol. 1982;9(2):289–91.
21. Smith V, Pizzorni C, De Keyser F, Decuman S, Van Praet JT, Deschepper E, et al. Reliability of the qualitative and semiquantitative nailfold videocapillaroscopy assessment in a systemic sclerosis cohort: a two-Centre study. Ann Rheum Dis. 2010;69(6):1092–6.
22. Cutolo M, Melsens K, Wijnant S, Ingegnoli F, Thevissen K, De Keyser F, et al. Nailfold capillaroscopy in systemic lupus erythematosus: a systematic review and critical appraisal. Autoimmun Rev. 2018;17(4):344–52.
23. Melsens K, Leone MC, Paolino S, Elewaut D, Gerli R, Vanhaecke A, et al. Nailfold capillaroscopy in Sjogren's syndrome: a systematic literature review and standardised interpretation. Clin Exp Rheumatol. 2020;38 Suppl 126(4):150–7.
24. Melsens K, Cutolo M, Schonenberg-Meinema D, Foeldvari I, Leone MC, Mostmans Y, et al. Standardized nailfold capillaroscopy in children with rheumatic diseases: a worldwide study. Rheumatology. 2023;62(4):1605–15.
25. Vanhaecke A, Cutolo M, Distler O, Riccieri V, Allanore Y, Denton CP, et al. Nailfold capillaroscopy in SSc: innocent bystander or promising biomarker for novel severe organ involvement/progression? Rheumatology. 2022;61(11):4384–96.
26. Sulli A, Secchi ME, Pizzorni C, Cutolo M. Scoring the nailfold microvascular changes during the capillaroscopic analysis in systemic sclerosis patients. Ann Rheum Dis. 2008;67(6):885–7.

Quantitative Analysis

Michael Berks and Chris Taylor

Key Messages

- The need for subjective judgement can limit the value of nailfold capillaroscopy
- There is a large body of evidence to support the use of quantitative methods
- Fully automated quantitative analysis systems are here and have been clinically validated

Introduction

Nailfold capillaroscopy is an established clinical investigation that plays an important role in the diagnosis of Systemic Sclerosis (SSc), with abnormal nailfold capillaries scoring two of the nine points required to fulfil the ACR/EULAR classification for SSc [1, 2]. Most patients with SSc first present to primary care with Raynaud's phenomenon (RP) [3], providing an opportunity for early diagnosis. Nailfold capillaroscopy plays a critical role in differentiating patients with SSc from those with Primary (idiopathic) RP. It may also be key to very early diagnosis [4].

M. Berks (✉)
University of Manchester, Manchester, UK
e-mail: Michael.Berks@manchester.ac.uk

C. Taylor
School of Engineering and School of Health Sciences, University of Manchester, Manchester, UK
e-mail: Michael.Berks@manchester.ac.uk

A. L. Herrick et al. (eds.), *Nailfold Capillaroscopy in Rheumatological Diseases*,
https://doi.org/10.1007/978-3-032-03970-5_5

Nailfold capillary patterns characteristic of SSc ('scleroderma pattern') were first described more than 50 years ago in the seminal work of Hildegard Maricq [5, 6], but interpretation of nailfold images remains challenging. The ACR/EULAR classification criteria refer to 'enlarged capillaries and/or capillary loss with or without pericapillary haemorrhages', whilst Maricq describes 'disruption of the normal capillary architecture'. Applying these criteria involves subjective judgement, which is demanding given the highly variable appearance of nailfold images. As a result, the level of agreement in assessing vessel abnormality is poor, even for nailfold capillaroscopy experts [7]. Interpretation is even more challenging for the general rheumatologist.

As a result, there has been great interest in quantifying vessel abnormality, providing an objective basis for assessing nailfold capillary images and, potentially, for tracking disease progression. Building on the classification criteria, most of this work has focused on quantifying vessel morphology—vessel width, vessel density and vessel shape/architecture—but functional characteristics such as blood flow and oxygenation have also been investigated. Methods have also been developed to combine measurements to provide an overall assessment of vessel abnormality.

In this chapter we review the development of quantitative capillaroscopy (see Fig. 1). We begin by discussing the acquisition of nailfold images suitable for quantitative analysis. Then we show how quantitative measures of vessel abnormality have been developed and validated starting from the qualitative descriptions provided by Maricq and the ACR/EULAR classification for SSc. We discuss semi-quantitative methods for detecting disease-related abnormalities or predicting risk that apply these measurement concepts to reduce subjectivity, whilst aiming for practicality in the clinical setting. We then discuss the development of fully automated systems that aim to measure vessel abnormality directly from nailfold images and present two state-of-the-art systems that use artificial intelligence to achieve disease detection results that are at least as good as those obtained by human experts. Finally, we discuss some of the future challenges for the field.

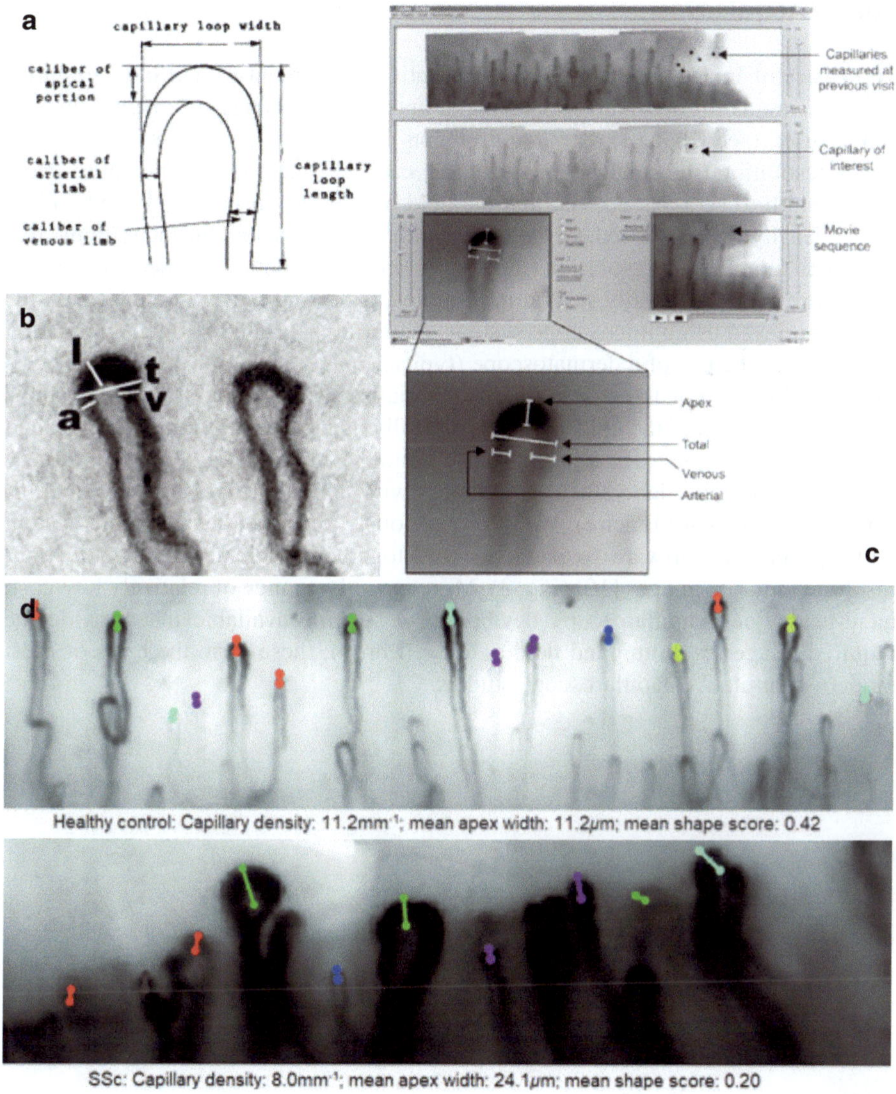

Fig. 1 Advances in quantification: (**a**) Schematic representation of capillary measurement (Maricq [6]); (**b**) Manually measuring arterial ***a***, venous ***v***, apical loop ***l*** diameters and total loop width ***t*** using Capiflow software (Bukhari et al. [8]); (**c**) Manual measurements from enhanced panoramic mosaic images, allowing comparison to previous images (Anderson et al. [9]); (**d**) Fully automated measurements across the whole nailfold (Berks et al. [10]). (Reproduced with permission from [11])

Image Acquisition

The basics of image acquisition for quantitative assessment of nailfold capillaries are the same as for qualitative assessment, and a similar range of imaging devices can be used (see Chap. 3). Key requirements for quantitative assessment are that image resolution (the smallest structure that can be resolved) is sufficient to allow vessel width to be assessed, and that the field of view is sufficiently large to allow vessel density to be assessed. Given typical values for vessel width and spacing, this translates to an image resolution of 2.5 micrometres or better and field width of 1 millimetre or more (ideally several millimetres, capturing the entire nailfold). This can be achieved using microscope systems operating at around x200 magnification but rules out the use of a dermatoscope (typical image resolution 10–15 micrometres), see Fig. 2. For the past 30 years, specialised video capillaroscopy systems have been considered the gold standard, typically using green light illumination and capturing digital images at a resolution of around 1 micrometre per pixel. Initially these were complex laboratory instruments with a limited field of view (significantly less than 1 millimetre). We have previously described using such a system with specialised software to patch images together to create large-field, high-resolution mosaic images [10] (Fig. 3). More recently a range of relatively low-cost, hand-held video capillaroscopy devices have become available that provide the required image resolution and field of view (Fig. 4); these form the basis of most modern quantitative capillaroscopy studies.

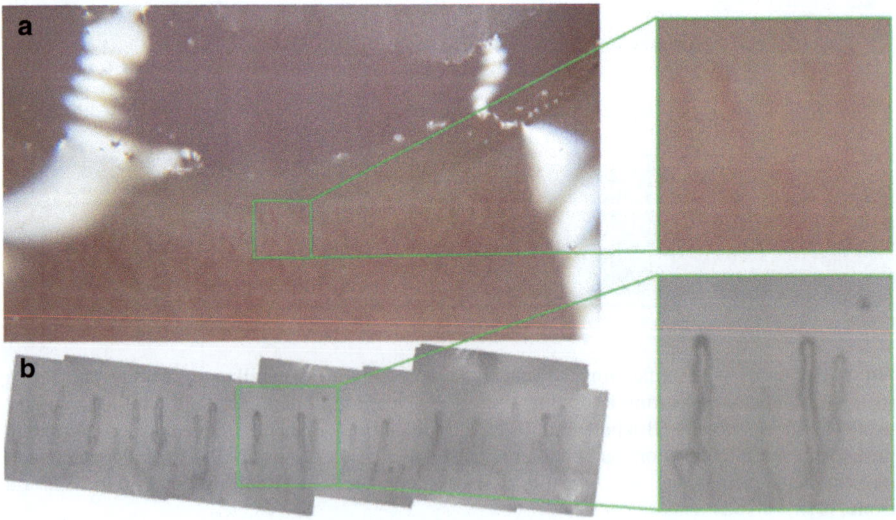

Fig. 2 (**a**) An image of the nailfold captured through a dermatoscope, which permits a wide-field visual inspection of the whole nailfold, but when zoomed in has too low resolution to adequately define and measure individual capillary morphology; (**b**) a mosaic image of the nailfold with spatial resolution of approximately 1 micron per pixel, with vessel limbs of the capillaries well resolved in the zoomed-in image allowing accurate quantification of morphology

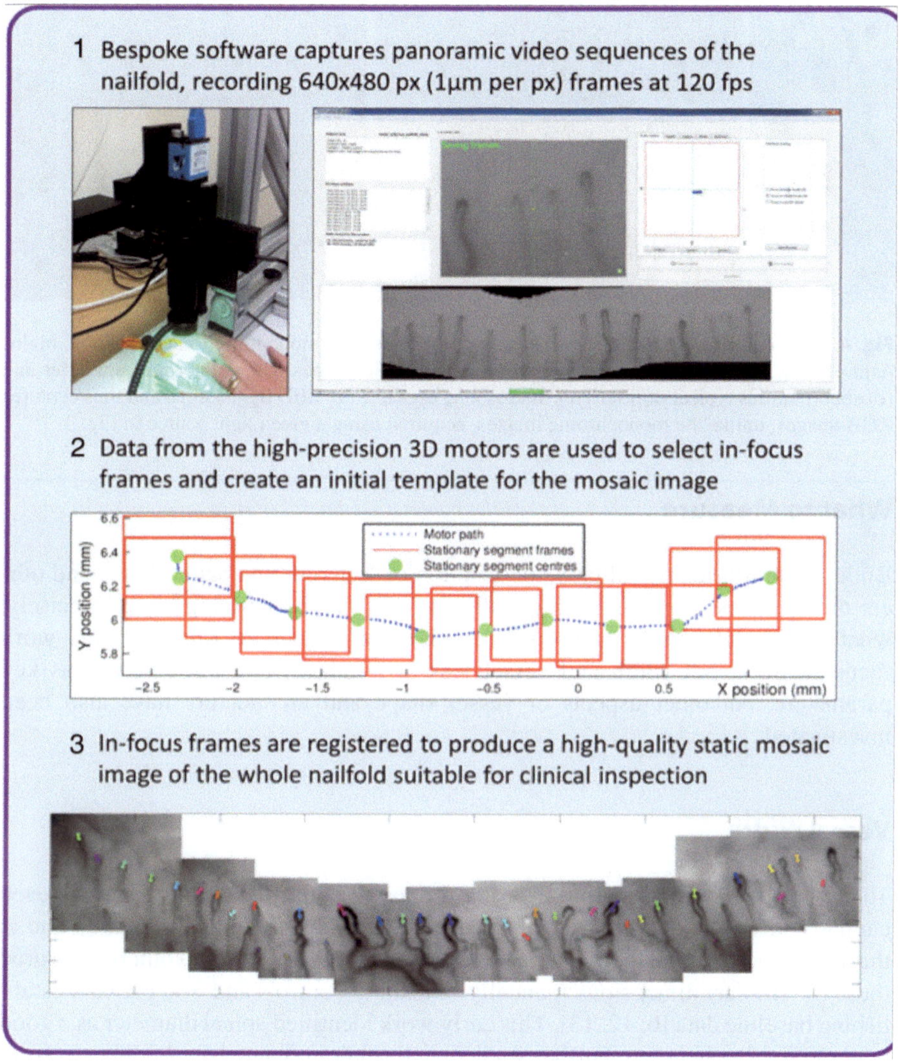

Fig. 3 Schematic of the specialised lab-based videocapillaroscopy system developed by Berks et al. [10], for automatically generating high-quality, high-magnification images of the nailfold. As well as acquiring video images and generating static mosaics, the system computes automated estimates of vessel morphology and red blood cell velocity

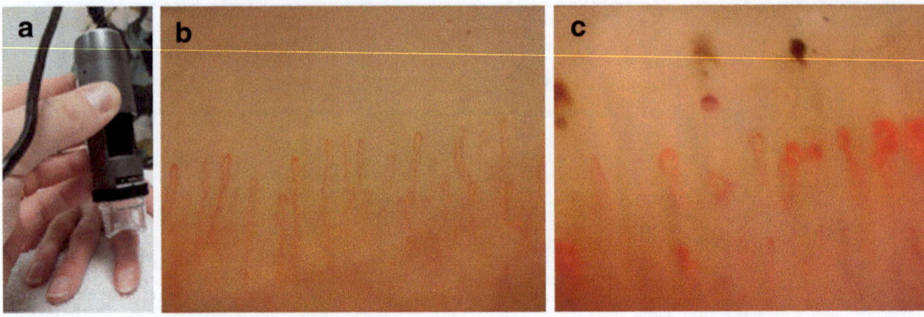

Fig. 4 (**a**) Acquiring a nailfold capillaroscopy image using a modern high-magnification, hight-field-of-view, handheld digital USB microscope; example images with (**b**) normal capillaries and (**c**) abnormalities typical of SSc. This microscope uses a white LED light source and thus captures RGB images, unlike the monochrome images, acquired using a green light source in Fig. 3

What to Measure

Building on Maricq's qualitative description of 'scleroderma pattern', she and others took the first steps towards quantitative analysis by defining, more precisely, what aspects of capillary appearance might be measured. Much of this work focussed on vessel width and vessel loss (avascularity), which emerged as key parameters, but other aspects of vessel shape and architecture have also been investigated.

Vessel Width

To further define vessel width, Maricq proposed a set of measurements for each capillary loop—vessel diameter in the arterial and venous limbs of the loop and at the apex, together with loop width and length (see Fig. 1a). She and others measured these (or similar) dimensions manually in healthy controls and SSc patients establishing baseline data [6, 12, 13]. This early work identified apical diameter as a good predictor of disease state. Further studies used semi-automated methods to measure the apical diameter of manually selected vessels, allowing larger sample sizes and establishing normal ranges [8, 9, 14] (Fig. 1b, c). The concept of giant capillaries emerged at an early stage, defined as vessels with an apical diameter of greater than 50 micrometres, the presence or absence of which could be assessed relatively easily by eye. Capillaries with an apical diameter > 30 micrometres are generally considered to be enlarged [15].

Vessel Density

In Maricq's initial quantitative work she measured vessel loss as the fraction of the imaged nailfold that was avascular [6], but this was still very much dependant on subjective judgement. Most subsequent work has focussed on vessel density—primarily defined as the number of vessels per millimetre in the distal row of capillaries. This definition begs the question of which capillaries should be treated as belonging to the distal row. Many investigators have adopted the 90 degree rule—a capillary is only counted if the angle between its apex and the two adjacent apices is greater than 90 degrees [16–18]. Another challenge is how to treat angiogenic capillaries, which can have a 'ramified' or 'bushy' appearance with multiple apices. Barth et al. [19] excluded such vessels from density estimation. Karbalaie addressed the problem by fitting an ellipse to each vessel and taking the most distal end of its major axis as the apex—giving a single apex even for complex vessels and improving inter-observer agreement [20]. These and other studies [8, 13, 14, 21], generally based on manual mark-up of apices in computerised images, established vessel density as a good predictor of disease state. Emrani et al. reviewed this literature and found reported capillary densities for healthy controls in the range 7–10 capillaries per millimetre, with reduced densities for SSc patients [22].

Vessel Shape

While it is not mentioned in the ACR/EULAR classification criteria, from Maricq onward other aspects of vessel morphology have been proposed as indicative of disease. Abnormally shaped vessels described variously as ramified, bushy, tortuous, arborized, meandering, branching or bizarre have been implicated [17, 23, 24] (see Fig. 5). The presence or absence of abnormally shaped vessels can be assessed relatively easily by eye, but there is disagreement regarding predictive value, with Cutolo et al. suggesting that any vessel with a concave apex should be counted as abnormal [24] but others claiming that tortuous, even bushy, capillaries are seen in health controls [13, 25, 26]. Unlike vessel width and density, quantitative definitions of vessel shape only became possible with the advent of semi- or fully-automated analysis. For example, Murray et al. and Berks et al. measured the orientation at every point on the vessel pathway and defined tortuosity as the circular variance of orientations [10, 14], with normal (hairpin-like) vessels producing a very narrow distribution of orientations and tortuous vessels producing a flatter distribution (see Fig. 6). The mean of this value over all vessels observed for an individual proved a good stand-alone predictor of SSc with an area under the ROC of 0.85 [10].

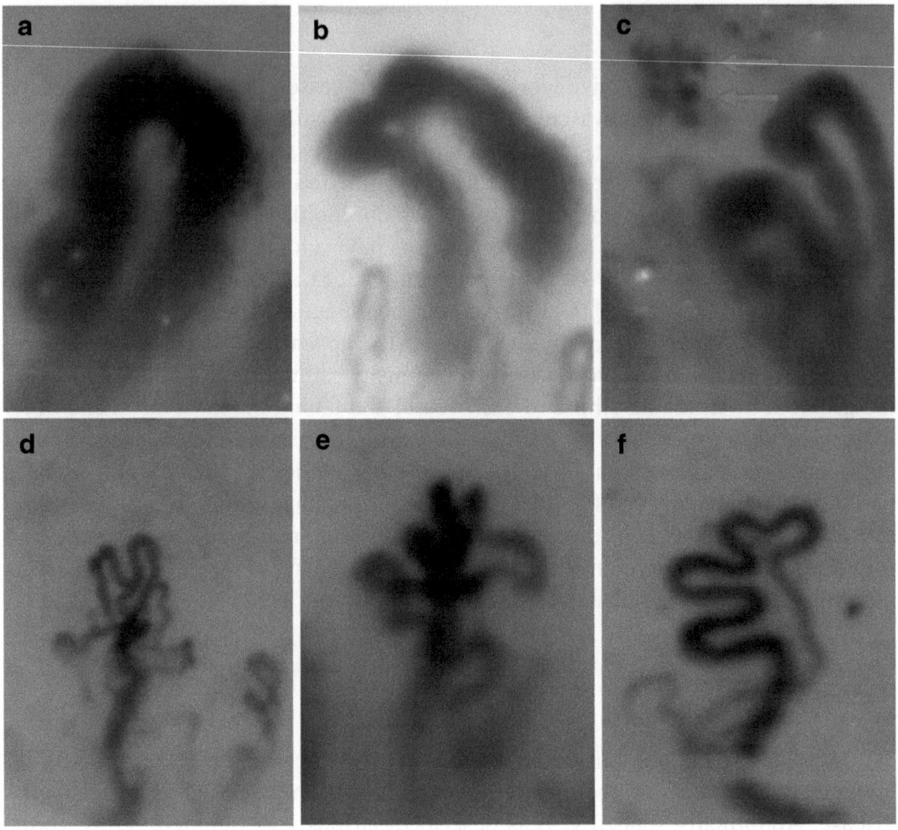

Fig. 5 Examples of the major capillaroscopic abnormalities: (**a**) Giant capillary; (**b**) Irregularly enlarged capillary; (**c**) Microhaemorrhages (arrowheads); (**d**–**f**) Different appearance of neoangiogenesis in capillaries: branching (**d**), coiled (**e**), and ramified (**f**)

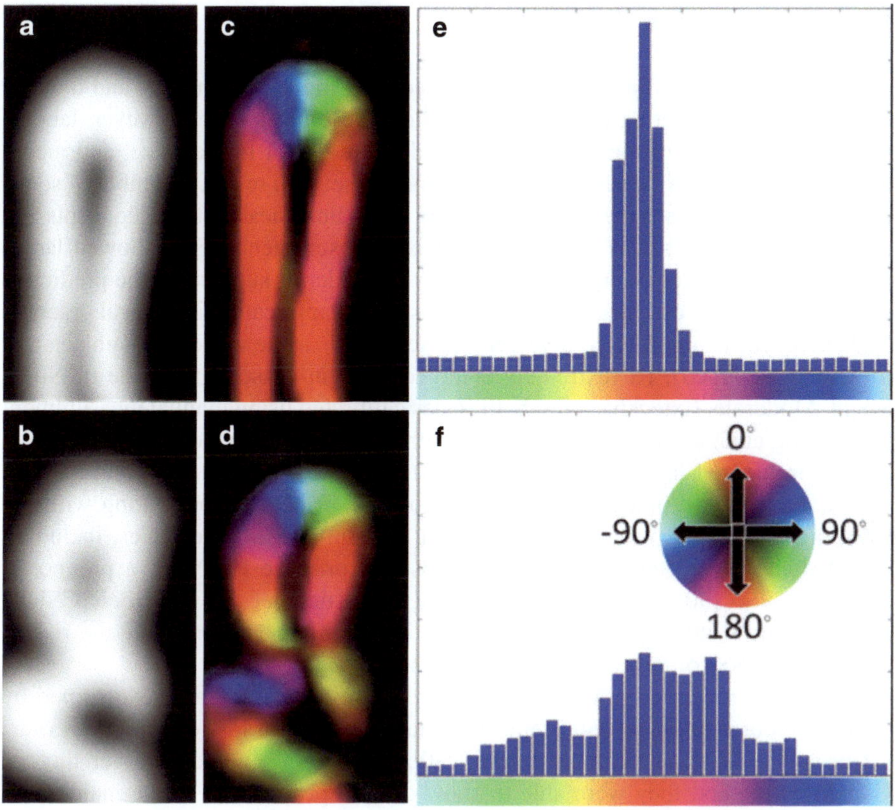

Fig. 6 Quantifying vessel shape (**a–b**) capillaries are segmented from the background to produce binary masks; (**c–d**) vessel orientation is estimated using the masks. Here colour depicts angle on the half-circle (orientations 180 degrees apart are considered identical); (**e–f**) taking histograms over the vessel orientation allows us to estimate the distribution of angles present in each capillary. A normal hairpin capillary as shown in (**a**) generates a highly peaked histogram, while the more tortuous capillary shown in (**b**) shows a much greater spread over angle. Summary measures of the distribution (*eg* circular variance or histogram entropy) can be used to assign a shape score to each capillary, which has been shown to be a strong differentiator of SSc vs non-SSc [27, 28] (see also Fig. 9a)

Semi-quantitative Methods

The body of work outlined above established measurement standards and demonstrated value in detecting disease. The methods developed were, however, labour-intensive and time-consuming. This resulted in studies of limited size, and meant the approach was not suitable for routine clinical use. As a result, a number of semi-quantitative methods were developed using the same measurement concepts but applying subjective scales rather than precise measurements. This allowed larger studies to be undertaken, adding to the body of evidence supporting the predictive value of capillaroscopy, and held out the prospect of application in clinical practice.

Maricq, for example used a vessel size scale of I (same as healthy subjects), II (definitely enlarged), III (extremely enlarged) and an avascularity scale of None, Slight, Moderate, Extensive, with both scales calibrated using manual measurement [6]. Koenig et al. used Maricq's method (with a slightly expanded vessel size scale) in their influential large-scale prospective study which showed abnormal nailfold capillaries to be an independent predictor of SSc in patients presenting with RP [29]. Ingegnoli et al. used an expanded set of semi-quantitative scales, including vessel shape descriptors, combining a subset to produce PRINCE, a prognostic Index for SSc [30, 31]. More specifically, Sebastiani et al. with their CSURI approach and Cutolo et al. used semi-quantitative methods to evaluate the risk in patients with SSc of developing ulcers [23, 24, 32].

Sulli et al. described a Microangiopathy Evolution Score that was obtained by summing scores on three-point semi-quantitative scales for loss of capillaries (vessel density), disorganization and ramification, averaging the scores over fingers. Using this method they were able to show disease progression in the majority of patients [33]. Smith et al. also applied Suli's method to predicting the risk of developing trophic lesions in patients with SSc [34].

More recently, Smith et al. proposed the semi-quantitative Fast Track algorithm for detecting SSc from capillaroscopy images. The aim was to provide a simple-to-apply set of rules that could be used widely to classify patients into SSc and not-SSc groups. They proposed that the presence in a 1 millimetre section of nailfold of either a vessel density less than 3 capillaries per millimetre or a giant capillary was sufficient to classify a case as positive for SSc, particularly if low vessel density was accompanied by clearly abnormal vessel shapes, with all other cases classified as not-SSc (see Fig. 7). They reported excellent inter-rater agreement in a large group of mixed experience [35], but they did not report the performance of the method classifying the true disease state of patients. The method is likely to be specific but not sensitive, given that other investigators have reported vessel densities of >3 capillaries per millimetre in patients with SSc [36–39] with densities of >7 capillaries per millimetre in early stage disease [40].

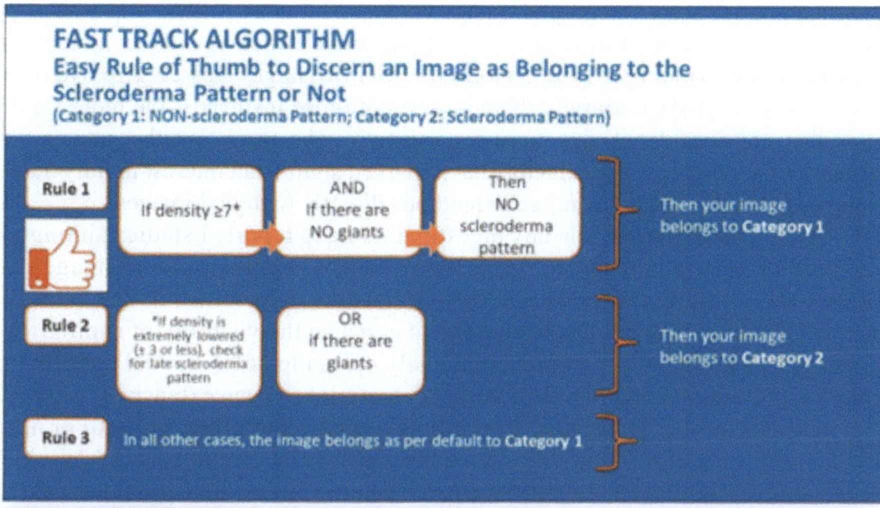

Capillaroscopic characteristics	CATEGORY 1					CATEGORY 2		
	Non-scleroderma pattern					Scleroderma Pattern		
	Normal	Non-Specific Abnormalities: If any of the capillaroscopic characteristics are abnormal (alone or in any combination) as highlighted in grey				Early	Active	Late
Density (/mm)	≥ 7	↓				≥ 7	Lowered density (4-6)	Further lowered density (≤3)
Dimension (µm)	Normal		20-50			> 50 (giant)	> 50 (giant)	-
Abnormal morphology	-			+		-	+	++
Haemorrhages	-				+	+/-	+/-	-

Fig. 7 Schematic of the Fast-Track Algorithm and associated standardized evaluation chart for semi-quantitative scoring of nailfold images. (Adapted and reproduced from [35] under CC by 4.0)

Automated Analysis of Vessel Mophology

Semi-quantitative methods have played an important role in characterising disease-related vessel abnormalities and demonstrating the potential of nailfold capillaroscopy to support early diagnosis of SSc. There are, however, limitations to this approach: they still depend on subjective judgement, where comparison is available they do not perform as well as fully quantitative methods [7, 14], they are generally difficult to apply and, as a result, they have not found their way into general clinical practice. It is worth unpacking the first of these points—not only is there subjective judgement involved in deciding, for each parameter under consideration, to which semi-quantitative scale category an image belongs, but there is generally a need to select an area of nailbed to image and, often, select which vessels to include in assessing vessel width (e.g. most abnormal vessel [8], largest vessel [16], five consecutive vessels [14]). Generally there is a compromise involved—the more capillaries that are considered, the more representative the result but the greater the burden for the observer. These factors have sparked significant interest in fully automated systems that apply quantitative methods directly to digital images.

Over the past 20 years, various investigators have reported studies aiming to automate or semi-automate the analysis of nailfold capillaroscopic images in patients with different diseases, including diabetes, hypertension, and SSc. At the most basic level, work has been done to enhance the visibility of capillaries, sometimes as a precursor to automated analysis, using color, spatial pattern, or temporal pattern filtering [41–46]. Vessel detection has been extensively studied with methods aiming either to extract whole vessels/centrelines [47–50] or apices [51–54]. Few of these systems have been clinically evaluated at scale, with the notable exception of the AUTOCAPI system [54], which provides vessel density results in good agreement with experts for a manually selected region. Both fully automated [43, 51] and semi-automated [8, 55] measurements of vessel width and shape have been described, but again, with very limited clinical validation. There has also been work to explore the potential for texture analysis to detect disease in whole nailfold images [44, 56], but only very preliminary results have been presented.

We previously described what was probably the first fully automated system to make clinically validated predictions of disease state [10, 27]. The system used a motorised microscope to acquire a set of images across the full width of a given nailfold and combined these to create a panoramic mosaic image of the nailfold. It made automated measurements of capillary density, mean capillary width, maximum capillary width, vessel tortuosity (as described above), and vessel derangement for each finger studied (Fig. 1d). These measurements were averaged across fingers and combined to give an abnormality score that allowed patients with SSc to be distinguished from healthy controls and patients with primary RP, with an area under the ROC of 0.92 (SE 0.26). This system was the forerunner of the Capilytics system which we describe below.

State-of-the-Art Systems

In this section we bring things up-to-date by describing two state-of-the-art fully automatic quantitative capillaroscopy systems. Both systems exploit recent advances in machine learning, in particular Convolutional Neural Networks (CNNs) [57] to learn from annotated training images and predict disease status—though in slightly different ways.

Capilytics System

The Capilytics system [7, 28] builds on the earlier work described above [10, 27] which also used machine learning (Random Forest classification and regression [58]). The current system uses a pipeline of specialised CNNs: U-Net [59] applied to the whole nailfold image to generate apex candidates and segment vessels, ResNet34 [60] applied to a small patch around each apex candidate for candidate classification (apex/distal-apex/non-apex) and width estimation (Fig. 8). This allows apical width and tortuosity (using the method of Berks et al. [27]) to be measured for each capillary, and maximum apical width and vessel density to be measured for each image. To evaluate the system, images were acquired with a hand-held USB microscope (Dino-Lite CapillaryScope 200 Pro, and other devices less relevant to this discussion). Five (mainly) non-overlapping images were selected automatically from the video stream for each of four fingers using a ResNet34 trained on image quality (see below for more detail). The morphological measurements were averaged over all images per finger and all fingers and were used in a logistic regression model to provide a probability of SSc. The system was evaluated using images from 175 subjects, 88 with a clinical diagnosis of SSc, 87 healthy controls and primary RP. Data from none of the subjects had been used in training. The system achieved a sensitivity and specificity of 91% (5th–95th centile 87%–94%) with an area under the ROC of 96% (5th–95th centile 94%–98%) in detecting SSc from the images alone (Fig. 9).

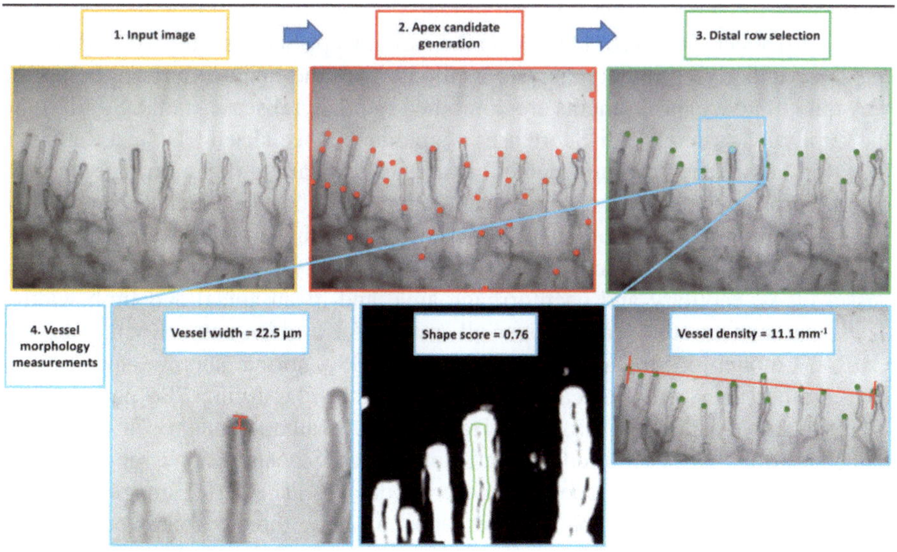

Fig. 8 Schematic of the Capilytics system for automated estimation of vessel morphology [28]. The measures of vessel width (mean and max across all fingers), shape score and vessel density are combined to compute an overall SSc-score (see Fig. 9)

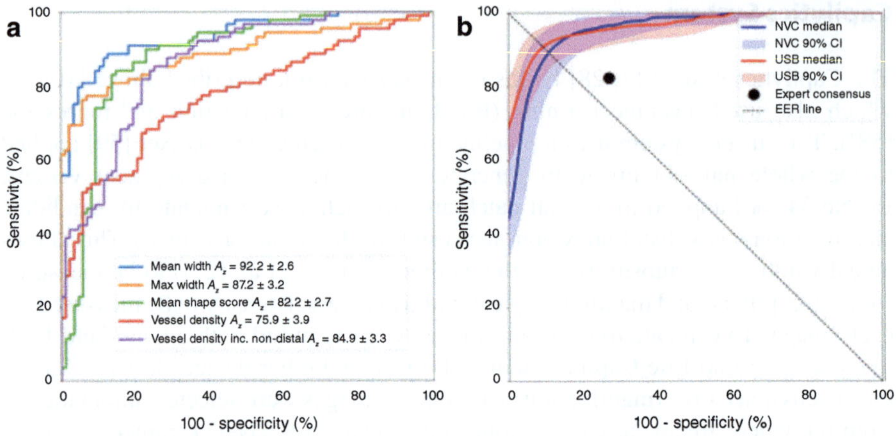

Fig. 9 ROC curves differentiating between non-SSc (healthy controls and primary Raynauds phenomenon) and SSc subjects using the Capilytics system [28]: (**a**) for individual measures of capillary morphology; (**b**) for the combined SSc score—here results are shown for images acquired on a lab-based videocapillarosocpy system (NVC, as see Fig. 3) and the handheld USB microscope (see Fig. 4), with the latter achieving an area-under-the-curve of 96% (5th–95th centile 94%–98%) and equal-error rate (EER) sensitivity and specificity of 91% (5th–95th centile 87%–94%). SSc-scores for both systems significantly outperform an estimate expert human consensus

Capi-Detect System

The Capi-Detect system [61] builds on the earlier Capi-Score system [62]. Both use the same underlying image analysis methods, with the main difference being the way quantitative measurements are combined to predict disease status. Similarly to the Capilytics system, Capi-Score uses a pipeline of specialised CNNs: a Retinanet [63] for vessel/haemorrhage detection and classification (haemorrhage/normal-capillary/tortuous-capillary/ramified-capillary) and a Stacked Dense Net [64] to measure capillary dimensions. This allows the following parameters to be measured for each image: capillary density, capillary density by type of vessel, distribution of vessel types, capillary and haemorrhage area, and mean apical and limb widths. These parameters are averaged over all images for a given subject and used in a CatBoost model [65] to categorise subjects into SSc, normal and non-specific patterns (rather than actual disease state), and further classifying SSc patterns into 'early', 'active' and 'late' disease. Training and evaluation has been performed using nailfold images acquired at nine Spanish and US hospitals on a range of high-magnification, handheld videocapillaroscopy devices. The set of images for each subject in the data was assigned a pattern label by either three or four expert observers blinded to the subject's diagnosis. Subjects were included in the data if at least two out of three, or three out of four, observers agreed on the label, resulting in a final dataset of 1490 subjects, of which 1192 were used for training and 298 for evaluation (83 normal; 114 non-specific; 45 early SSc; 39 active SSc; 17 late SSc). On these data, Capi-Detect achieved 5-way classification accuracies of 66% for

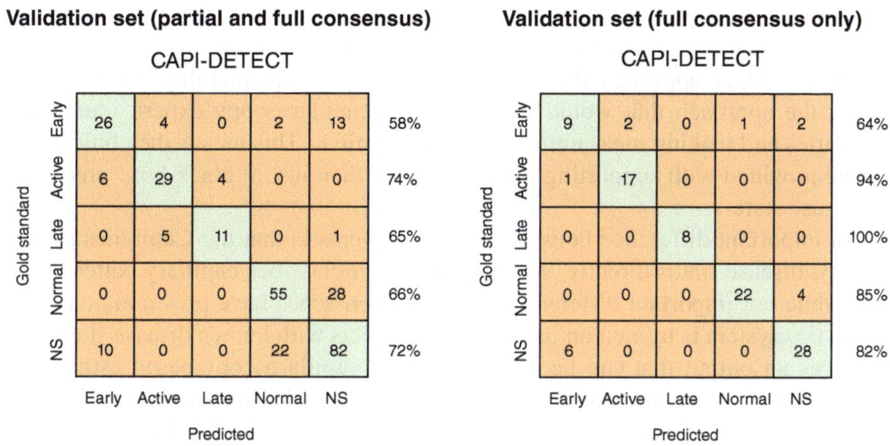

Fig. 10 5-way confusion matrices for Capi-Detect's [62] classification of nailfold images into normal, non-specific and early, active and late SSc patterns: (**a**) using images with (at least) partial agreement between on the ground truth label between experts; (**b**) using only images with full agreement between experts. (Amended with permission from [62], under CC by 4.0)

normal patterns, 72% for non-specific, and 58%, 74% and 65% for early, active and late SSc patterns respectively (see Fig. 10a for the full 5-way classification table). Restricting the classification to a binary decision between SSc pattern (101 subjects) vs non-SSc pattern (normal + non-specific, 197 subjects), Capi-Detect achieved a sensitivity of 84% and specificity of 95% (confidence intervals not provided). Using only subjects for whom all observers agreed on the label (100 out of 298) improved class-wise accuracies to 85% (normal), 82% (non-specific), 64% (early), 94% (active) and 100% (late) (Fig. 10b), with corresponding SSc vs non-SSc sensitivity and specificity of 93% and 90%. Evaluation on subjects with no-consensus between the three expert observers (comprising approximately 15% of the original data) was not performed as it was ambiguous which label should be assigned as ground truth.

State-of-the-Art Discussion

Both state-of-the-art systems use a two-stage approach, first detecting vessels (plus haemorrhages for Capi-Detect) then making measurements. This is important for two main reasons: it makes better use of training data, and it provides a human-accessible explanation of disease status prediction.

Deep learning methods that take images as their input require very large training sets (typically >1000) to avoid over-fitting, leading to poor generalisation. Whilst capillaroscopy datasets typically contain images for a few hundred subjects, there are usually multiple images for each subject and many capillaries for each image—so a dataset with 100 subjects would typically include tens of thousands of capillaries. This is exploited by both systems by training second-stage models on small image patches centred on candidate capillaries detected in the first stage, providing the very large training sets required for effective model training.

The two-stage approach also has the advantage of explainability. Both systems mirror the approach that would be taken by a capillaroscopy expert, identifying capillaries and making measurements that are familiar. This means the clinical user can be provided with supporting evidence rather than just a 'black-box' prediction of disease state.

An important difference between the two systems is that the Capilytics system predicts disease status directly, whilst Capi-Detect classifies capillary pattern. This is a subtle but important difference and both approaches have pros and cons. The Capilytics system is trained on images from subjects with known disease status and produces an output that can be interpreted as a capillaroscopy-based estimate of disease risk. By design, the system provides a disease risk estimate for every subject imaged, without reference to expert opinion on capillary pattern. This provides an 'honest' estimate of 'real-world' performance, as long as test data is representative of the population that will be encountered in clinical practice. It is a major concern that this may not be the case, because the need to recruit subjects with known disease status for training and testing is likely to bias towards patients with established SSc.

In contrast, Capi-Detect attempts to predict capillary pattern, from which disease status can be inferred. Training and testing are based on expert classification of capillary pattern into SSc pattern and non-SSc pattern, with further subdivision of SSc pattern into early, active and late and non-SSc pattern into normal and non-specific. Thus the system can be considered a virtual expert, which may be closer to normal clinical practice where a generalist might seek an expert opinion on a particular investigation. There are, however, two issues with this approach. First, in both training and testing only subjects for which there was an expert consensus were considered, this resulted in a significant proportion of subjects studied being excluded. Thus it is not clear what the real-world performance of the system would be in clinical practice where all subjects would need to be assessed. This is particularly concerning because the cases excluded from testing through lack of expert consensus are, by definition, likely to be 'difficult'—exactly those where quantitative analysis would be most valuable in resolving ambiguity. The second issue is that a system trained on expert opinion can, by definition, never be better than the experts, and will be unable to exploit subtle changes in appearance that human experts have failed to recognise. For example, evidence from the Capilytics system suggests that small but consistent increases in vessel width, that are difficult for experts to quantify, are a powerful indicator of disease.

A final point to consider is that machine learning systems are sensitive to the characteristics of the data on which they are trained and tested—in this case, the noise, contrast and optical resolution characteristics of the imaging systems used. It is thus important to recognise that a system that works well with data from one imaging device will not necessarily work as well with data from another. In fact, although we have not provided details here, both the Capilytics and Capi-Detect systems have been trained and evaluated on data from a range of imaging systems and have shown the ability to generalise well. This is no guarantee, however, that they will work with data from a previously unseen device, and additional training may be required to adapt these systems to new devices.

Quantifying Image Quality

For a fully automated quantitative capillaroscopy system to be applied in a clinical setting, it is important to accompany any assessment of disease status with an indication of its reliability. Image quality plays a key role in determining reliability. Image quality is determined by a range of factors including: intrinsic visibility of capillaries (e.g. in dark skin), focus, position of the distal row in the field of view (roughly central, horizontal, apices pointing up), glare (reduced by using a polarizing filter), and appropriate use of coupling fluid. The Capilytics system includes a subsystem for estimating image quality. This is used to select good-quality images from the microscopy video stream, and to provide an assessment of image quality in the clinical report generated by the system.

The task of image quality assessment is nuanced. Given that SSc causes significant disruption to the normal appearance of nailfold capillaries, often resulting in 'messy' images, it is important to base assessment of image quality on diagnostic quality rather than visual quality (which would favour normal capillary patterns). To address the problem, the Capilytics system uses a machine learning approach (previously unpublished). We assembled a training set of images of varying quality including images from SSc patients, healthy controls and patients with primary RP. We selected thousands of pairs of images at random from this set and presented them to expert human observers, asking them to select from each pair the image that had higher diagnostic value. The results were used to form a ranking over the dataset, which in turn was normalised to provide a quality score from 0 to 100 for each image. The images and associated quality score data were used to train a ResNet regressor which can be used to assess the quality of previously unseen images (see Fig. 11).

We are using this model not only to support post-analysis reporting, but also to improve image acquisition itself. We are working on a nailfold capillaroscopy system in which models of quality and position make predictions on frames from the video stream from a video microscope in real time, so that feedback and guidance can be given to the operator and the best frames (i.e. those with highest diagnostic value) can be automatically selected for quantitative analysis. The system is still in development and is currently being trialled in several frontline rheumatology clinics in the UK, but we are hopeful it will significantly improve the quality of capillaroscopy images acquired in clinical settings while simultaneously solving the problem of having an objective measure to determine the evaluability of images for quantitative analysis.

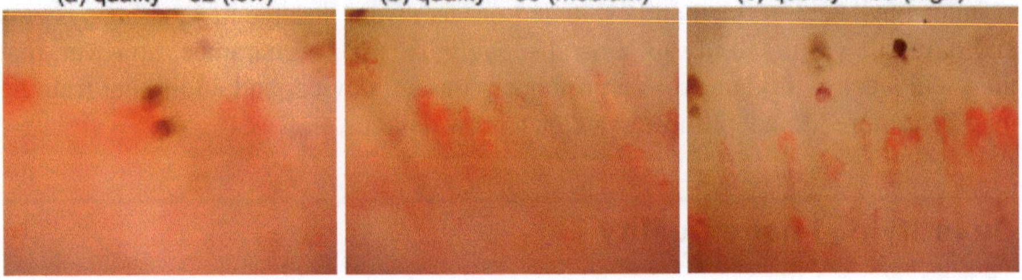

Fig. 11 Estimating the quality of nailfold images using a model trained on human experts. The model assigns each frame a score out of 100 comprising elements of focus, positioning and diagnostic information and is capable of running in real-time while video frames are recorded: (**a**) a low quality frame with poorly visualised capillaries; (**b**) a medium quality frame—capillaries are visible and the positioning is good, however some vessels are out-of-focus making accurate quantification of morphology difficult; (**c**) a high-quality frame, with excellent positioning and well-focused vessels, providing high diagnostic information for clinicians and enabling accurate quantification of morphology

Measuring Capillary Function

Thus far we have focussed on methods for measuring capillary morphology. There is, however, the exciting possibility of measuring changes in capillary function, which are likely to be more responsive/sensitive to disease progression and intervention. We describe briefly initial work on quantifying two aspects of capilliary function: blood flow and oxygenation.

Quantifying Red Blood Cell Velocity (Flow)

Capillaries are designed to transport red blood cells (RBCs), enabling the delivery of oxygen to tissues. Although changes in vessel morphology are easy to observe, alterations in RBC flow may be more sensitive to disease processes and treatment. For example: initial studies of RBC velocity in patients with SSc-spectrum disorders assessed the 'stop-flow' time in response to a cooling stimulus [66]; Mugii et al. reported that RBC velocity was reduced in patients with SSc and dermatomyositis compared to healthy controls, although in dermatomyositis differences were not significant [67, 68]; in seven patients with SSc, RBC velocity increased after treatment with alprostadil [67]; increased RBC velocity has also been reported in response to vasoactive treatment in other conditions [69, 70].

RBC velocity can, in principle, be measured from videocapillaroscopy sequences if the spatial and temporal resolution of the imaging device is sufficient to visualise and track individual RBCs. This is the case for many modern videocapilloscopy devices. Methods to quantify RBC velocity include manual frame-by-frame analysis measuring the displacement of plasma gaps [71], cross-correlation between manually selected windows on the same capillary [71, 72], oblique trace extraction

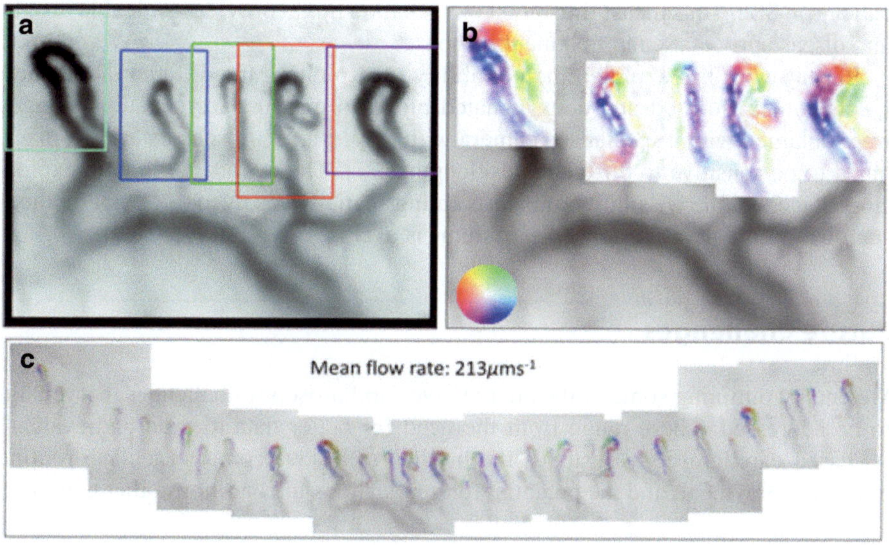

Fig. 12 Estimating red blood cell velocity (flow rate) in nailfold video images. (**a**) Video sequences are computed from a lab-based, videocapillaroscopy system when the motorised platform is stationary and frames are in-focus (see Fig. 3), with automated detection of apices used to extract localised videos about each capillary; (**b**) a regularised optical flow algorithm is used to estimated the flow velocity along each capillary—here the colour represents flow direction and the brightness its magnitude; (**c**) projecting estimates of flow for all capillaries across the nailfold and combining to compute a mean flow rate [27]

from spatio-temporal images formed by taking image intensity along the vessel at successive timepoints [73, 74], and optical flow [75].

We extended the fully automated quantitative capillaroscopy system developed by Berks et al., described previously [27], to include average RBC velocity across all capillaries in a nailfold using an optical flow method [10, 76] (Fig. 12). We found that adding flow to morphological measurements improved discrimination between patients with SSc and patients with primary RP plus healthy controls, increasing the area under the ROC curve from 92% (SE 2.6%) to 93% (SE 2.4%). The approach was methodologically challenging, and would be difficult to translate directly into clinical practice, but these initial findings show promise and merit further investigation.

Quantifying Oxygenation

A second form of functional information that researchers have attempted to quantify using capillaroscopy is the oxygenation of nailfold capillaries. Because capillaries represent the point at which oxygen is delivered from blood vessels to the tissue, they carry oxygenated blood on the arterial limb and deoxygenated blood on the venous limb. Ultimately, it is the breakdown in oxygen delivery to tissue that harms patients in SSc. Thus measuring blood oxygenation might provide invaluable insight into disease processes and treatment response.

Recent work has explored the possibility of exploiting the different absorption spectra of oxygenated and deoxygenated blood to measure oxygenation. Images were obtained with a specialised camera with a 3 x 3 array of sensors at each pixel, tuned to be sensitive to different wavelengths [77]. This work is still at an exploratory stage, but the possibility of incorporating spatially-resolved oxygenation measurement into videocapillaroscopy systems is exciting.

Future Challenges

We end by outlining some of the quantitative capillaroscopy challenges that remain to be addressed. These range from the need for better data to train and evaluate AI-based capillaroscopy systems, the hurdles to be overcome to achieve routine clinical deployment, and the potential for applications in conditions other than SSc.

Reference Data

Well curated datasets with expert annotation are critical to the development and evaluation of AI-based quantitative capillaroscopy. The Capilytics and Capi-Detect teams have both built such resources, but neither is ideal. The fact that it is impossible to make a like-for-like comparison of the performance of the two systems is telling, and potentially problematic for the future of the field. The creation of ImageNet [https://www.image-net.org] as a resource that can be used for training and comparing the performance of general image classification and object recognition systems has been transformational, and quantitative capillaroscopy would benefit from a similar initiative, with a very large database of annotated images and agreed, standardised methods of comparing the performance of different systems. This is an important opportunity for international collaboration.

Clinical Deployment

Quantitative capillaroscopy has developed significantly over the past 25 years to the point there are now fully automated analysis systems that measure capillary structure and make predictions of the presence of abnormalities indicative of disease in a fast, objective manner. There are, however, still challenges to be overcome before such systems can be deployed for routine use in frontline clinical settings.

While regulations differ between jurisdictions, in most major medical markets (including the US, EU and UK), if an automated image analysis system generates results that support the diagnosis of a patient, then the system is deemed to be a medical device and must be certified for regulatory compliance before it can be distributed commercially. Typically, this requires demonstrating that the system, and especially the software within it, has been designed and developed to a rigorous standard. Such standards are not usually required of software used in research and thus, even though a system may have been shown to generate very promising results in published research, there may still be significant work to be done in translating the system into a certified medical device.

A second key requirement for certifying a system as a medical device is that it has been shown to work in its target clinical population. As discussed earlier, this population may differ from the study cohorts used in published research, so these evaluations may again require significant further work and resources.

Other Clinical Applications

Nailfold capillaroscopy has primarily been developed and evaluated for application in the diagnosis of SSc. It has potential applications, however, in other conditions where distinctive damage to the microcirculation may be present. These include the following.

- Other connective tissue diseases
  - Lupus
  - Dermatomyositis
  - Polymyositis
  - Mixed Connective Tissue Disease
- Rheumatoid Arthritis
- Type 2 Diabetes
- Hypertension and Cardiovascular Disease
- COVID-19 and Post-COVID syndromes

Detailed discussion of these applications is beyond the scope of this chapter, but this is an important area of research that merits further investigation.

Summary

In summary, nailfold capillaroscopy has progressed from its purely observational beginnings, through a range of investigations and developments, to a mature field where objective criteria can be used to detect the presence of disease-related capillary abnormalities, and this process can be fully automated. Its importance in the early diagnosis of SSc has been firmly established. There are still challenges to meet, but fully automated analysis has the potential to bring reliable capillaroscopy investigation to the general rheumatology clinic. There are also exciting opportunities to explore applications in other disease areas.

References

1. Van den Hoogen F, Khanna D, Fransen J, et al. Classification criteria for systemic sclerosis: an American College of Rheumatology/European league against rheumatism collaborative initiative. Arthritis Rheum. 2013;65:2737–47.
2. Van den Hoogen F, Khanna D, Fransen J, et al. 2013 classification criteria for systemic sclerosis: an American College of Rheumatology/European league against rheumatism collaborative initiative. Ann Rheum Dis. 2013;72:1747–55.
3. Walker UA, Tyndall A, Czirják L, et al. Clinical risk assessment of organ manifestations in systemic sclerosis: a report from the EULAR scleroderma trials and research group database. Ann Rheum Dis. 2007;66:754–63.
4. Bellando-Randone S, Del Galdo F, Lepri G, et al. Progression of patients with Raynaud's phenomenon to systemic sclerosis: a five-year analysis of the European scleroderma trial and research group multicentre, longitudinal registry study for very early diagnosis of systemic sclerosis (VEDOSS). Lancet Rheumatol. 2021;3(12):e834–43.
5. Maricq HR, LeRoy EC. Patterns of finger capillary abnormalities in connective tissue diseases by 'widefield' microscopy. Arthritis Rheum. 1973;16:619–28.
6. Maricq HR. Comparison of quantitative and semiquantitative estimates of nailfold capillary abnormalities in scleroderma spectrum disorders. Microvasc Res. 1986;32:271–6.
7. Gurunath-Bharathi P, Berks M, Dinsdale G, et al. A deep learning system for quantitative assessment of microvascular abnormalities in nailfold capillary images. Rheumatology. 2023;62(6):2325–9.
8. Bukhari M, Herrick AL, Moore T, Manning J, Jayson MIV. Increased nailfold capillary dimensions in primary Raynaud's phenomenon and systemic sclerosis. Br J Rheumatol. 1996;35:1127–31.
9. Anderson ME, Allen PD, Moore T, et al. Computerised nailfold video capillaroscopy—a new tool for assessment of Raynaud's phenomenon. J Rheumatol. 2005;32:841–8.
10. Berks M, Dinsdale G, Murray A, et al. Improved diagnosis of systemic sclerosis using nailfold capillary flow. In: Ourselin S, Joskowicz L, Sabuncu M, Unal G, Wells W, editors. Medical image computing and computer-assisted intervention—MICCAI 2016, Lecture notes in computer science, vol. 9902. Cham: Springer; 2016. p. 344–52.
11. Herrick AL, Berks M, Taylor CJ. Quantitative nailfold capillaroscopy—update and possible next steps. Rheumatology. 2021;60(5):2054–65.
12. Lefford F, Edwards JC. Nailfold capillary microscopy in connective tissue diseases: a quantitative morphological analysis. Ann Rheum Dis. 1986;45:741–9.
13. Kabasakal Y, Elvins DM, Ring EF, McHugh NJ. Quantitative nailfold capillaroscopy findings in a population with connective tissue disease and in normal healthy controls. Ann Rheum Dis. 1996;55:507–12.
14. Murray AK, Feng K, Moore TL, et al. Preliminary clinical evaluation of semi-automated nailfold capillaroscopy in the assessment of patients with Raynaud's phenomenon. Microcirculation. 2011;18:440–7.
15. Trombetta AC, Smith V, Pizzorni C, et al. Quantitative alterations of capillary diameter have a predictive value for development of the capillaroscopic systemic sclerosis pattern. J Rheumatol. 2016;43:599–606.
16. Hofstee HM, Serne EH, Roberts C, et al. A multicentre study on the reliability of qualitative and quantitative nailfold videocapillaroscopy assessment. Rheumatology. 2012;51:749–55.
17. Guillen-Del-Castillo A, Simeon-Aznar CP, CallejasMoraga EL, et al. Quantitative videocapillaroscopy correlates with functional respiratory parameters: a clue for vasculopathy as a pathogenic mechanism for lung injury in systemic sclerosis. Arthritis Res Ther. 2018;20:281.
18. Wildt M, Wuttge DM, Hesselstrand R, Scheja A. Assessment of capillary density in systemic sclerosis with three different capillaroscopic methods. Clin Exp Rheumatol. 2012;30:S50–4.

19. Barth Z, Witczak BN, Flato B, et al. Assessment of microvascular abnormalities by nailfold capillaroscopy in juvenile dermatomyositis after medium- to long-term followup. Arthritis Care Res. 2018;70:768–76.
20. Karbalaie A, Abtahi F, Fatemi A, et al. Elliptical broken line method for calculating capillary density in nailfold capillaroscopy: proposal and evaluation. Microvasc Res. 2017;113:1–8.
21. Scheja A, Akesson A, Niewierowicz I, et al. Computer based quantitative analysis of capillary abnormalities in systemic sclerosis and its relation to plasma concentration of von Willebrand factor. Ann Rheum Dis. 1996;55:52–6.
22. Emrani Z, Karbalaie A, Fatemi A, Etehadtavakol M, Erlandsson BE. Capillary density: an important parameter in nailfold capillaroscopy. Microvasc Res. 2017;109:7–18.
23. Sebastiani M, Manfredi A, Colaci M, et al. Capillaroscopic skin ulcer risk index: a new prognostic tool for digital skin ulcer development in systemic sclerosis patients. Arthritis Rheum. 2009;61:688–94.
24. Cutolo M, Herrick AL, Distler O, et al. CAP study investigators. Nailfold videocapillaroscopic features and other clinical risk factors for digital ulcers in systemic sclerosis. A multicenter, prospective cohort study. Arthritis. Rheumatol. 2016;68:2527–39.
25. Andrade LE, Gabriel A, Assad RL, Ferrari AJ, Atra E. Panoramic nailfold capillaroscopy: a new reading method and normal range. Semin Arthritis Rheum. 1990;20:21–31.
26. Ingegnoli F, Gualtierotti R, Lubatti C, et al. Nailfold capillary patterns in healthy subjects: a real issue in capillaroscopy. Microvasc Res. 2013;90:90–5.
27. Berks M, Tresadern P, Dinsdale G, et al. An automated system for detecting and measuring nailfold capillaries. Med Image Comput Comput Assist Interv. 2014;17:658–65.
28. Berks M, Gurunath Bharathi P, Murray A, et al. Automated analysis of Nailfold capillaries using a low-cost USB microscope—a route to increasing uptake of Nailfold Capillaroscopy in the out-patient clinic? Ann Rheum Dis. 2024;83(S1):1057–8.
29. Koenig M, Joyal F, Fritzler MJ, Roussin A, et al. Autoantibodies and microvascular damage are independent predictive factors for the progression of Raynaud's phenomenon to systemic sclerosis. Arthritis Rheum. 2008;58:3902–12.
30. Ingegnoli F, Boracchi P, Gualtierotti R, et al. Prognostic model based on nailfold capillaroscopy for identifying Raynaud's phenomenon patients at high risk for the development of a scleroderma spectrum disorder. Arthritis Rheum. 2008;58:2174–82.
31. Ingegnoli F, Boracchi P, Gualtierotti R, et al. Improving outcome prediction of systemic sclerosis from isolated Raynaud's phenomenon: role of autoantibodies and nailfold capillaroscopy. Rheumatology. 2010;49:797–805.
32. Sebastiani M, Manfredi A, Vukatana G, et al. Predictive role of capillaroscopic skin ulcer risk index in systemic sclerosis: a multicentre validation study. Ann Rheum Dis. 2012;71:67–70.
33. Sulli A, Secchi ME, Pizzorni C, Cutolo M. Scoring the nailfold microvascular changes during the capillaroscopic analysis in systemic sclerosis patients. Ann Rheum Dis. 2008;67:885–7.
34. Smith V, De Keyser F, Pizzorni C, et al. Nailfold capillaroscopy for day-to-day clinical use: construction of a simple scoring modality as a clinical prognostic index for digital trophic lesions. Ann Rheum Dis. 2011;70:180–3.
35. Smith V, Ickinger C, Hysa E, et al. Nailfold capillaroscopy. Best Pract Res Clin Rheumatol. 2023;37(1):101849.
36. Wildt M, Hesselstrand R, Scheja A, Akesson A. Capillary density in patients with systemic sclerosis, as determined by microscopy counts and compared with computer-based analysis. Clin Exp Rhematol. 1999;17:219–22.
37. Bukhari M, Hollis S, Moore T, Jayson MIV, Herrick AL. Quantitation of microcirculatory abnormalities in patients with primary Raynaud's phenomenon and systemic sclerosis by video capillaroscopy. Rheumatology. 2000;39:506–12.
38. Correa MJ, Andrade LE, Kayser C. Comparison of laser Doppler imaging, fingertip lacticemy test, and nailfold capillaroscopy for assessment of digital microcirculation in systemic sclerosis. Arthritis Res Therapy. 2010;12:R157.

39. Avouac J, Lepri G, Smith V, et al. Sequential nailfold videocapillaroscopy examinations have responsiveness to detect organ progression in systemic sclerosis. Sem Arthritis Rheum. 2017;47:86–94.
40. Smith V, Herrick AL, Ingegnoli F, et al. Standardisation of nailfold capillaroscopy for the assessment of patients with Raynaud's phenomenon and systemic sclerosis. Autoimmun Rev. 2020;19:102458.
41. Allen PD, Taylor CJ, Herrick AL, Moore T. Image analysis of nailfold capillary patterns from video sequences. In: Taylor C, Colchester A, editors. Medical image computing and computer-assisted intervention. Berlin/Heidelberg: Springer; 1999. p. 698–705.
42. Hamar G, Horvath G, Tarjan Z, Virag T. Markov chain based edge detection algorithm for evaluation of capillary microscopic images. In: Jarm T, Kramar P, Zupanic A, editors. 11th Mediterranean conference on medical and biomedical engineering and computing. IFMBE proceedings, vol. 16. Berlin/Heidelberg: Springer; 2007. p. 818–21.
43. Riao-Rojas JC, Prieto-Ortiz FA, Morantes LJ, SanchezCamperos E, Jaramillo-Ayerbe F. Segmentation and extraction of morphologic features from capillary images. In: 2007 Sixth Mexican International Conference on Artificial Intelligence, Special Session (MICAI); 2007. p. 148–59.
44. Doshi NP, Schaefer G, Merla A. An evaluation of image enhancement techniques for capillary imaging. In: 2012 IEEE international conference on systems, man, and cybernetics (SMC). IEEE; 2012. p. 1428–32.
45. Goffredo M, Schmid M, Conforto S, et al. Quantitative color analysis for capillaroscopy image segmentation. Med Biol Eng Comput. 2012;50:567–74.
46. Ingegnoli F, Ughi N, Dinsdale G, et al. EULAR study group on microcirculation in RheumaticDiseases. An international SUrvey on non-iNvaSive tecHniques to assess the mIcrocirculation in patients with RayNaud's phEnomenon (SUNSHINE survey). Rheumatol Int. 2017;37:1879–90.
47. Wen C-H, Hsieh T-Y, Liao W-D, Lan J-L, Chen D-Y, Li K-C, et al. A novel method for classification of highresolution nailfold capillary microscopy images. In: First IEEE international conference on Ubi-media computing. IEEE; 2008. p. 513–8.
48. Doshi NP, Schaefer G, Zhu SY. An improved binarisation algorithm for nailfold capillary skeleton extraction. In: 2013 IEEE international conference on systems, man, and cybernetics. IEEE; 2013. p. 2565–9.
49. Cheng C, Lee CW, Daskalalakis C. A reproducible computerized method for quantitation of capillary density using nailfold capillaroscopy. J Vis Exp. 2015;104:e53088.
50. Suma KV, Rao B. Quantification of capillary density and inter-capillary distance in nailfold capillary images using scale space capillary detection and ordinate clust. Int J Biomed Clin Eng. 2017;6:32–49.
51. Vucic V. Image analysis for nail-fold capillaroscopy. Masters thesis, KTH Stockholm; 2015. http://urn.kb.se/resolve?urn¼urn:nbn:se:kth:diva-174868
52. Sainthillier J-M, Gharbi T, Muret P, Humbert P. Skin capillary network recognition and analysis by means of neural algorithms. Skin Res Technol. 2005;11:9–16.
53. Kwasnicka H, Paradowski M, Borysewicz K. Capillaroscopy image analysis as an automatic image annotation problem. In: 2007 6th international conference on computer information systems and industrial management applications. IEEE; 2007. p. 266–71.
54. Cutolo M, Trombetta AC, Melsens K, et al. Automated assessment of absolute nailfold capillary number on videocapillaroscopic images: proof of principle and validation in systemic sclerosis. Microcirculation. 2018;25:e12447.
55. Hu Q, Mahler F. New system for image analysis in nailfold capillaroscopy. Microcirculation. 1999;6:227–35.
56. Urwin SG, Griffiths B, Allen J. Quantification of differences between nailfold capillaroscopy images with a scleroderma pattern and normal pattern using measures of geometric and algorithmic complexity. Physiol Meas. 2017;38:N32–41.
57. Lecun L, Bottou L, Bengio Y, Haffner P. Gradient-based learning applied to document recognition. Proc IEEE. 1998;86(11):2278–324.

58. Breiman L. Random forests. Mach Learn. 2001;45:5–32.
59. Ronneberger O, Fischer P, Brox T. U-net: convolutional networks for biomedical image segmentation. In: Navab N, Hornegger J, Wells W, Frangi A, editors. International conference on medical image computing and computer-assisted intervention—MICCAI 2015, Lecture notes in computer science, vol. 9351. Springer; 2015. p. 234–41.
60. He K, Zhang X, Ren S, Sun J. Deep residual learning for image recognition. In: Proceedings of the IEEE conference on computer vision and pattern recognition (CVPR); 2016. p. 770–8.
61. Lledó-Ibáñez GM, Comet LS, Dapena MF, et al. CAPI-detect: machine learning in capillaroscopy reveals new variables influencing diagnosis. Rheumatology. 2025;64(6):3667–75.
62. Gracia Tello BC, Saez Comet L, Lledo G, et al. CAPI-SCORE: a quantitative algorithm for identifying disease patterns in nailfold videocapillaroscopy. Rheumatology. 2024;63(12):3315–21.
63. Lin T, Goyal P, Girshick R, et al. Focal loss for dense object detection. IEEE Trans Pattern Anal Mach Intell. 2020;42:318–27.
64. Graving JM, Chae D, Naik H, et al. DeepPoseKit, a software toolkit for fast and robust animal pose estimation using deep learning. elife. 2019;8:e47994.
65. Prokhorenkova L, Gusev G, Vorobev A, et al. CatBoost: unbiased boosting with categorical features. Adv Neural Inf Process Syst (NeurIPS). 2018;31:6638–48.
66. Mahler F, Saner H, Boss C, Annaheim M. Local cold exposure test for capillaroscopic examination of patients with Raynaud's syndrome. Microvasc Res. 1987;33:422–7.
67. Mugii N, Hasegawa M, Hamaguchi Y, et al. Reduced red blood cell velocity in nail-fold capillaries as a sensitive and specific indicator of microcirculation injury in systemic sclerosis. Rheumatology. 2009;48:696–703.
68. Mugii N, Hasegawa M, Matsushita T, et al. Association between nail-fold capillary findings and disease activity in dermatomyositis. Rheumatology. 2011;50:1091–8.
69. Henriksson P, Diczfalusy U, Freyschuss A. Microvascular reactivity in response to smoking and oral antioxidants in humans. Microcirculation. 2012;19:86–93.
70. Martina B, Surber C, Jakobi C, Sponagel L, Gasser P. Effect of moxonidine and cilazapril on microcirculation as assessed by finger nailfold capillaroscopy in mild-tomoderate hypertension. Angiology. 1998;49:897–901.
71. Mawson DM, Shore AC. Comparison of CapiFlow and frame by frame analysis for the assessment of capillary red blood cell velocity. J Med Eng Technol. 1998;22:53–63. Ariane L. Herrick et al. 2064 https://academic.oup.com/rheumatology
72. Klyscz T, Junger M, Jung F, Zeintl H. Cap image—ein neuartiges computerunterstutztes Videoanalysessystem fur die dynamische Kapillarmikroskopie. Biomed Tech. 1997;42:168–75.
73. Sato Y, Chen J, Zoroofi R, et al. Automatic extraction and measurement of leukocyte motion in microvessels using spatiotemporal image analysis. IEEE Trans Biomed Eng. 1997;44:225–36.
74. Chen Y, Zhao Z, Liu L, Li H. Automatic tracking and measurement of the motion of blood cells in microveessels based on analysis of multiple spatiotemporal images. Meas Sci Technol. 2011;22:045803.
75. Wu C-C, Zhang G, Huang T-C, Lin K-P. Red blood cell velocity measurements of complete capillary in finger nail-fold using optical flow estimation. Microvasc Res. 2009;78:319–24.
76. Berks M, Dinsdale G, Murray A, et al. Automated structure and flow measurement—a promising tool in nailfold capillaroscopy. Microvasc Res. 2018;118:173–7.
77. Taylor-Williams M, Mead S, Sawyer TW, et al. Multispectral imaging of nailfold capillaries using light-emitting diode illumination. J Biomed Opt. 2022;27(12):126002.

Nailfold Capillaroscopy in Systemic Sclerosis (Including Associations)

Maurizio Cutolo and Vanessa Smith

Abbreviations

α-SMA	α-smooth muscle actin
aAbs	Autoantibodies
ACR	American College of Rheumatology
AECA	Anti-endothelial cell antibodies
AT1R	Autoantibodies against angiotensin II type 1 receptor
CTD	Connective tissue disease
DM	Dermatomyositis
EC	Endothelial cell
EndoMT	Endothelial-to-mesenchymal transition
ET-1	Endothelin-1
ETAR	Autoantibodies against endothelin type A receptor
EULAR	European Alliance of Associations for Rheumatology
GPCR	G protein-coupled receptor
IFN	Interferon
ILD	Interstitial lung disease

M. Cutolo (✉)
Laboratory of Experimental Rheumatology, Division of Rheumatology, Department of Internal Medicine and Medical Specialties (DiMI), University of Genova, IRCCS San Martino Polyclinic Hospital, Genova, Italy
e-mail: mcutolo@unige.it

V. Smith
Department of Internal Medicine/(Rheumatology) Ghent University (Hospital), and Unit for Molecular Immunology and Inflammation, VIB Inflammation Research Center (IRC), Ghent, Belgium
e-mail: vanessa.smith@ugent.be

A. L. Herrick et al. (eds.), *Nailfold Capillaroscopy in Rheumatological Diseases*,
https://doi.org/10.1007/978-3-032-03970-5_6

LDF	Laser doppler flowmetry
M2	Profibrotic/anti-inflammatory macrophage 2
MCTD	Mixed connective tissue disease
mm	Millimeter
NPV	Negative predictive value
NVC	Nailfold videocapillaroscopy
PAH	Pulmonary arterial hypertension
PPV	Positive predictive value
SCTC	Scleroderma Clinical Trials Consortium
SSc	Systemic sclerosis
Th2	Type 2 T helper cells
Treg	T regulatory cells
UCTD	Undifferentiated connective tissue disease
VEDOSS	Very early diagnosis of systemic sclerosis.
μm	Micrometer

Key Points

- The progressive damage of the microvasculature in SSc is mirrored by the NVC patterns (“Early”, “Active”, “Late”), and after 25 years of strict observations a possible pre-scleroderma signature has been suggested (i.e. “Very Early” NVC pattern).
- One of the driving mechanisms that follows the immune mediated damage of the ECs of microvessels in SSc, is represented by the endothelial-to-mesenchymal cells transition (EndoMT) process, by creating a bridge between the EC apoptosis and the development of dermal fibrosis.
- The progressive dilation of capillaries beyond the normal diameter (which is typically under 20 μm), may indicate a risk condition as “pre-scleroderma pattern signature” (particularly when the diameter ranges between 30 μm and 50 μm) reflecting ongoing EC damage at the level of microvascular wall. This process can eventually lead to formation of the giant capillary (over 50 μm), which is diagnostic for the “Early” SSc NVC pattern.
- In patients with dermatomyositis (DM) or overlap connective tissue diseases (CTDs) the “scleroderma-like” NVC pattern may exist, as well as scleroderma patterns.
- Long term follow-up clinical studies (up to 12 years of observation) have shown an association between the progression of the SSc NVC patterns and common clinical SSc manifestations and organ involvement.
- Several therapeutic trials evaluating vasodilators, immunosuppressive drugs and also antifibrotics (tyrosine kinase inhibitor [nintedanib]) have used NVC as an outcome measure.

Introduction

Systemic sclerosis is a rare and chronic autoimmune disease with vasculopathy, immune dysregulation, and fibrosis. It manifests in two main subsets: limited and diffuse cutaneous SSc [1, 2]. Raynaud's phenomenon is often the earliest symptom, sometimes preceding diagnosis by years. Early diagnosis is critical for preventing organ damage and initiating treatment. The modern NVC is born in 2000 and since then the progression of new achievements is increasing year by year at a very fast rate [3].

The introduction of NVC in the guidelines for the classification of SSc in 2013 by the American Collega of Rheumatology (ACR) and the European Alliance of Associations for Rheumatology (EULAR) taskforce, has reinforced the mandatory use of this safe and reliable imaging method, as important diagnostic tool. Also, important live (on site) and online (eLearning) EULAR courses, between 2004 and 2025 have enabled spreading the skill to execute NVC in the daily practice of rheumatologists attending from over the world. Centers of excellence on imaging including the capillaroscopy have been created by appointment of the EULAR Education Board and host young rheumatologists for training and research on NVC. This chapter discusses the most advanced topics regarding changes of capillaroscopic characteristics, observable by NVC and eventually by other devices, in SSc with brief mention in other CTDs. The other CTDs are covered more extensively in other chapters (see chapters "Nailfold Capillaroscopy in Idiopathic Inflammatory Myopathies" and "Nailfold Capillaroscopy in Other Rheumatological Diseases").

The main paragraphs are:

1. The quantitative analysis of capillaroscopic characteristics in the progression of the microvascular damage in SSc from "very early" to "very advanced".
2. Immune-pathophysiology of early and progressive microvascular damage in SSc.
3. The validated capillaroscopic nailfold scleroderma patterns ("Early", "Active", "Late") and the assessed very early NVC alterations.
4. The "scleroderma-like" pattern and the transition from "Active" to "Late" scleroderma pattern.
5. Association between the progression of the scleroderma pattern's severity and clinical manifestations.
6. Examples of therapeutical effects on both scleroderma pattern capillaroscopic parameters and associated clinical manifestations in SSc patients.

The Quantitative Analysis of Capillaroscopic Characteristics in the Progression of the Microvascular Damage in SSc from Very Early to Very Advanced

Nailfold videocapillaroscopy has become a prime example of how technology, with the continuous improvement of performance, has enabled to investigation of the capillaroscopic characteristics of the microvascular bed in a very detailed and informative manner [2]. To align interpretation of capillaroscopic images both in daily practice and worldwide research, the EULAR study group on capillaroscopy and microcirculation in rheumatic diseases and the Scleroderma Clinical Trials Consortium (SCTC) experts, published in 2020 a consensus framework to report capillaroscopic characteristics in a standard way [4] (see also chapter "Image Interpretation").

The following capillaroscopic characteristics in pathological conditions should always be reported: density (number of capillaries per linear mm), dimension of dilations (per default measured in the apical limb), number of abnormal shapes per linear mm and presence or absence of microhemorrahages [4] (Figs. 1, 2, 3, 4, 5 and 6). As matter of fact, the evaluations of the Figs. 1, 2, 3, 4, 5, 6 and 7 as well as Figs. 11, 12 and 13 have been done according to the EULAR/SCTC consensus (see text) [4].

Based on a combination of previous capillaroscopic images (Figs. 1-7) a capillaroscopic image can be categorised as a "scleroderma pattern", or a "non-scleroderma pattern" (stereotype normal and non-specific abnormalities [see chapter "Image Interpretation"]). Additionally, follow-up of capillary dimensions may let to detect a pre-SSc-pattern signature in certain Raynaud's phenomenon patients with dilations at first capillaroscopy (see below) [5, 6].

The earliest structural change in SSc on NVC is change in dimension (capillary dilations) that is at the beginning of the disease, the most important morphological parameter to be followed (see below). As a matter of fact, giant capillaries (diameter over 50 μm) are key in the "Early" and "Active" scleroderma patterns with the 200X magnification. In widefield technique the terminology "definite enlargement" had been used to refer to these SSc-specific dilations (see chapter "Image Interpretation"). The further progression of the capillary wall damage in SSc, includes the progression of more and more microvessel dilations over 50 μm (giant capillaries),

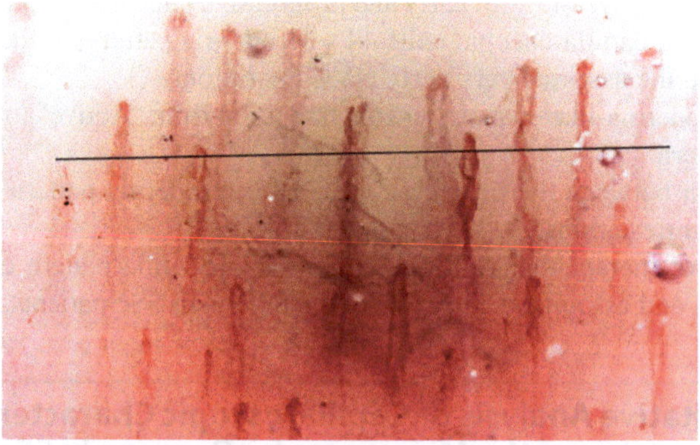

Fig. 1 The "Normal" NVC pattern is characterized by capillaries distributed in a regular manner along the nailfold first row. Report of the capillaroscopic image: density: 11 capillaries per linear mm; morphology: normal (in this case hairpin and crossing); dimension: within normal limits; microhaemorrhages: absent. Normal capillaroscopic findings. To consider that 0.01 mm is equivalent to 10 μm. Bar is 1 linear mm (1000 μm). Magnification 200x

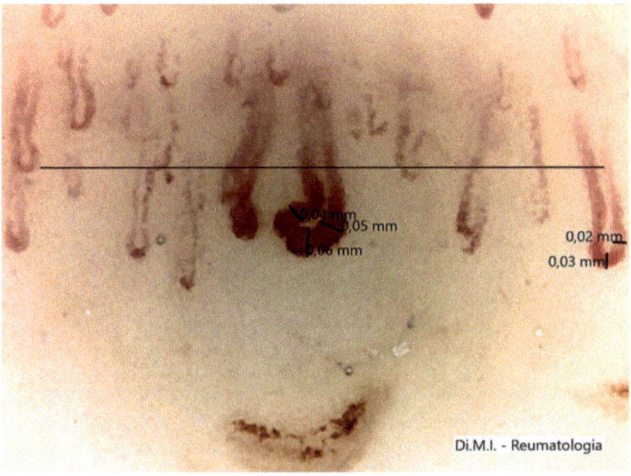

Fig. 2 "Early" NVC SSc pattern. Report of the present capillaroscopic image: density: 8 capillaries per linear mm; morphology: normal hairpin shaped capillaries; dimension: presence of dilatations of 30 μm (labeled as 0.03 mm on the picture) and a giant capillary 60 μm (labeled as 0.06 mm on the picture); microhaemorrhages: present. To consider that 0.01 mm is equivalent to 10 μm. Bar is 1 linear mm. Magnification 200x

followed by the critical disruption of the giant capillary structure and its final collaps and disappearence (Figs. 5 and 6).

The loss of capillaries (lowered density), in more advanced SSc stages, is associated, with an increase of branched and dilated neoangiogenetic new vessels (abnormal shapes) that creates a very altered and brand new microvascular status ("Late" NVC pattern) as originally defined by Cutolo M et al. [2] (Fig. 7).

In the most advanced stages, the predominance of progressive skin fibrosis leads to further loss of capillaries and tissue hypoxia. This manifests as a yellow or white background, also indicative of the "Late" NVC pattern. In very advanced cases, the extent of fibrosis may even obscure the visualization of residual angiogenesis [7].

More than 40 years of literature on capillaroscopy has enriched our knowledge on the role of changes in dimension in SSc. From the earliest studies on capillaroscopic parameters, dimensional changes (dilations) have been attested to discriminate from normal status (Figs. 1 and 2). In this way Maricq first described definite capillary dilations in SSc patients with the widefield technique [8].

Koenig et al. reported in their prospective follow-up study of patients affected by solely the Raynaud's phenomenon, the predictive role of "definitely enlarged", specific capillary dilations (at least four times normal loop dilation) for the development of SSc. Of note, this fundamental work also used the widefield microscopy (magnification of 8X–50X), which is less sensitive than the currently used 200X magnification [9].

In 2000, Cutolo et al. for the first time described the actual used scleroderma patterns (see below) with the 200X magnification technique, with the giant capillary (homogeneously enlarged capillary with apical diameter of at least 50 μm) being central feature to the "Early" scleroderma pattern [2].

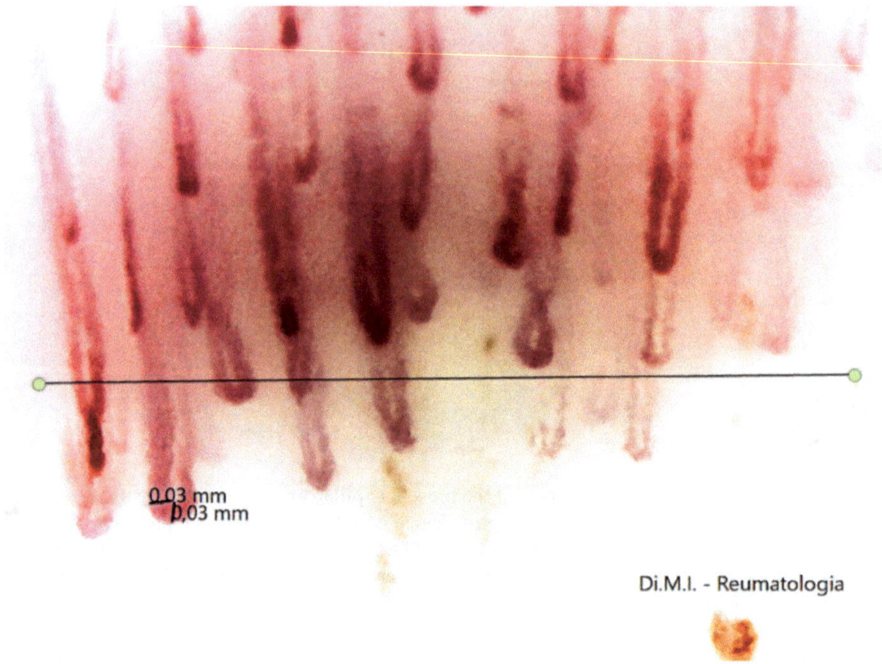

Fig. 3 Non-specific abnormalities. Report of the capillaroscopic image: density: 7 capillaries per linear mm; morphology: normal hairpin shaped capillaries; dimension: presence of dilatations (30 μm); microhaemorrhages: present. Non-specific abnormalities. Bar is 1 linear mm. To consider that 0.01 mm is equivalent to 10 μm. Magnification 200x

More recently, a prognostic index (PRINCE INDEX) was developed, assessing the risk of development of SSc in patients with isolated Raynaud's phenomenon. Giant loops, capillary density and microhemorrhages were used to construct this weighed prognostic index [10] (Fig. 2).

Recently the school of Cutolo studied the meaning of non-specific dilations. In a first retrospective study they attested that NVC capillary average diameter ≤ 30 μm had an independent negative predictive value (NPV) for not developing a scleroderma pattern [5] (Fig. 3). In this way, the evolution from isolated Raynaud's towards 'scleroderma pattern' is unlikely when NVC capillary dilations have a 20–30 μm average diameter. In a subsequent case control study, with a study population selected on having at least one capillary with a dilation of 30 μm, utolo et al. attested that a cut-off of a mean of 1.7 capillary dilations (>30 μm) per linear mm was a predictive variable for 'scleroderma pattern' (positive predictive value [PPV] 75%). This led the authors to state that the presence of frequent capillary dilations in a patient with Raynaud's may be regarded as a 'pre-scleroderma pattern signature' [6].

This retrospective study established for the first time, the PPV/role of non-specific capillary dilations (over 30 μm and under 50 μm dilated capillaries) for the possible 'scleroderma pattern' development (as mentioned above, a cut-off of a

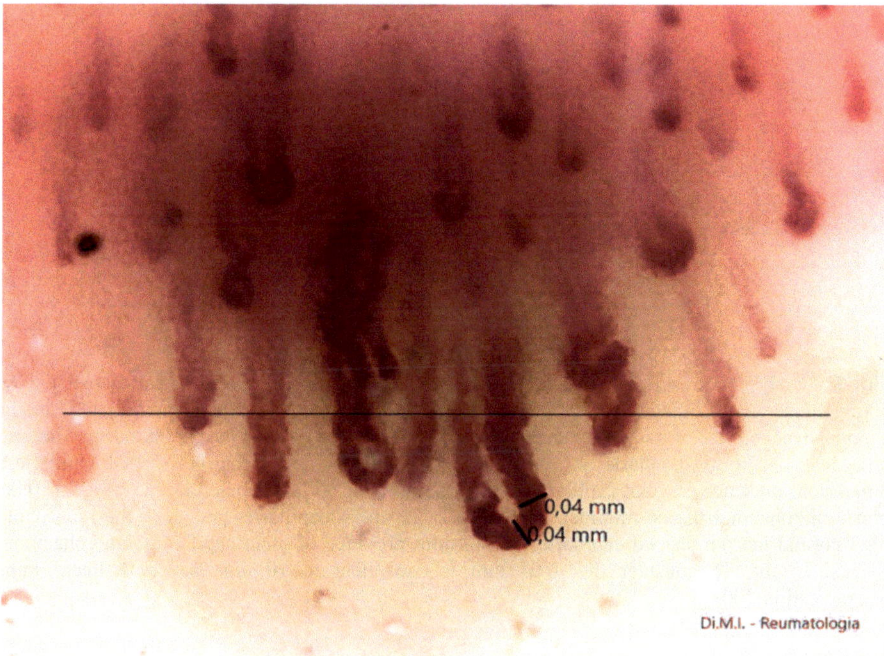

Fig. 4 Pre-scleroderma pattern signature (very early signature under 50 μm, labeled on this image as 0.05 mm) in a NVC image with non-specific findings. This image is an example of non-specific capillary dilations over 0.03 mm (30 μm) but under 0.05 mm (50 μm). This is not yet a giant, it may become over time. When a mean of 2 or more dilations over 0.03 mm (30 μm), but under 0.05 mm (50 μm) are present in 1 linear mm, this condition might be a "Very Early" NVC pattern (pre-scleroderma signature) [5]. Report of the capillaroscopic image: density: 8 capillaries per linear mm; morphology: normal (hairpin shaped capillaries); dimension: presence of dilation (40 μm, labeled on this image as 0.04 mm); microhaemorrhages: absent. The pre-scleroderma signature ("Very Early" pattern) should be followed-up over time. Bar is 1 linear mm. To consider that 0.01 mm is equivalent to 10 μm. Magnification 200x

mean of 1.7 capillary dilations/linear mm, PPV 75%), in a Raynaud's phenomenon population preselected on having dilations over 30 μm already [6] (Fig. 4).

Of course, a pre-scleroderma signature on capillaroscopy is not to be interpreted as having pre-scleroderma, but a biomarker of risk of progression to pre-SSc.

However, indeed, this study might have limitations as every advanced and exploratory investigation. In this way within a retrospective cohort of 273 patients who developed a scleroderma pattern over time (n = 273) it selected only those patients with Raynaud's phenomenon already having an enlarged diameter of 30 μm (only 18 patients form the cohort of 273) at baseline. Therefore and expectedly, this studied population may not be representative for all patients developing in the future a scleroderma pattern.

Accordingly and correctly, also the comparative groups (Raynaud's patients developing other CTDs or no CTDs at all) had also been preselected on having dilated capillary diameter.

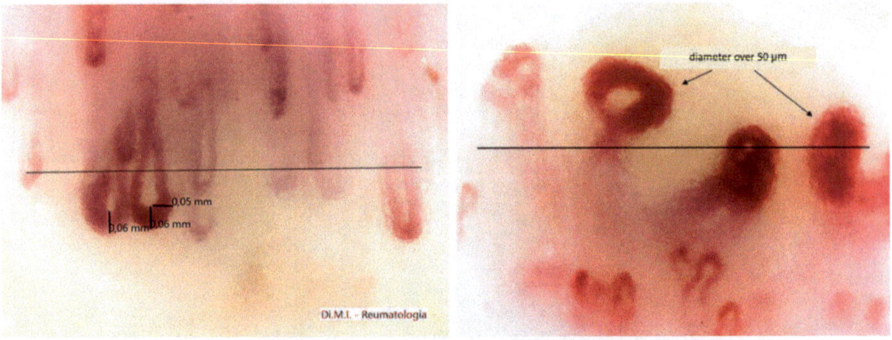

Fig. 5 "Early" NVC scleroderma pattern. Example of giant capillaries (apical diameter over 50μm, labeled in this image as 0.05 mm) in "Early" NVC SSc pattern at the beginning (left) and in a more advanced step of microvascular damage in SSc (right). Report of the capillaroscopic image: left panel: density: 6 capillaries per linear mm; morphology: normal hairpin shaped capillaries; dimension: presence of giant capillaries with a diameter of 60 μm (labeled in this image as 0.06 mm); microhaemorrhages: minimal. Right panel: density: 4 capillaries per linear mm; morphology: normal hairpin shaped capillaries; dimension: presence of giant capillaries; microhaemorrhages: absent. To consider that 0.01 mm is equivalent to 10 μm. Bar is 1 linear mm. Magnification 200x

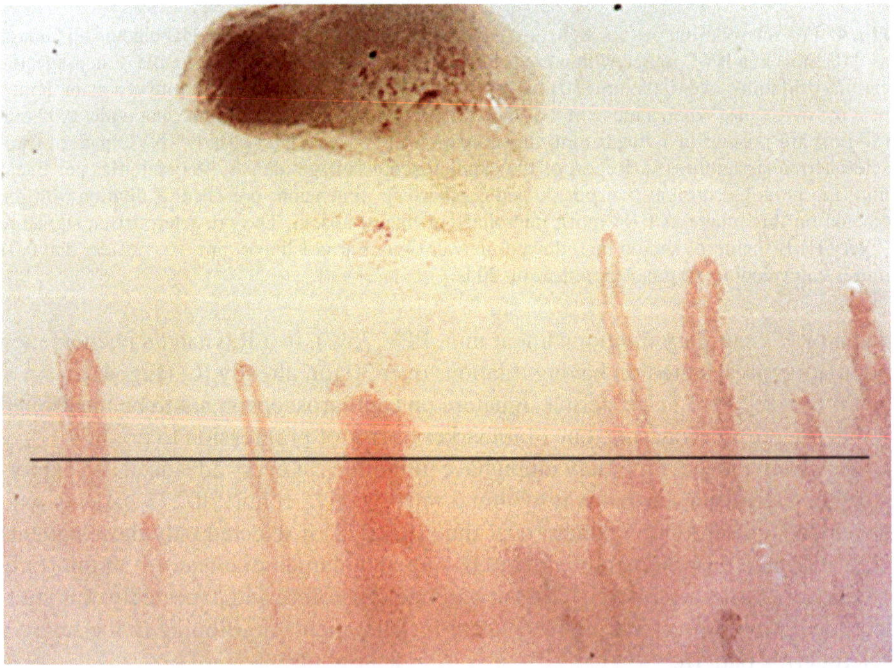

Fig. 6 "Active" scleroderma NVC pattern. Example of a giant capillary collapsing in an "Active" NVC SSc pattern and originating a microhemorrhages. Report of the capillaroscopic image: density: 6 capillaries per linear mm; morphology: normal hairpin shaped capillaries; dimension: a giant capillary; microhaemorrhages: present. To consider that 0.01 mm is equivalent to 10 μm. Bar is 1 linear mm. Magnification 200x.

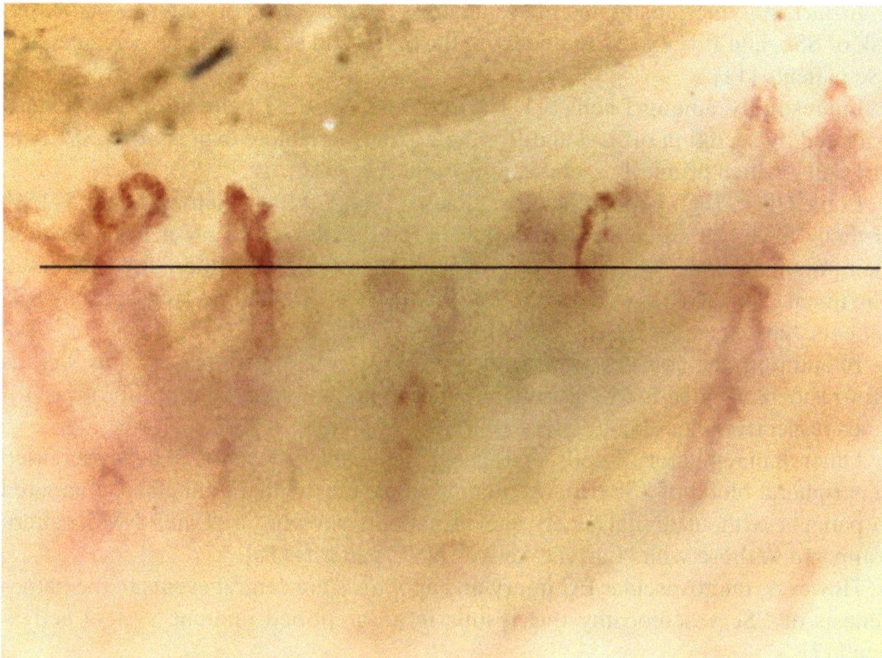

Fig. 7 "Late" scleroderma NVC pattern. Example of "Late" NVC SSc pattern, with presence of neoangiogenesis (abnormal capillary shapes) and intense fibrosis (yellow background). Report of the capillaroscopic image: density: 4 capillaries per linear mm; morphology: presence of an abnormal shape (neoangiogenesis [left part of capillaroscopic image]); dimension: within normal limits; microhaemorrhages: absent. To consider that 0.01 mm is equivalent to 10 µm. Bar is 1 linear mm. Magnification 200x

Actually, as matter of ongoing long-term analysis, large prospective cohorts of unselected Raynaud's phenomenon patients are followed-up prospectively to evaluate if the range 30 µm–50 µm is a discriminatory cut-off indicating a risk of development of SSc or whether it remains a non-specific change of dimension present in patients who will later develop SSc and also other CTDs.

Contrarily, in the prospective cohort of Koenig, evaluating patients with only the Raynaud's phenomenon at baseline "enlargements" were not discriminatory, but as mentioned before that study has the great limitation that was executed by a less sensitive and advanced technique.

Immune-Pathophysiology of Early and Progressive Microvascular Damage in Systemic Sclerosis

In clinical overt SSc the alteration of both innate and adaptive immune responses play a prominent role in the pathophysiology and includes the increased presence and altered functions of inflammatory cells and products in target tissues, such as the skin and lungs, together with a prominent type I interferon (IFN) signature.

In fact, polymorphisms in IFN-regulatory factors seem to confer an increased risk of SSc, and IFN excess is evident in the blood and skin of a large percentage of SSc patients [11].

Interestingly, among T cells ($CD4^+$ T cells), the type 2 T helper (Th2) cells characterized by secretion of IL-4 and IL-13 cytokines, are more expressed in SSc than Th1 cells, which primarily secrete antifibrotic IFNγ [12].

In the $CD4^+$ Tcell population, T regulatory (Treg) cells, which represent 5–15% of them, have started being studied during the last decade in order to understand their possible role in the development of SSc. Therefore, in the literature, decreased functional capacity, as well as the low number of circulating Treg cells in SSc patients, have been described [13, 14].

In addition, the conversion of circulating Treg cells into Th17 cells, as well as skin-resident Treg cells to Th2 cells producing inflammatory and profibrotic cytokines respectively, has been observed in SSc [15].

Other than regulatory T cells angiogenic T cells, have been found to be increased in peripheral blood of SSc patients, mainly in patients with digital ulcers compared to patients without digital ulcers and in patients showing a "Late" NVC pattern compared to those with "Early"/"Active" NVC patterns [16].

However, microvascular EC injury and apoptosis are central events in the pathogenesis of SSc vasculopathy that results in an amplified immune system activation [17].

Of real interest, functional autoantibodies (aAbs) have been observed also in SSc patients and are mainly directed against G protein-coupled receptor (GPCR), tyrosine kinase receptors, or other proteins like matrix metalloproteinases [18].

Those aABs seem mainly in association with both the "Early" and "Active" NVC patterns in SSc.

Of note, aAbs binding the platelet-derived growth factor receptor have been the first functional aAbs described in SSc and have been shown to contribute to the pathogenesis of the disease via activation of fibroblasts and fibroblast-like cells [19].

In addition, aAbs against angiotensin II type 1 receptor (AT1R) and endothelin type A receptor (ETAR) are GPCRs that appear widely expressed on cells of the vascular system and have also been detected in sera of SSc patients [20].

Interestingly, AT1R and ETAR aAbs have been found in nearly all SSc patients and high levels are associated with severe SSc manifestations, such as digital ulcers and pulmonary arterial hypertension (PAH), predicting cardiovascular complications and mortality, especially in SSc-related PAH [21].

Both anti-AT1R and anti-ETAR aAbs act agonistically on their receptors, as demonstrated by the induction of ERK 1/2 phosphorylation and increased transforming growth factor β messenger RNA expression in ECs [20] and act as functional (pathogenetic) autoantibodies.

Finally, anti-endothelial cell aAbs (AECA) have been detected in 25–85% of patients with SSc and were found to be associated with severe microvascular involvement. An increased ability of AECA to adhere to ECs and to induce EC activation, followed by Ab-dependent cell-mediated cytotoxicity and endothelial apoptosis has been demonstrated in several in vitro studies [21].

These effects can be linked to SSc pathogenesis, especially to ECs altered function. The existence of functional aAbs also among the heterogeneous AECA group has been demonstrated; in particular AECA targeting ICAM-1 that have been shown to induce the inflammatory reaction at the level of the ECs [22].

A further important aspect is that the detection and identification of functional aAbs, together their molecular targets, might represent a possible way for specific treatments, especially during the early (very early) steps of SSc, before the overt clinical manifestations of disease progression.

On the other hand, the immune mediated damage of the ECs of microvessels in SSc, creates a bridge between the endothelial apoptosis and the development of dermal fibrosis, through the mechanism represented by the Endothelial-to Mesenchymal cell Transition (EndoMT) process [23, 24].

The EndoMT is a trans-differentiation process by which ECs lose the ability to express their phenotype markers, as well as their morphology, and express mesenchymal cell products, such as α-smooth muscle actin (α-SMA) and collagen type I, acquiring mesenchymal/myofibroblast features and functions [25] (Fig. 8).

The EndoMT process seems to be mediated by vasoconstrictor molecules and growth factors, including ET-1 and transforming growth factor beta (TGFβ), probably as a consequence of the imbalance of vasoactive factors due to the altered function of the endothelium itself [26, 27].

The EndoMT process seems highly responsible for the presence of an abnormal microvascular architecture, which is characterized in SSc patients by capillary loss and mainly by progressive tissue fibrosis (NVC patterns: "Active" and "Late").

An increased interest for innate immunity in SSc is also focused on the role of macrophage activation (M1) at the beginning and in association with the development of microvascular damage [28].

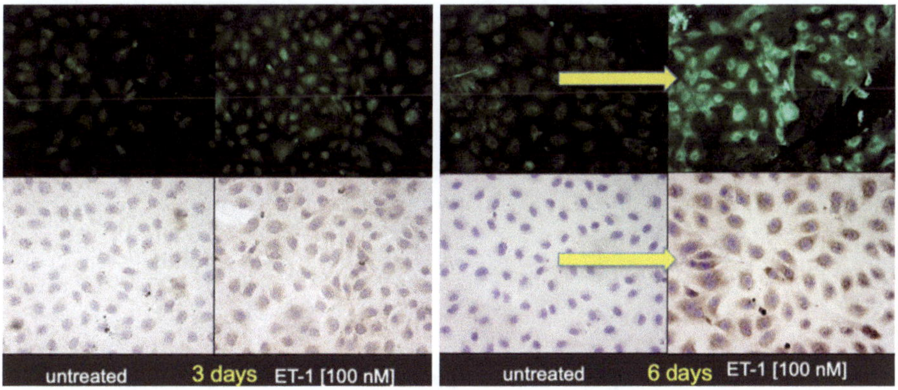

Fig. 8 Fluorescence microscopy images showing cellular response to Endothelin-1 (ET-1) treatment over time. The top row displays fluorescence images, while the bottom row shows corresponding brightfield images Hematoxylin & Eosin stained. The first and third columns represents untreated cells, and the second and fourth columns show the ECs treated with 100 nM ET-1 for 3 and 6 days, respectively. Yellow arrows indicate progression over time

Indeed, M2 macrophages are considered as inducers of tissue fibrosis in SSc especially at the peak of the profibrotic immune response, like what is observed during the tissue wound healing. Therefore, M2 macrophages partially dowregulate the proinflammatory M1 responses (by their polarization and transition in M2) and promote extracellular matrix protein synthesis, including profibrotic cytokine release, as well as potentiate the anti-inflammatory response by enhancing Th2 effector activities [29] (Fig. 9).

Interestingly, ET-1 seems to induce the M2 polarization in cultured human macrophages, from the beginning of the microvascular damage, a process apparently contrasted by the action of the ET-1 receptor antagonism, suggesting possible clinical implications in those fibrotic diseases characterized by increased ET-1 serum concentrations, such as in SSc but also in type 2 diabetes [30].

The increased and sustained release of cytokines, and growth factors, especially from M2 macrophages (M2a, M2c) and Th2, induces in SSc a progressive fibrotic state that involves tissues and organs with concomitant and severe further microvascular damage (capillary loss) [31].

In addition, a recent preliminary study demonstrated significantly higher percentages of circulating hybrid M1/M2 monocytes/macrophages in SSc patients compared to healthy subjects [32].

Importantly, major gene signatures related to hybrid phenotype, activation and migration of macrophages, have been shown to be significant for the progressive pulmonary fibrosis, considering macrophages as key players in SSc lung involvement and interstitial lung disease (ILD) [33, 34].

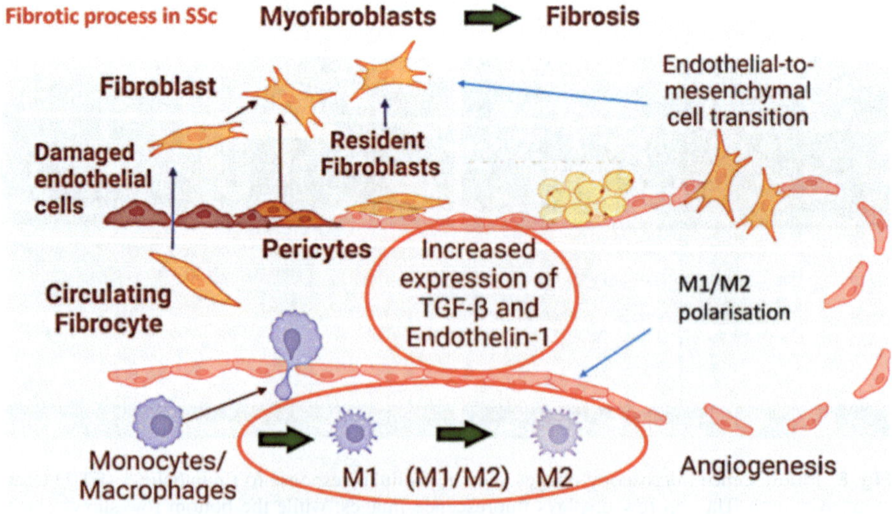

Fig. 9 Flow chart summarizing the fibrotic process in systemic sclerosis (SSc). It shows the transition from damaged endothelial cells to fibroblasts and myofibroblasts, leading to fibrosis. Key elements include also circulating fibrocytes, pericytes, and monocytes/macrophages (transition from M1 to profibrotic M2) and the effects of TGF-β and Endothelin-1

However, classifications based on a wider spectrum of phenotypes of which M1 and M2 subsets would constitute only the two extremes have been reported [35].

The Validated Capillaroscopic Nailfold Scleroderma Patterns ("Early", "Active", "Late") and the Very Early NVC Alterations

As mentioned, in 2000 the first comprehensive classification system for NVC patterns in SSc was published as related to the SSc progression and was categorized as "Early"," Active" and "Late" patterns (at a suggested magnification of 200X) [7].

The "Early" NVC pattern in SSc is characterized by some different level of dilated capillaries (<33%) that must include homogeneously dilated 'giant' capillaries (diameter > 50 μm) and some microhaemorrhages (<33%), whereas the "Active" NVC pattern is characterized by several giant capillaries (>66%), several microhaemorrhages and moderate capillary loss (<33%), finally, the "Late" NVC pattern is characterized by the presence of several irregular non-specific capillary dilations (NOTE: that are not giant capillaries, but represent dilations of the neoangiogenetic branches [abnormal shapes]), severe capillary loss (>66%) with evident avascular areas and ramified or bushy capillaries indicative of angiogenesis (abnormal shapes) [3, 36] (Fig. 10).

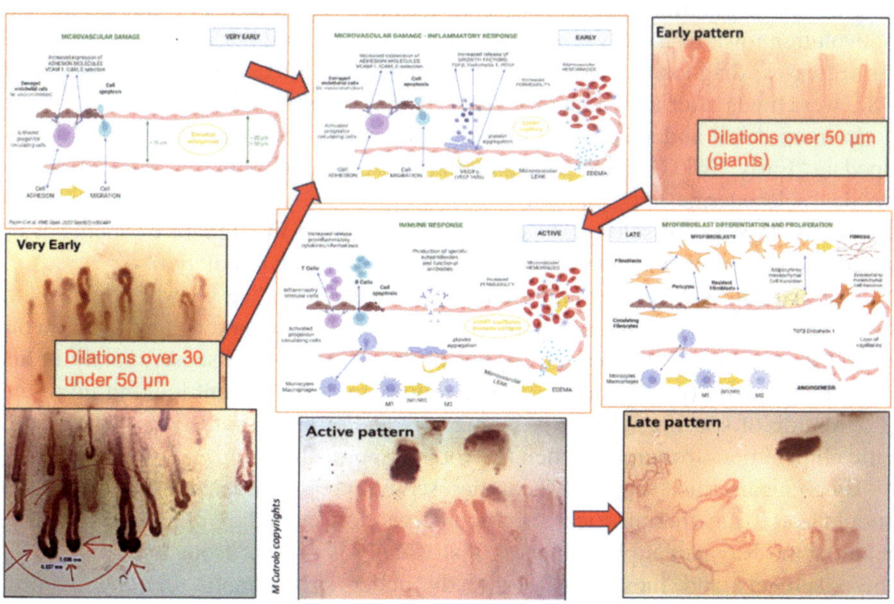

Fig. 10 Flow chart summarizing the progression of microvascular damage and inflammatory response in SSc tissues. The chart is divided into stages: "Very Early," "Early," "Active," and "Late." Each stage includes diagrams and text boxes explaining the progression of the process. Arrows connect stages, showing progression from microvascular damage to immune response and tissue changes with progressed fibrosis

Following the publication by the EULAR Study Group on Capillaroscopy and Microcirculation and concerning the classification system of microvascular status in CTDs, the terminology for reporting NVC findings in autoimmune rheumatic diseases was clearly re-defined and a scoring system for microvascular changes was also re-introduced [37].

As mentioned before, and more recently, an investigation described for the first time, in a Raynaud's phenomenon population selected on presence of capillary dilations (>30 μm) on capillaroscopy at baseline visit, the PPV for non-specific capillary dilations (over 30 μm and under 50 μm) as "pre-scleroderma" pattern signature ("Very Early" NVC pattern/biomarker) for the possible further "Early" scleroderma NVC pattern development. Such images, seem to intercept the SSc microvascular damage at a very early and totally preclinical stage, but including of course the presence of the Raynaud's phenomenon, as hallmark to suspect an incoming CTD [5].

This investigation has shown the progressive homogeneous capillary dilation (at the beginning >30 μm and under 50 μm dilations), involving all the capillary branches, which is at first, more evident at the apical capillary limb, then involves both the arterial and venous branches up to the classical giant capillary shape. More specifically in patients with a cut-off of a mean of 1.7 capillary dilations (>30 μm) per linear mm, a median transition time of 13 months was needed to convert to an "Early" scleroderma pattern (previous pages text). Of note, only giants, when finally full diameter is over 50 μm, are specific for SSc [5].

Specifically, at the stepwise logistic regression analysis, for each increase in a single over 30 μm dilated capillary per linear mm, there was a 24% additional risk of evolution towards the NVC scleroderma pattern (OR 1.24, 95% CI 1.17 to 1.32). As for cases, diagnosis of both "Early" scleroderma NVC pattern and associated SSc, were made after a median of 4 years (IQR 2–8) from RP onset [5].

In more detail and specifically, 78% of Raynaud's phenomenon patients developed an "Early" NVC scleroderma pattern (only one was "Active") and 22% developed a "scleroderma-like" pattern.

At this stage a "pre-scleroderma" (or "Very Early") NVC signature is being evaluated in a prospective unselected Raynaud's phenomenon population.

It is mandatory at this point, to underline that the term "very early SSc" should be accomplished with just in presence of "very early biomarkers", since in medicine, the concept of "very early" applies to the suspect of a disease, mainly in his pre-clinical phase (pre-disease). A close follow-up of the patient looking up to the progression of specific very early biomarkers and/or at the detection of early specific clinical manifestations is then the correct approach.

By no means this "very early" capillaroscopic (pre-scleroderma) NVC signature should lead to any therapeutical specific intervention, excluding of course, the treatment of the Raynaud's phenomenon, that usually is present from long time in all these subjects and mostly, it is already under symptomatic therapy. A pre-scleroderma signature on NVC is not to be interpreted as having pre-scleroderma diagnosis, but a condition of NVC biomarker risk of progression.

Definite predictive factors for SSc in a patient with Raynaud's are the specific SSc NVC pattern and SSc auto-antibodies.

Puffy fingers (considered red flags) in itself are not frequent (16% in the VEDOSS validation study and also a red but clinical diagnostic criterium for other CTDs such as mixed connective tissue disease [MCTD]) (see chapter "Image Interpretation") [38–40].

The Differences Between the "Scleroderma-like" Pattern and the Transition from "Active" to "Late" Scleroderma Pattern

The importance of endothelial injury, perivascular immune and inflammatory reaction, together with capillary loss, mirrored at NVC by several associated and progressive abnormal morphological findings, is common in patients with CTDs [41, 42].

A complex severe microangiopathy is often present from baseline in patients with dermatomyositis (DM) labeled as "scleroderma-like" NVC pattern. The "scleroderma-like" pattern is defined as a capillary pattern showing mixed microvascular markers of the different scleroderma NVC patterns, but not fully fitting the definition for the single "Early", "Active" or "Late" scleroderma pattern. In this regard all NVC characteristics observed in SSc, including giant capillaries, some microhaemorrhages, severe capillary loss and neoangiogenesis (abnormal shapes) may occur simultaneously in the "scleroderma-like" pattern [43] (Fig. 12).

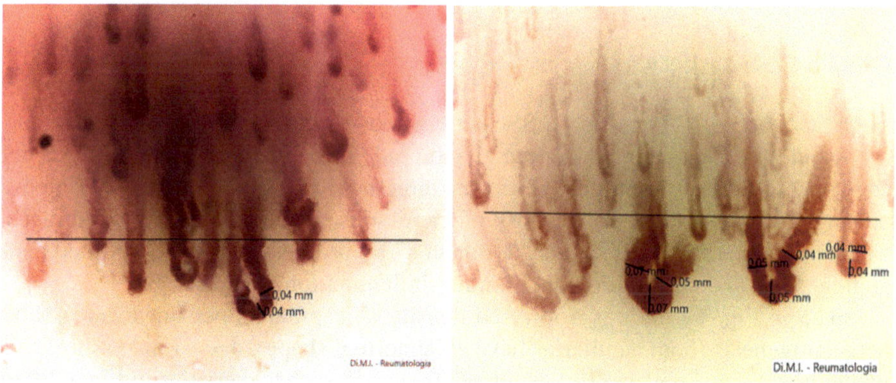

Fig. 11 Pre-scleroderma pattern NVC signature versus "Early" scleroderma pattern. Left panel: example of a pre-scleroderma NVC signature ("Very Early" pattern, see text for explanations) showing capillary dilations of 40 μm (labeled in this figure as 0.04 mm). Density: left: 8 capillaries per linear mm. In the "Early" NVC SSc pattern (right panel), dilations of 50 μm (giant capillaries) together with 40 μm dilations co-exists. Density: left: 8 capillaries per linear mm. The transition from non-specific dilations (under 50 μm) up to giant capillaries (over 50 μm) is progressive. Final report of the capillaroscopic images: Left panel: morphology: presence of normal shapes (all hairpin shapes) and dilations; dimension: dilations; microhaemorrhages: absent. Non-specific abnormalities of dimension. To be followed-up. Right panel: morphology: presence of normal shapes (all hairpin shapes); dimension: dilations and giant capillaries present; microhaemorrhages: absent. To consider that 0.01 mm is equivalent to 10 μm. Bar is 1 linear mm. Magnification 200x

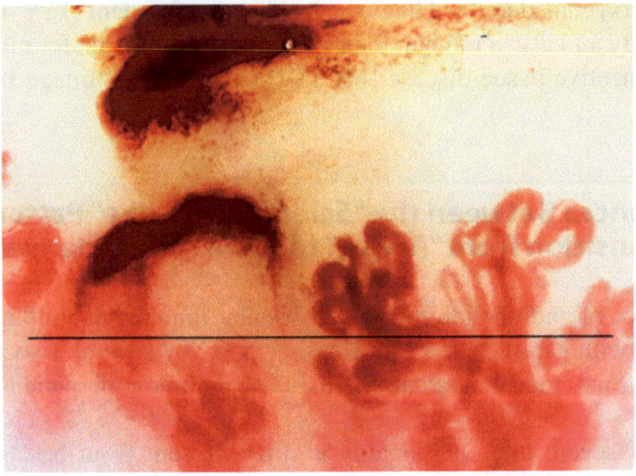

Fig. 12 A "scleroderma-like" pattern". The "scleroderma-like" pattern is defined as a NVC pattern showing mixed microvascular morphological biomarkers of the different SSc scleroderma NVC patterns, but not fully fitting the definition for the single "Early", "Active" or "Late" scleroderma pattern. Report of the capillaroscopic image: density: 2 capillaries per linear mm; dimension: dilations present; morphology: 2 abnormal shapes (neoangiogenesis); microhaemorrhages: present. Since microhaemorrhages are not expected in the classical images of the "Late" scleroderma pattern, we call this a "scleroderma like" NVC pattern. To consider that 0.01 mm is equivalent to 10 μm. Bar is 1 linear mm. Magnification 200x

In fact, the full "Active" NVC SSc pattern shows giant capillaries, microhaemorrages and loss of capillaries. Conversely, the full "Late" NVC SSc pattern, does not show any more giants, but only severe asymmetrical notable dilations, with intense neoangiogenesis and of course loss of capillaries, but never microhaemorrages, since the field at this final step is "dominated" by progressive fibrosis, limited neoangiogenesis and no further local immuno-inflammation.

Since in Fig. 12 there is a lowered density (2 capillaries per linear mm), with neoangiogenesis (both capillaries have an abnormal shape), one would assume this would be a "Late" pattern. But, as there are also SSc characteristics in Fig. 12 that do not fit in the "Late" SSc NVC pattern, but meet criteria for the "Active" pattern (more specifically microhaemorrhages) we call this a "scleroderma like" NVC pattern.

Of course, the clinical and laboratory findings in DM (showing the "scleroderma-like" NVC pattern), will help to indicate the correct diagnosis.

However, it is possible in SSc, that the transition from "Active" to "Late" NVC pattern shows images with also a limited angiogenesis (abnormal shapes), but always in presence of very few giant capillaries (before to become a true "Late" SSc pattern), microhaemorrhages and collaps of the dilated giant capillaries (Fig. 13).

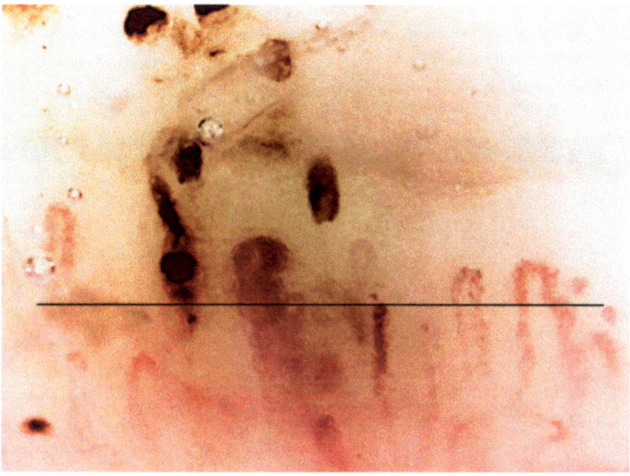

Fig. 13 Advanced "Active" SSc NVC pattern. The picture shows limited angiogenesis (abnormal shapes) that may characterize the incoming "Late" SSc NVC pattern in a SSc patient already showing and "Active" pattern. Presence of giants, microhaemorrages, still some normal capillaries. The number of capillaries is 6 per linear mm. To consider that 0.01 mm is equivalent to 10 μm. Bar is 1 linear mm. Magnification 200x

Also in CTD overlap syndromes, "scleroderma-like" as well as other scleroderma patterns may occur.

In a study of patients with auto-immune rheumatic diseases in which half of patients were affected by the Raynaud's phenomenon, a clear NVC "scleroderma-like" pattern was identified, from the beginning, in 18.3% of patients with undifferentiated connective tissue diseases (UCTD) and 26.9% of patients with DM [42].

In a recnt study 70% of patients with MCTD showed a "scleroderma-like pattern" at first NVC. No statistically significant variation of the observed NVC parameters was detected during the 3-year follow-up, and no statistically significant correlation was observed between capillary parameters and MCTD clinical findings at first visit and during the follow-up [42].

In fact, in patients with UCTD, MCTD or DM, the "scleroderma-like" pattern may occur, as well as the "Early", "Active" and "Late" scleroderma NVC patterns, but we need long term and large cohort follow-up studies to define the prevalence and evolution of certain patterns in those diseases. As mentioned, a small long-term study of ten patients with MCTD suggested that nailfold microvascular damage does not seem to progress during 3 years of follow-up [42].

Of note, the identification of the "scleroderma-like" pattern in MCTD, can support for a differential diagnosis from other auto-immune rheumatic diseases in all of the above mentioned pathological conditions.

Clinical Manifestations of Systemic Sclerosis Are Associated with the Progression of the Scleroderma Patterns Severity

Several clinical studies over the years have shown how, at least the most common clinical manifestations of SSc are associated with the progression of the SSc NVC patterns severity with associated tissue and organ damage (Fig. 14).

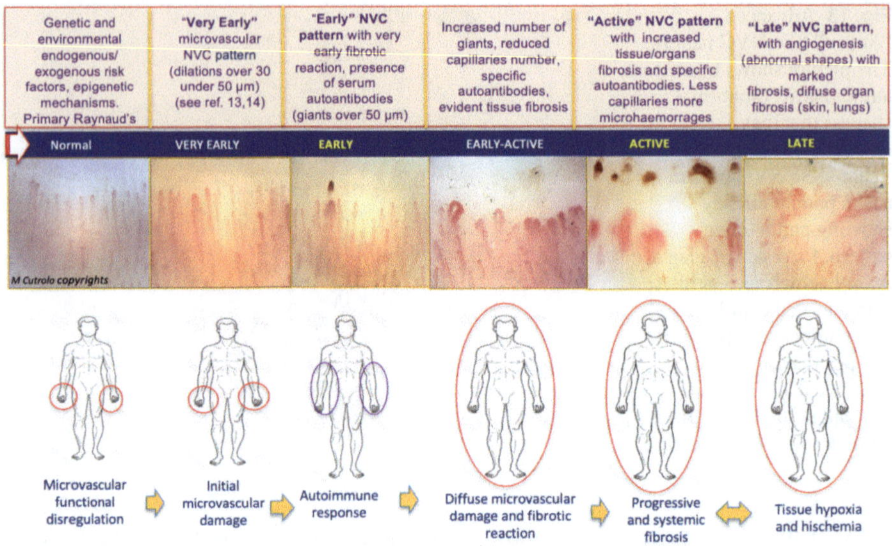

Fig. 14 Diagram illustrating the association between NVC patterns and clinical manifestations of SSc, including the pathophysiological steps (top row). Several clinical studies over the years (up to 12 years) have shown how, at least the most common, clinical manifestations of SSc are linked with the progression of the SSc patterns severity (see central bar with NVC images) and associated tissue with progressive involvement and organ damage (bottom row) [44]

Recently, a comprehensive observational longitudinal NVC study, analysed over a twelve-year follow-up the progression of nailfold microvascular damage in a cohort of SSc patients showing the "Early" NVC pattern at baseline and collecting all data in a therapeutic care setting [44].

The results of this large study showed a transition of NVC pattern from the "Early" to either the "Active" or "Late" pattern in 64% of SSc patients. Interestingly, the "Early" pattern did not change in 24% of SSc patients over 12 years of observations and even reversed to normal (showing only non-specific capillary abnormalities) in 4 patients (12%).

In 2012, a previous study had already demonstrated the progression from the "Early" to either the "Active" or "Late" NVC pattern in 47% of SSc patients after a 5-year follow-up [45].

However, by extending the observation regarding the NVC pattern progression at the 12-years study, a larger number of SSc patients were found to progress from the "Early" to a further NVC pattern ("Active" 26%, "Late" 38%), suggesting that despite treatment, the disease and at least the microvascular damage, still progresses over long time.

The time of progression to a next pattern of nailfold microangiopathy was found to be 24 months from the "Early" to the "Active" NVC pattern and 59 months from the "Active" to the "Late" pattern. However, by considering only the cohort of patients who progressed to the "Late" pattern, their time of progression from an "Early" to the "Active" NVC pattern was found to be only 11 months [45].

This observation is of great interest, since the SSc patients that during the follow-up showed a fast progression (<1 year) from the "Early" to the "Active" NVC pattern might be at higher risk to quickly progress to the most advanced "Late" NVC pattern [44, 45].

Of note and in parallel, the clinical severity of the disease appeared to increase at the highest level in presence of the "Late" NVC pattern. As a matter of fact, higher loss of capillaries is correlated to the increased tissue fibrosis, several studies have clearly demonstrated also the higher prevalence of internal organ involvement [46–48].

Finally, by considering skin involvement, the prevalence of the "Active" NVC SSc pattern was found to be higher in limited cutaneous SSc patients, while 75% of patients with diffuse cutaneous SSc progressed more frequently to the "Late" pattern [44].

In addition, the single NVC pattern at baseline, may be of great value to predict novel future SSc organ involvement, as recently demonstrated, suggesting capillaroscopy to be a biomarker for disease progression [49–52].

Examples of Therapeutical Effects on Scleroderma Patterns Parameters and Associated Clinical Manifestations in Systemic Sclerosis Patients

It is well described that NVC parameters have been used to evaluate responses to treatment in patients with SSc. In the last 10 years, several investigations have monitorized the follow-up of the disease by NVC, looking at the effects of vasodilators, immunosuppressive drugs and also the antifibrotic tyrosine kinase inhibitor (nintedanib) on microvascular status.

One of the earliest studies showed that the long-term treatment of patients with SSc with an ET-1 receptor antagonist (bosentan) in combination with the vasodilator drug iloprost, reduced the progression of NVC damage over a 3-years follow-up period [53].

A further study evaluated the long-term effects of ET-1 antagonism on both capillary morphology (evaluated by NVC) and peripheral blood perfusion (evaluated by laser doppler flowmetry [LDF]) in patients with SSc [54].

The results showed, as effect of treatment, and by using concomitant morphological and functional microvascular analysis, an increase in capillary number, as well as increased fingertip blood perfusion in the SSc patients [54].

Similar results for NVC qualitative analysis (scleroderma patterns) were observed in a study of patients with SSc, who were treated with bosentan and the phosphodiesterase inhibitor sildenafil, in which the progression to the advanced NVC scleroderma patterns ("Active" and "Late") was found reduced after 6 months of treatment [55].

A further study quantified in patients with SSc, the absolute nailfold capillary number per linear mm on NVC images and detected fingertip blood flow by LDF during long-term therapy with bosentan and iloprost [56]. In this study, patients with SSc who had received >4 years of combined therapy (bosentan and iloprost) showed a progressive recovery in both microvascular morphology and function, as well as improved clinical outcomes, independent of disease severity, suggesting that the combined analysis (morphological and functional) might increase the precision of evaluation of the treatment's effect.

To be considered, how a contribution exerted by the above drugs (bosentan or macitentan) on to improved NVC status in SSc, may be also explained by the inhibitory effects induced by the same drugs on cultures of human microvascular EC by downregulating the EndoMT [57].

A very seminal and interestingly pilot study evaluating the links between immunomodulation and microvascular damage in SSc patients, that has also used NVC evaluation, showed the improving effects of treatment courses of the immunosuppressive drug rituximab, in patients with early diffuse cutaneous SSc who were receiving stable background therapy with methotrexate [58]. In particular, the study showed at NVC analysis, that rituximab was able to stabilize and reduce the progression of microvascular damage over 12 months, particularly the loss of capillaries.

More recently, a prospective study cohort evaluated capillary density (measured over 3 x linear mm) in 80 newly diagnosed SSc patients who, in a retrospective review, had at least two NVC tests. As result, mycophenolate mofetil treatment was associated with a significant lower number of fingers that had worsened in terms of capillary density from baseline [59].

Finally, and very interestingly, a recent investigation involved 120 SSc patients, as NVC sub-study of the SENSCIS trial (safety and efficacy of nintedanib in SSc associated ILD) and 68 of them had risk factors for rapid FVC decline at baseline, whereas 24 had ILD progression over 52 weeks [60]. Among 35 patients with risk factors for rapid FVC decline who had NVC data at baseline, mean (SD) capillary density at baseline was 5.2 (1.9) capillaries per linear mm.

A numerical reduction in mean capillary density over 52 weeks, was observed only in patients with risk factors for rapid FVC decline at baseline who received placebo, but not in those who received nintedanib. In the subgroup with ILD progression, a numerical stabilization in mean capillary density was seen in the placebo group and a numerical augmentation in the nintedanib group. Therefore, the antifibrotic treatment at least in SSc-ILD, might be over the time evaluated in indirectly manner also by NVC.

In conclusion and overall, imaging of the microcirculation (in particular by NVC) especially in SSc, like the last studies comparing limited with diffuse cutaneous SSc, offers an important non-invasive and safe complementary tool in diagnosing and monitoring the progression and organ involvement in SSc, as well as in other CTDs. Increased availability of imaging technologies will enable larger intercentre investigations to be carried out [61–63].

Research Agenda

- Longterm prospective follow-up with 200X magnification technique in an unselected Raynaud's phenomenon cohort with solely Raynaud's phenomenon at baseline to describe with EULAR/SCTC consensus capillaroscopic characteristics over time in those who develop SSc and those who do not.
- Other CTDs (ie. Systemic Lupus Erythematosus or Psoriatic arthritis) must be evaluated with the standardised reporting and validated nomenclature presented at the yearly EULAR eLearning and on site courses, as well as EULAR/SCTC Study Groups in large prospective cohorts.
- A carefull observation with standardised evaluation of the NVC characteristics according to the EULAR/SCTC consensus, should be applied to all the SSc patients who are currently being monitored and treated, since this offers important information about the progression of the microvascular damage and in turn of the organ/tissue damage (i.e. ILD severity).

Acknowledgements Our gratitude goes to Drs. Carmen Pizzorni, Sabrina Paolino, Emanuele Gotelli, Alberto Sulli, Elvis Hysa, Rosanna Campitiello, Tamara Vojinovic, Elisa Alessandria, Stefano Soldano, Giulia Bernard, and several other postgraduate fellows for providing NVC images analysed and commented as contributors of the EULAR study group on Capillaroscopy and microcirculation in rheumatic diseases (Chair Vanessa Smith). Maurizio Cutolo, as chairman of the "Capillaroscopy and Microcirculation in RMD Study Group" (CAPSIR) of the Italian Society of Rheumatology and he thanks the national board for the continous support. Vanessa Smith is Chair of the EULAR study group on Capillaroscopy and Microcircaulation in Rheumatic Diseases. Our gratitude equally goes to Melissa De Decker for the editing of this manuscript.

References

1. Volkmann ER, Andreasson K, V. Systemic sclerosis. Lancet. 2023;401(10373):304–18.
2. Cutolo M, Smith V. Detection of microvascular changes in systemic sclerosis and other rheumatic diseases. Nat Rev Rheumatol. 2021;17(11):665–77.
3. Cutolo M, Sulli A, Pizzorni C, Accardo S. Nailfold videocapillaroscopy assessment of microvascular damage in systemic sclerosis. J Rheumatol. 2000;27(1):155–60.
4. Smith V, Herrick AL, Ingegnoli F, Damjanov N, De Angelis R, Denton CP, et al. Standardisation of nailfold capillaroscopy for the assessment of patients with Raynaud's phenomenon and systemic sclerosis. Autoimmun Rev. 2020;19(3):102458.
5. Trombetta AC, Smith V, Pizzorni C, Meroni M, Paolino S, Cariti C, et al. Quantitative alterations of capillary diameter have a predictive value for development of the Capillaroscopic systemic sclerosis pattern. J Rheumatol. 2016;43(3):599–606.
6. Pacini G, Pogna A, Pendolino M, Pizzorni C, Carmisciano L, Gotelli E, et al. Understanding the value of non-specific abnormal capillary dilations in presence of Raynaud's phenomenon: a detailed capillaroscopic analysis. RMD Open. 2022;8(2):e002449.
7. Cutolo M, Soldano S, Smith V. Pathophysiology of systemic sclerosis: current understanding and new insights. Expert Rev Clin Immunol. 2019;15(7):753–64.
8. Maricq HR. Wide-field capillary microscopy: technique and rating scale for abnormalities seen in scleroderma and related disorders. Arthritis Rheum. 1981;24(9):1159–65.
9. Koenig M, Joyal F, Fritzler MJ, Roussin A, Abrahamowicz M, Boire G, et al. Autoantibodies and microvascular damage are independent predictive factors for the progression of Raynaud's

phenomenon to systemic sclerosis: a twenty-year prospective study of 586 patients, with validation of proposed criteria for early systemic sclerosis. Arthritis Rheum. 2008;58(12):3902–12.
10. Ingegnoli F, Boracchi P, Gualtierotti R, Lubatti C, Meani L, Zahalkova L, et al. Prognostic model based on nailfold capillaroscopy for identifying Raynaud's phenomenon patients at high risk for the development of a scleroderma spectrum disorder. Arthritis Rheum. 2008;58(7):2174–82.
11. Skaug B, Assassi S. Type I interferon dysregulation in systemic sclerosis. Cytokine. 2020;132:154635.
12. Boin F, De Fanis U, Bartlett SJ, Wigley FM, Rosen A, Casolaro V. T cell polarization identifies distinct clinical phenotypes in scleroderma lung disease. Arthritis Rheum. 2008;58(4):1165–74.
13. Slobodin G, Rimar D. Regulatory T cells in systemic sclerosis: a comprehensive review. Clin Rev Allergy Immunol. 2017;52(2):194–201.
14. Chizzolini C, Boin F. The role of the acquired immune response in systemic sclerosis. Semin Immunopathol. 2015;37(5):519–28.
15. MacDonald KG, Dawson NAJ, Huang Q, Dunne JV, Levings MK, Broady R. Regulatory T cells produce profibrotic cytokines in the skin of patients with systemic sclerosis. J Allergy Clin Immunol. 2015;135(4):946. e9
16. Manetti M, Pratesi S, Romano E, Bellando-Randone S, Rosa I, Guiducci S, et al. Angiogenic T cell expansion correlates with severity of peripheral vascular damage in systemic sclerosis. PLoS One. 2017;12(8):e0183102.
17. Arends SJ, Damoiseaux JGMC, Duijvestijn AM, Debrus-Palmans L, Vroomen M, Boomars KA, et al. Immunoglobulin G anti-endothelial cell antibodies: inducers of endothelial cell apoptosis in pulmonary arterial hypertension? Clin Exp Immunol. 2013;174(3):433–40.
18. Cabral-Marques O, Riemekasten G. Functional autoantibodies targeting G protein-coupled receptors in rheumatic diseases. Nat Rev Rheumatol. 2017;13(11):648–56.
19. Dragun D, Distler JHW, Riemekasten G, Distler O. Stimulatory autoantibodies to platelet-derived growth factor receptors in systemic sclerosis: what functional autoimmunity could learn from receptor biology. Arthritis Rheum. 2009;60(4):907–11.
20. Riemekasten G, Philippe A, Nather M, Slowinski T, Muller DN, Heidecke H, et al. Involvement of functional autoantibodies against vascular receptors in systemic sclerosis. Ann Rheum Dis. 2011;70(3):530–6.
21. Carvalho D, Savage CO, Black CM, Pearson JD. IgG antiendothelial cell autoantibodies from scleroderma patients induce leukocyte adhesion to human vascular endothelial cells in vitro. Induction of adhesion molecule expression and involvement of endothelium-derived cytokines. J Clin Invest. 1996;97(1):111–9.
22. Wolf SI, Howat S, Abraham DJ, Pearson JD, Lawson C. Agonistic anti-ICAM-1 antibodies in scleroderma: activation of endothelial pro-inflammatory cascades. Vasc Pharmacol. 2013;59(1–2):19–26.
23. Soldano S, Montagna P, Brizzolara R, Ferrone C, Parodio A, Sulli A, et al. Endothelin receptor antagonists: effects on extracellular matrix synthesis in primary cultures of skin fibroblasts from systemic sclerosis patients. Reumatismo. 2012;64(5):326–34.
24. Piera-Velazquez S, Jimenez SA. Endothelial to mesenchymal transition: role in physiology and in the pathogenesis of human diseases. Physiol Rev. 2019;99(2):1281–324.
25. Piera-Velazquez S, Mendoza FA, Jimenez SA. Endothelial to mesenchymal transition (EndoMT) in the pathogenesis of human fibrotic diseases. J Clin Med. 2016;5(4):45.
26. Cipriani P, Di Benedetto P, Ruscitti P, Campese AF, Liakouli V, Carubbi F, et al. Impaired endothelium-mesenchymal stem cells cross-talk in systemic sclerosis: a link between vascular and fibrotic features. Arthritis Res Ther. 2014;16(5):442.
27. Soldano S, Paolino S, Pizzorni C, Trombetta AC, Montagna P, Brizzolara R, et al. Dual endothelin receptor antagonists contrast the effects induced by endothelin-1 on cultured human microvascular endothelial cells. Clin Exp Rheumatol. 2017;35(3):484–93.
28. Campitiello R, Soldano S, Gotelli E, Hysa E, Montagna P, Casabella A, et al. The intervention of macrophages in progressive fibrosis characterizing systemic sclerosis: a systematic review. Autoimmun Rev. 2024;23(10):103637.

29. Cutolo M, Campitiello R, Gotelli E, Soldano S. The role of M1/M2 macrophage polarization in rheumatoid arthritis synovitis. Front Immunol. 2022;13:867260.
30. Soldano S, Pizzorni C, Paolino S, Trombetta AC, Montagna P, Brizzolara R, et al. Alternatively activated (M2) macrophage phenotype is inducible by Endothelin-1 in cultured human macrophages. PLoS One. 2016;11(11):e0175238.
31. Christmann RB, Lafyatis R. The cytokine language of monocytes and macrophages in systemic sclerosis. Arthritis Res Ther. 2010;12(5):146–52.
32. Soldano S, Trombetta AC, Contini P, Tomatis V, Ruaro B, Brizzolara R, et al. Increase in circulating cells coexpressing M1 and M2 macrophage surface markers in patients with systemic sclerosis. Ann Rheum Dis. 2018;77(12):1842–5.
33. Gotelli E, Soldano S, Feghali-Bostwick C, Montagna P, Campitiello R, Contini P, et al. Prevalence of hybrid TLR4(+)M2 monocytes/macrophages in peripheral blood and lung of systemic sclerosis patients with interstitial lung disease. Front Immunol. 2024;15:1488867.
34. Trombetta AC, Soldano S, Contini P, Tomatis V, Ruaro B, Paolino S, et al. A circulating cell population showing both M1 and M2 monocyte/macrophage surface markers characterizes systemic sclerosis patients with lung involvement. Respir Res. 2018;19(1):186.
35. Cutolo M, Soldano S, Smith V, Gotelli E, Hysa E. Dynamic macrophage phenotypes in autoimmune and inflammatory rheumatic diseases. Nat Rev Rheumatol. 2025;21(9):546–565. https://doi.org/10.1038/s41584-025-01279-w. Epub 2025 Jul 28.
36. Cutolo M, Trombetta AC, Melsens K, Pizzorni C, Sulli A, Ruaro B, et al. Automated assessment of absolute nailfold capillary number on videocapillaroscopic images: proof of principle and validation in systemic sclerosis. Microcirculation. 2018;25(4):e12447.
37. Cutolo M, Paolino S, Smith V. Nailfold capillaroscopy in rheumatology: ready for the daily use but with care in terminology. Clin Rheumatol. 2019;38(9):2293–7.
38. Bellando-Randone S, Del Galdo F, Lepri G, Minier T, Huscher D, Furst DE, et al. Progression of patients with Raynaud's phenomenon to systemic sclerosis: a five-year analysis of the European scleroderma trial and research group multicentre, longitudinal registry study for very early diagnosis of systemic sclerosis (VEDOSS). Lancet Rheumatol. 2021;3(12):e834–43.
39. Tanaka Y, Kuwana M, Fujii T, Kameda H, Muro Y, Fujio K, et al. 2019 diagnostic criteria for mixed connective tissue disease (MCTD): from the Japan research committee of the ministry of health, labor, and welfare for systemic autoimmune diseases. Mod Rheumatol. 2021;31(1):29–33.
40. Avouac J, Fransen J, Walker UA, Riccieri V, Smith V, Muller C, et al. Preliminary criteria for the very early diagnosis of systemic sclerosis: results of a Delphi consensus study from EULAR scleroderma trials and research group. Ann Rheum Dis. 2011;70(3):476–81.
41. Pizzorni C, Ferrari G, Schenone C, Hysa E, Carmisciano L, Gotelli E, et al. Capillaroscopic analysis of the microvascular status in mixed versus undifferentiated connective tissue disease. Microvasc Res. 2022;142:104367.
42. Paolino S, Ferrari G, Pizzorni C, Patane M, Smith V, Cutolo M, et al. Long-term follow-up of nailfold videocapillaroscopic microvascular parameters in mixed connective tissue disease versus systemic sclerosis patients: a retrospective cohort study. Clin Exp Rheumatol. 2019;37(Suppl 119):102–7.
43. Smith V, Pizzorni C, De Keyser F, Decuman S, Van Praet JT, Deschepper E, et al. Reliability of the qualitative and semiquantitative nailfold videocapillaroscopy assessment in a systemic sclerosis cohort: a two-Centre study. Ann Rheum Dis. 2010;69(6):1092–6.
44. Sulli A, Paolino S, Pizzorni C, Ferrari G, Pacini G, Pesce G, et al. Progression of nailfold capillaroscopic patterns and correlation with organ involvement in systemic sclerosis: a 12 year study. Rheumatology (Oxford). 2020;59(5):1051–8.
45. Sulli A, Pizzorni C, Smith V, Zampogna G, Ravera F, Cutolo M. Timing of transition between capillaroscopic patterns in systemic sclerosis. Arthritis Rheum. 2012;64(3):821–5.
46. Caramaschi P, Canestrini S, Martinelli N, Volpe A, Pieropan S, Ferrari M, et al. Scleroderma patients nailfold videocapillaroscopic patterns are associated with disease subset and disease severity. Rheumatology (Oxford). 2007;46(10):1566–9.

47. Smith V, Decuman S, Sulli A, Bonroy C, Piettte Y, Deschepper E, et al. Do worsening scleroderma capillaroscopic patterns predict future severe organ involvement? A pilot study. Ann Rheum Dis. 2012;71(10):1636–9.
48. Ingegnoli F, Ardoino I, Boracchi P, Cutolo M, Airò P, Ananieva LP, et al. Nailfold capillaroscopy in systemic sclerosis: data from the EULAR scleroderma trials and research (EUSTAR) database. Microvasc Res. 2013;89:122–8.
49. Smith V, Riccieri V, Pizzorni C, Decuman S, Deschepper E, Bonroy C, et al. Nailfold Capillaroscopy for prediction of novel future severe organ involvement in systemic sclerosis. J Rheumatol. 2013;40(12):2023–8.
50. Markusse IM, Meijs J, de Boer B, Bakker JA, Schippers HPC, Schouffoer AA, et al. Predicting cardiopulmonary involvement in patients with systemic sclerosis: complementary value of nailfold videocapillaroscopy patterns and disease-specific autoantibodies. Rheumatology (Oxford). 2017;56(7):1081–8.
51. Kasser C, Boleto G, Allanore Y, Avouac J. Nailfold videocapillaroscopy findings and associations with organ involvement in mixed connective tissue disease. Clin Exp Rheumatol. 2025;43(3):418–24.
52. Vanhaecke A, Cutolo M, Distler O, Riccieri V, Allanore Y, Denton CP, et al. Nailfold capillaroscopy in SSc: innocent bystander or promising biomarker for novel severe organ involvement/progression? Rheumatology. 2022;61(11):4384–96.
53. Cutolo M, Zampogna G, Vremis L, Smith V, Pizzorni C, Sulli A. Longterm effects of endothelin receptor antagonism on microvascular damage evaluated by Nailfold Capillaroscopic analysis in systemic sclerosis. J Rheumatol. 2013;40(1):40–5.
54. Cutolo M, Ruaro B, Pizzorni C, Ravera F, Smith V, Zampogna G, et al. Longterm treatment with endothelin receptor antagonist Bosentan and Iloprost improves fingertip blood perfusion in systemic sclerosis. J Rheumatol. 2014;41(5):881–6.
55. Bellando-Randone S, Lepri G, Bruni C, Blagojevic J, Radicati A, Cometi L, et al. Combination therapy with Bosentan and sildenafil improves Raynaud's phenomenon and fosters the recovery of microvascular involvement in systemic sclerosis. Clin Rheumatol. 2016;35(1):127–32.
56. Trombetta AC, Pizzorni C, Ruaro B, Paolino S, Sulli A, Smith V, et al. Effects of Longterm treatment with Bosentan and Iloprost on Nailfold absolute capillary number, fingertip blood perfusion, and clinical status in systemic sclerosis. J Rheumatol. 2016;43(11):2033–41.
57. Corallo C, Cutolo M, Kahaleh B, Pecetti G, Montella A, Chirico C, et al. Bosentan and macitentan prevent the endothelial-to-mesenchymal transition (EndoMT) in systemic sclerosis: in vitro study. Arthritis Res Ther. 2016;18(1):228.
58. Smith V, Pizzorni C, Riccieri V, Decuman S, Brusselle G, De Pauw M, et al. Stabilization of microcirculation in patients with early systemic sclerosis with diffuse skin involvement following rituximab treatment: an open-label study. J Rheumatol. 2016;43(5):995–6.
59. Wildt M, Andreasson K, Hamberg V, Hesselstrand R, Wuttge DM. Treatment with mycophenolate mofetil is associated with improved nailfold vasculature in systemic sclerosis. Rheumatology (Oxford). 2024;63(2):385–91.
60. Smith V, Denton C, Herrick A, Ittrich C, Alves M, Cutolo M. Nailfold videocapillaroscopy in patients with systemic sclerosis associated interstitial lung disease (SSc-ILD). RMD Open. RMD Open. 2025;11(4):e005704.
61. Smith V, Vanhaecke A, Herrick AL, Distler O, Guerra MG, Denton CP, et al. Fast track algorithm: how to differentiate a "scleroderma pattern" from a "non-scleroderma pattern". Autoimmun Rev. 2019;18(11):102394.
62. Cutolo M, Vojinovic T, Paolino S, Campitiello R, Smith V. Cerebrovascular involvement in systemic sclerosis. ACR Open Rheumatol. 2025;7(4):e70032.
63. Correia AM, Campitiello R, Pizzorni C, Gotelli E, Sulli A, Paolino S, Smith V, Cutolo M. Differences in nailfold capillaroscopy findings between limited and diffuse cutaneous systemic sclerosis: a detailed analysis. RMD Open. 2025 Jul 5;11(3):e005716.

Nailfold Capillaroscopy in Idiopathic Inflammatory Myopathies

Liza J. McCann and Ariane L. Herrick

Abbreviations

ACR	American College of Rheumatology
ASynS	Anti-synthetase syndrome
CADM	Clinically amyopathic dermatomyositis
CAJDM	Clinically amyopathic juvenile dermatomyositis
DM	Dermatomyositis
EULAR	European Alliance of Associations for Rheumatology
IBM	Inclusion body myositis
IIM	Idiopathic inflammatory myopathy
ILD	Interstitial lung disease
IMNM	Immune mediated necrotising myopathy
JIA	Juvenile idiopathic arthritis
JIIM	Juvenile onset idiopathic inflammatory myopathy
JDM	Juvenile dermatomyositis
JPM	Juvenile onset polymyositis

L. J. McCann (✉)
Alder Hey Children's NHS Foundation Trust, Liverpool, UK
e-mail: Liza.McCann@alderhey.nhs.uk

A. L. Herrick
Centre for Musculoskeletal Research, Division of Musculoskeletal and Dermatological Sciences, The University of Manchester, Manchester Academic Health Science Centre, Manchester, UK

Northern Care Alliance NHS Foundation Trust, Salford, UK

National Institute for Health and Care Research (NIHR) Manchester Biomedical Research Centre, Manchester, UK

Department of Rheumatology, Aberdeen Royal Infirmary, NHS Grampian, Aberdeen, UK

Centre for Arthritis and Musculoskeletal Health, University of Aberdeen, Aberdeen, UK

A. L. Herrick et al. (eds.), *Nailfold Capillaroscopy in Rheumatological Diseases*,
https://doi.org/10.1007/978-3-032-03970-5_7

jSLE	Juvenile onset systemic lupus erythematosus
jSSc	Juvenile onset systemic sclerosis
MAA	Myositis associated antibody
MCTD	Mixed connective tissue disease
MSA	Myositis specific antibody
NFC	Nailfold capillaroscopy
PM	Polymyositis
SLE	Systemic lupus erythematosus
SSc	Systemic sclerosis

Key Points

- Vasculopathy is key to the pathogenesis of idiopathic inflammatory myopathies (IIM) with involvement of both the microvasculature and microvasculature.
- Loss of capillary end row loops on nailfold capillaroscopy can reflect the small vessel destruction associated with IIM that is apparent on skin and muscle biopsies.
- Nailfold capillaroscopy is increasing recognised as a useful tool to aid diagnosis and monitoring of disease activity and/or risk of organ involvement in IIM.
- NFC assessment is one of the potential items to include when revising classification criteria in skin predominant IIM.
- Many studies have shown that 'bushy' capillaries tend to be a distinctive feature of IIM, particularly juvenile and adult-onset dermatomyositis, but also anti-synthetase syndrome.
- Scleroderma pattern, recognised in systemic sclerosis and mixed connective tissue disease, is common in juvenile and adult onset dermatomyositis, clinically amyopathic dermatomyositis and overlap myositis but rarely seen in polymyositis.
- Nailfold capillaroscopy has potential as an outcome measure in clinical trials in patients with IIM.

Introduction

Idiopathic Inflammatory Myopathies (IIM)

Idiopathic inflammatory myopathies (IIM) are a heterogenous group of rare acquired autoimmune diseases, historically described as dermatomyositis (DM) or polymyositis (PM), but now best defined within a number of disease sub-types. The incidence and prevalence of disease may vary with age, gender, ethnicity, and geographical region but IIM has an estimated incidence of 0.2–2 per 100,000 person-years and a prevalence of 2–25 per 100,000 people [1]. Juvenile-onset IIM (JIIM) has a reported incidence of between 1.6 and 4 cases per million children per year [2].

IIM are typically characterised by muscle weakness and involvement of other organs, including the skin, joints, lungs, heart, and gastrointestinal tract [3]. Based on clinical, serological, and histopathological, features, they can be classified into DM/juvenile dermatomyositis (**JDM**), which includes clinically amyopathic dermatomyositis (**CADM**), PM/juvenile polymyositis (**JPM**), overlap myositis, anti-synthetase syndrome (**ASynS**), immune-mediated necrotising myopathy (**IMNM**), inclusion body myositis (**IBM**) and cancer-associated myositis [2, 3]. PM/JPM is characterised by moderate to severe weakness with characteristic histological findings without cutaneous features. With the increasing use of myositis-specific antibodies (**MSA**) and advances in histopathology, a proportion of patients previously classified as PM/JPM, are now best classified as adult or juvenile-onset ASynS or IMNM, IBM or genetic muscle disease, decreasing the proportion of patients classified as PM or JPM [3, 4].

Indications for Nailfold Capillaroscopy in IIM

Nailfold capillaroscopy (**NFC**) has a number of clinical and research applications in IIM. Clinically, NFC can aid diagnosis of IIM, particularly in sub-types where NFC changes are common, including JDM, DM and overlap myositis. In addition, the loss of capillary end row loops on NFC can reflect the small vessel destruction associated with IIM. Therefore, NFC has the potential to be used to monitor disease activity/severity, and to predict risk of complications such as lung disease or calcinosis, as described in more detail within this chapter.

Research applications include the possibility of using NFC to help determine treatment response in clinical trials, mainly in DM, to examine pathogenesis and to look for associates. Importantly, some of the NFC literature examines NFC appearances in different IIM subtypes (and in patients with different autoantibodies) and this can provide insights into pathogenesis. This is an evolving field, and for this reason a brief description of different IIM subtypes is given below.

IIM Subtypes

Dermatomyositis (DM) and Clinically Amyopathic Dermatomyositis (CADM)

DM is defined by the presence of characteristic cutaneous manifestations and myositis. Heliotrope rash and Gottron's papules are pathognomonic (Figs. 1 and 2). In childhood-onset disease, DM is by far the most common disease sub-type (JDM), affecting 81–91% of children with JIIM [5, 6]. In contrast, fewer than half of patients with adult-onset IIM fall within the DM sub-type [6]. Children are more likely to develop calcinosis, ulceration and vasculopathy than those with adult onset DM, but are less likely to have Raynaud's phenomenon particularly when onset of disease is before 5 years of age [6, 7]. Patients with characteristic DM skin rashes who do not have weakness of myositis are considered to have CADM or clinically amyopathic

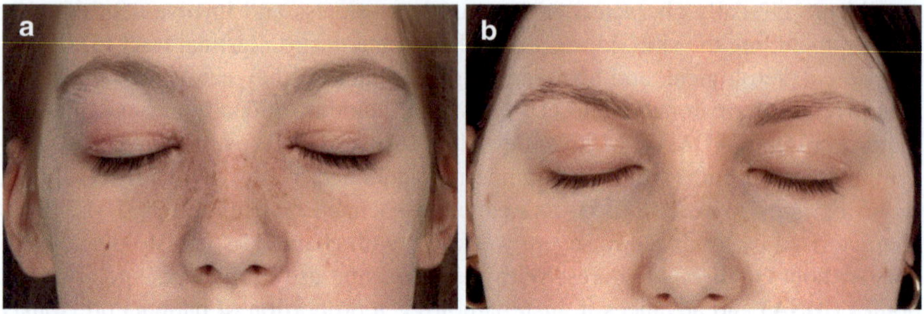

Fig. 1 Heliotrope rash over eyelids in a 12-year-old girl with juvenile dermatomyositis at time of disease diagnosis (**a**) and during a disease flare at 18 years of age (**b**)

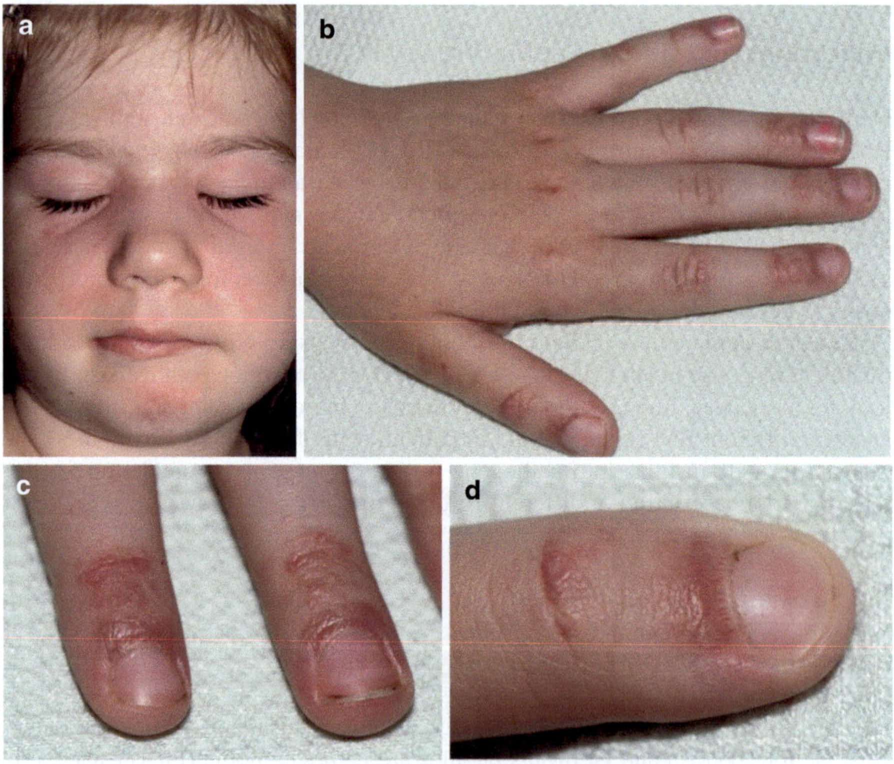

Fig. 2 Heliotrope rash over eyelids and malar rash over the cheeks (**a**) of a 3-year-old girl at the time of diagnosis of juvenile dermatomyositis. In the same patient, Gottron's papules seen over metacarpophalangeal and interphalangeal joints of the hands (**b**) and nailfold changes apparent to the naked eye in the periungual areas of the fingers (**c**) and thumbs (**d**)

juvenile dermatomyositis (**CAJDM**). **CADM** is recognised in adult-onset IIM as a distinct phenotype, highly associated with the presence of anti-MDA5 autoantibodies and rapidly progressive interstitial lung disease (ILD), characterised by severe cutaneous rashes without objective muscle weakness. In contrast, this phenotype is seen only in about 1% of childhood IIM, often associated with anti-transcriptional intermediary factor-gamma (anti-TIF1ɣ) antibody or anti-MDA5 [8]. Manifestations recognised in adult-onset CADM, such as calcinosis, ulcerations, ILD or malignancy, are infrequent in CAJDM [8].

Overlap Myositis

There is currently no internationally agreed definition of overlap myositis, but it is recognised as a distinct clinical sub-type of IIM that may be associated with increased risk of extra-muscular manifestations including Raynaud's phenomenon, arthritis/arthralgia, sclerodactyly and ILD [6, 9]. Overlap myositis is described when DM/JDM or PM/JPM is associated with other autoimmune diseases, most commonly systemic sclerosis (SSc), systemic lupus erythematosus (**SLE**), arthritis, or as part of mixed connective tissue disease (**MCTD**) with anti-U1RNP autoantibodies [6, 10]. Raynaud's phenomenon is particularly common in patients with RNP-positive MCTD (more than 90% of patients) and anti-Pm-Scl positive myositis-scleroderma overlap (78–100%) compared to DM/PM where it is seen in around 40% of cases [11].

Anti-synthetase Syndrome

ASynS is less common in children than adults, seen in approximately 5% of JIIM cases compared to more than 25% of those with adult-onset IIM [10, 12]. Disease phenotype is similar across juvenile and adult age groups, with the presence of moderate to severe weakness, arthritis, frequent ILD, "mechanic's hands", fever, and Raynaud's phenomenon [10]. Disease characteristics differ between Jo-1 positive and non-Jo-1 ASynS, the latter associated with more severe ILD, milder weakness, and higher mortality [12]. Raynaud's phenomenon is seen in approximately one-third of patients with ASynS and can be a relevant feature to aid diagnosis and classification [11]. The prevalence of Raynaud's phenomenon may vary according to anti-synthetase antibody specificities and is particularly common in those with anti-PL12 and anti-PL7 antibodies [11]. These two antibody subtypes are also associated with early, severe and more rapidly progressive ILD [13].

Immune Mediated Necrotising Myositis

IMNM, also referred to as necrotising autoimmune myopathy, includes individuals with anti-signal recognition particle (**SRP**) and anti-3-hydroxy-3-methylglutaryl--coenzyme A reductase (**HMGCR**) autoantibodies as well those without a known MSA [14]. Patients typically have moderate to severe proximal muscle weakness with frequent distal weakness and significantly elevated creatinine kinase. IMNM is characterised by muscle fibre necrosis with absent or minimal lymphocytic infiltration on muscle biopsy, which, along with MSA profile, may help to confirm the diagnosis [14]. Extra-muscular manifestations, including skin rashes, arthralgia, Raynaud's phenomenon or ILD, are recognized in a minority of cases [14].

Inclusion Body Myositis

IBM is characterised by asymmetrical muscle weakness of both proximal and distal muscles, including finger flexors, that progresses slowly and shows a poor response to immunotherapy [15]. Dysphagia is common but extra muscular manifestations are rare. IBM can be associated with other autoimmune disorders [15]. IBM does not tend to occur in childhood and is mostly seen in individuals over 50 years of age [15].

Polymyositis

Historically PM has been described as a myositis phenotype with chronic muscle weakness without cutaneous involvement, involving predominant T-cell mechanisms [3]. As mentioned above, most patients previously described as PM can now best be classified as ASynS, IBM, IMNM or genetic muscle disease. However, there remains a small subset of patients who have classical clinical and pathological findings of PM without the characteristic features or MSA allowing them to be classified differently and thus remain classified as PM.

Cancer Associated Myositis

Increased risk of malignancy compared to the general population is recognised in all adult-onset IIM subtypes, with the exception of ASynS and IBM [3, 15]. Risk is particularly high within the 3 years prior to and 3 years after myositis onset, with other high risk factors including DM phenotype, being greater than 40 years of age at time of myositis onset, having anti-TIF1ɣ or anti-nuclear matrix protein 2 (anti-NXP2) antibody positivity, having features of persistent high disease activity despite immunosuppression, having moderate to severe dysphagia, or cutaneous ulceration [16]. Cancer associated myositis is extremely rare in children, described only in occasional case reports [17] and hence routine cancer screening is not required in juvenile onset IIM [16].

Other forms of myositis, including focal myositis, orbital myositis, eosinophilic myositis and macrophagic myofasciitis, are exceedingly uncommon, particularly in children [18].

Pathogenesis of IIM and Importance of Vasculopathy

The exact mechanisms causing IIM are unknown, but evidence supports the concept of an environmental trigger in a genetically susceptible individual [3]. Vasculopathy and endothelial dysfunction are thought to play a key role in the pathogenesis of IIM [19, 20]. In DM/JDM in particular vasculopathy is a prominent feature, manifest by erythematous heliotrope rash, nailfold erythema, frequent nailfold capillary changes, and elevated serum vascular markers. It is thought that an inflammatory small vessel vasculitis during the acute stages of the disease is followed by a noninflammatory occlusive vasculopathy with capillary drop out later in the disease process [19].

Vascular involvement in IIM impacts both the microvasculature and the macrovasculature. Microvascular changes can be appreciated by histopathological analysis of skin or muscle biopsies. Capillary drop out is seen in muscle biopsies, with extent of capillary loss associated with the severity of muscle disease and thought to be related to clinical features suggestive of vasculopathy such as limb oedema [11]. Histopathology in DM/JDM skin specimens shows evidence of vasculopathy with interface dermatitis, mucin deposition and perivascular inflammation [20]. The small vessel destruction in skin and muscle is also apparent in the loss of nailfold capillary end row loop that can be captured using high power microscopy.

The impact of IIM on macrovasculature can be appreciated by the increased risk of myocardial infarction or venous thromboembolism seen in IIM relative to the general population [11]. Vascular injury has also been postulated to have a role in the development of calcinosis, which can occur at ischaemic foci in the extensor surfaces of the joints [11, 21]. Important associates for risk of calcinosis include duration of disease and also periungual capillary changes [22, 23].

Genetic risk factors influencing disease phenotype may differ across the world or in different races, and there are specific differences in HLA risk factor alleles between children and adults with particular MSAs [24, 25]. The presence of MSA and their association with distinct phenotypes strongly implicate a role for B cells in the disease, but it is unclear whether these antibodies are pathogenic or reflective of a T-cell driven immune pathology, as T cells have been found to be dysfunctional in IIM [26].

IIM subtypes distinguished by MSA may differ in the degree of vasculopathy that is apparent, and some studies (described later in this chapter) have explored this using NFC. Individuals with anti-MDA5 antibodies have been found to be significantly more likely to have vasculopathy than those without this MSA in an analysis of 42 skin biopsies from 22 patients with DM/CAMD [27]. In a study of 121 anti-MDA5 positive patients compared with 201 anti-MDA5 negative patients, Allenbach et al. confirmed that anti-MDA5 patients more frequently had signs of skin vasculopathy with a DM skin rash, skin ulcers, calcinosis, and mechanic's hands, as well as ILD, arthritis/arthralgia and a higher mortality rate compared to those who were MDA5 negative [28].

A strong interferon type 1 signature has been extensively implicated in IIM [29–31]. In parallel to the interferon pathway, both adaptive and innate immune pathways are proposed to contribute to IIM. Recent studies have supported a role for cell death via neutrophil extracellular traps (NETosis), mitochondrial dysfunction, and endoplasmic reticulum stress in the pathogenesis of disease, which also may contribute to increased type 1 interferon production [32–35].

Possible environmental triggers for IIM in susceptible individuals include ultraviolet light, vaccinations, medications (in particular statin exposure in adult onset anti-HMGCR associated IMNM), immunostimulatory herbal supplements, smoking, environmental pollutants and infection [1, 20, 36, 37]. SARS-CoV-2 can induce an acute viral myositis but has also been associated with the onset of classical DM and worsening of disease in patients with established JDM, DM and IMNM [38]. It is interesting to note that similarities have been found between SARS-CoV-2 infection and anti-MDA5 autoantibody-positive DM, including interstitial pneumonia, vasculopathy, and thrombosis, suggesting a common pathogenic link [39].

Capillary Loss (Which Can Be Assessed by NFC) as a Key Element of Pathogenesis

Capillary loss on muscle biopsy has been identified in both adult and juvenile onset DM, but has been found to be more prominent in juvenile onset disease, with hypoxia-related mechanisms as well as interferon-related pathways leading to perifascicular myofibre atrophy [40]. In JDM, non-necrotizing vasculitis and extensive loss of capillary bed on muscle biopsy has long been recognised to associate with NFC changes [41]. Severe vascular changes on muscle biopsy have been found to be predictive of a more chronic disease course and persistent vasculopathy is thought to be a poor prognostic factor [19]. Capillary drop out on muscle biopsy and clinical features of vasculopathy have been found to be associated with disease severity [42]. Vasculopathy has also been found to be associated with severe extra-muscular manifestations such as ulcerative skin disease, calcinosis, gastrointestinal, cardiac and respiratory manifestations [19, 29].

In a study of 90 patients with JDM, increased circulating endothelial cells and microparticles, as markers of vasculopathy, were found to be increased in patients with JDM, and correlated with disease activity and nailfold capillary abnormalities [19, 29]. Endothelial soluble adhesion molecules and biomarkers related to type 1 interferon signature such as galectin-9, CXCL-10 and Siglec-1, which have been shown to track disease activity, are under investigation as biomarkers of vasculopathy in IIM, but are not yet available in routine clinical practice [43, 44]. The association of elevated circulating endothelial cell counts with NFC changes found by Papadopoulou et al., supports the use of NFC as a marker of JDM vasculopathy [19].

Kubo et al. found that patients with NFC scleroderma pattern had more severe lymphocytic infiltration on skin biopsy than those without scleroderma NFC changes, and severe lymphocytic infiltration was noted only in those with scleroderma spectrum abnormalities on NFC [45]. This would suggest that NFC can be a useful marker of the skin disease activity.

Diagnostic and Classification Criteria for IIM

Diagnostic criteria for IIM published by Bohan and Peter in 1975 are still commonly used, with modification in the clinical setting, to confirm the diagnosis of IIM [46, 47]. There has been a move away from using EMG or muscle biopsy for all cases of IIM, and increasing dependence on muscle magnetic resonance imaging (**MRI**) and use of an MSA profile to aid diagnosis, leading to numerous attempts to define better diagnostic or classification criteria [47]. The European Alliance of Associations for Rheumatology (**EULAR**)—American College of Rheumatology (**ACR**) classification criteria, developed more recently, can be used in clinical and research settings [48]. These criteria define the probability of a patient having IIM, either with or without muscle biopsy criteria, although a biopsy is recommended for patients without characteristic rashes. Items within the probability score include age of disease onset, patterns of weakness, the presence of skin and extra-muscular features including dysphagia or oesophageal dysmotility, and laboratory testing

[47]. Except for anti-Jo-1 autoantibodies, MSA was not documented in a sufficient number of subjects for the classification criteria to include other myositis autoantibodies within this data-driven approach. If a patient meets probable or definite criteria for IIM, an algorithm is used to determine the clinicopathologic subgroup. However, in children, a distinction for the non-JDM subgroups could not be determined, due to insufficient data in juvenile onset disease. Additional variables are currently being evaluated for incorporation into the EULAR/ACR classification criteria, with particular consideration of other myositis antibodies and cutaneous features.

A retrospective study of 211 adult patients with DM demonstrated that 26% of individuals with CADM would not be captured by the EULAR/ACR criteria [49]. Data are currently being collected within a multi-centre international effort to construct criteria to better categorise DM skin features to complement the EULAR/ACR criteria or to be used as standalone criteria in skin-predominant disease [20, 50]. NFC is not currently part of the EULAR/ACR classification criteria, but the presence of nailfold capillary loop changes by eye or microscopy has been proposed as a potential item for classification criteria by the Skin Myositis Delphi group, particularly in skin-predominant disease [20, 51].

The Role of NFC in Diagnosis of IIM

The diagnostic utility of NFC in the differentiation of individuals with primary Raynaud's phenomenon from those that may have secondary Raynaud's phenomenon due to an underlying connective tissue disease, particularly systemic sclerosis (**SSc**), has long been recognised (discussed in chapter "Clinical Indications"). In a similar way, routine use of NFC may improve diagnostic accuracy in DM/JDM described in more detail in sections below. In particular, NFC may be helpful for the diagnosis of JDM, where nailfold capillary changes are seen very frequently, and in CADM/CAJDM, where current classification criteria may not adequately capture individuals, as described above. In a study by Schmeling et al., all 28 JDM patients captured within an inception cohort at time of diagnosis had reduced nailfold capillary density suggesting that nailfold capillary density is a sensitive diagnostic marker for JDM [52].

In childhood, nailfold capillary density is reduced in patients with JDM, MCTD, juvenile-onset systemic sclerosis (jSSc), and juvenile-onset systemic lupus erythematosus (jSLE), but is typically normal in patients with primary Raynaud's phenomenon and juvenile idiopathic arthritis (JIA) [53]. Malar rash and erythema can be seen in both DM/JDM and SLE/jSLE, and skin biopsy findings can be indistinguishable on H&E [54]. In this context, it is interesting that studies have shown that scleroderma pattern (also termed 'SSc pattern' or 'scleroderma-spectrum pattern', although in this chapter we shall use 'scleroderma pattern') on NFC was more common in JDM, MCTD and SSc whereas patients with jSLE were more likely to have non-specific abnormalities [53, 55, 56]. Thus, when scleroderma pattern is present NFC may help differentiate between jSLE and JDM, particularly when muscle weakness is less prominent. Since Raynaud's phenomenon and arthritis can be seen in isolation, or in patients with IIM, NFC can help aid the diagnosis of JDM/DM or other causes of secondary Raynaud's phenomenon within a diagnostic pathway. Torrente-Segarra et al. evaluated 115 subjects, including 16 with JDM, aiming to assess NFC patterns in connective tissue disease, with or without Raynaud's phenomenon and related to ANA status. No associations reached statistical significance, but ANA negative patients were more likely to have normal NFC and none of the ANA negative patients had scleroderma pattern. The authors suggested that when ANA is positive, NFC may help as a diagnostic and prognostic tool, irrespective of the presence of Raynaud's phenomenon [57]. It is important to note that ANA can frequently be negative in IIM, particularly juvenile onset disease, and therefore ANA status should not be relied upon within a diagnostic pathway [58]. The importance of evaluating nailfold changes in IIM as part of diagnosis and ongoing monitoring, particularly for juvenile onset disease has been highlighted within consensus-based guidelines for JIIM in the United Kingdom and Europe [59, 60]. Although, as mentioned earlier, abnormal nailfold capillaries are not included in the classification criteria for IIM [48], in adults as in children they may add weight to a diagnosis, the patterns of abnormality being described in later sections. A review of the literature published in 2025 summarised findings from 37 papers including 346 patients with adult onset DM: the authors reported that 223/346 patients (64.5%) had an 'increase in vessel diameter', 94 (27.2%) had giant capillaries, 199 (57.5%) had decreased vascularity, and 156 (45.1%) had a scleroderma-spectrum pattern [61].

NFC Patterns in IIM

It has long been recognised that patients with IIM and especially those with DM can have very abnormal nailfold capillaries with capillary enlargement, and areas of avascularity, similar to those seen in patients with SSc [62]. Early studies also reported the finding of 'bushy' capillaries [63, 64] also variously termed 'arborised', 'ramified', 'angiogenic' or 'bizarre': these very abnormal capillaries have multiple apices or 'branches' all arising from a single arteriole (Fig. 3). Since then and as described below, several investigators have examined the patterns of abnormality which occur in IIM, comparing patterns between patients with IIM and healthy controls (and/or in those with primary Raynaud's phenomenon in whom nailfold capillaries should be structurally normal), between patients with IIM and SSc, and between the different subtypes of IIM. Many of these studies have confirmed that 'bushy' capillaries tend to be a distinctive feature of IIM - in particular DM/JDM [65, 66], and also ASynS [67].

Tables 1 and 2 summarise results of some of the studies which have examined nailfold capillaroscopic abnormalities in children and adults with IIM. They also demonstrate the changes over the years in the technique of examining nailfold capillaries—earlier studies tended to use a stereomicroscope, whereas later studies have tended to use videocapillaroscopy.

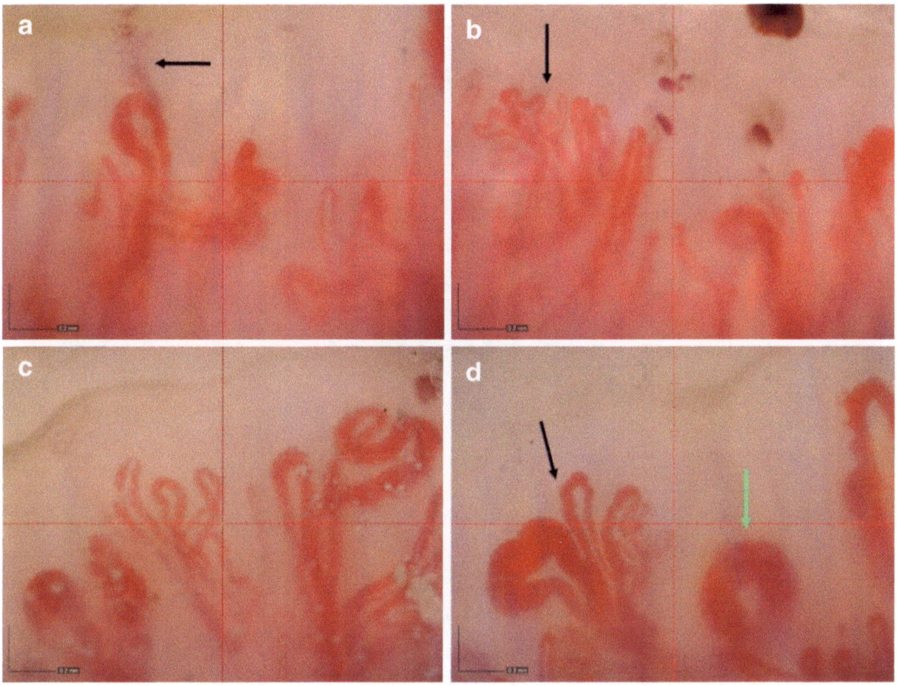

Fig. 3 Abnormal nailfold capillaries in a patient with dermatomyositis. Each image is from a different finger. All images show reduced capillary density and distortion of the capillary architecture. In addition, (**a**) shows new haemorrhage (arrow). (**b**) shows a good example of a ramified capillary (arrow) and haemorrhages of different ages. (**c**) shows ramified capillaries. (**d**) shows a good example of a giant ramified capillary (black arrow) and a giant capillary (green arrow). Some nailfold capillary changes are so abnormal that they can be appreciated by the naked eye (as shown in chapter "Clinical Indications", Fig. 2). (Images courtesy of Professor Hector Chinoy and Dr. Graham Dinsdale)

Comparing IIM with Healthy Controls/Primary Raynaud's Phenomenon

Studies in Children

Several studies have evaluated the NFC changes seen in patients with JDM compared to subjects with other paediatric rheumatic diseases and healthy controls [41, 55, 68, 70, 75]. Studies up until 2012 were summarised in a review of the literature [97]. Significant differences have been found in nailfold capillary changes, and in particular nailfold capillary density, between patients with JDM (and other connective tissues diseases such as jSSc) and healthy controls [55, 75]. More recent studies have confirmed that untreated children with JDM have a significantly lower mean end row loop density compared to healthy controls [53, 66, 80].

A project from the EULAR Study Group on Microcirculation in Rheumatic Diseases, evaluated 209 patients with juvenile rheumatic disease from 13 centres worldwide compared to 204 age and sex matched healthy controls [53]. Twenty-two

Table 1 Summary of some of the studies in paediatric patients examining nailfold capillaroscopic abnormalities in patients with idiopathic inflammatory myopathies

Reference	Number of subjects with IIM	Comparators if relevant—healthy controls/other disease	NFC technique used	Summary of methods	Summary of results	If longitudinal component, duration of follow up and key points	Associates	Key conclusions
Spencer-Green et al. 1982 [68]	19 JDM.	Between group comparisons:20 JIA, 20 HC.	Wide field stereo-microscope 25x or 40x magnification. Second and third fingers of each hand. Single blinded observer.	Cross sectional study, single centre. Qualitative assessments.	Abnormal NFC pattern noted in 11/19 (58%) JDM patients and none of the JIA/HCs.	Not applicable.	Most consistent NFC changes seen in patients with chronic disease type, (7/8 with abnormalities). Those with limited (monocyclic) disease tended to have normal NFC.	This was one of the earliest studies to demonstrate that NFC changes were common in JDM (more than 50% of cases), and related to chronic disease type. In contrast, NFC changes not seen in JIA or HCs.
Spencer-Green et al. 1983 [41]	32 JDM.	Between group comparisons:22 JIA, 9 SSc, 10 localised scleroderma, 7 SLE, 4 MCTD, 34 HC.	Stereo-microscope 25x or 40x magnification. Second and third fingers of each hand. Analysed by 2 independent observers.	Cross sectional study, 3 centres. Qualitative assessment.	NFC abnormalities found in 29/118 subjects - exclusively those with JDM or SSc. Similar findings in JDM and SSc but highly arborised loops seen more frequently in JDM.	Not applicable.	For those (n = 25) with muscle biopsy data, non-necrotizing vasculitis and extensive loss of capillary bed was seen only in patients with abnormal capillary patterns.	This was one of the earliest studies to show that NFC abnormalities seen in JDM and SSc but not SLE, HC, MCTD or localised scleroderma. In JDM, NFC changes found to associate with muscle biopsy findings.

Silver et al. 1989 [64]	9 JDM.	None.	Stereo-microscope, magnification x 12x - 14x. All 10 fingers examined. NFC images coded and analysed by 2 observers.	Longitudinal, single centre study. Qualitative assessment. Patients included had ≥2 NFC (range 2–11) during course of illness.	Dynamic changes in microvascular noted in all 9 children - thrombosis/haemorrhage, evolved over several months to characteristic capillary pattern (giant capillary loops/bushy capillary formations).	1.3–9 years (mean 4 years). Those with persistent disease had relatively severe NFC changes that did not return to normal. Those with monocyclic disease completely normalised.	Morphological change in NFC associates with clinical course.	This was one of the earliest studies to demonstrate dynamic changes in NFC in JDM patients, with persistently abnormal NFC associating with chronic disease course.
Dolezalova et al. 2003 [55]	8 JDM.	Between group comparison with HC (20 healthy adults, 17 healthy children), 9 RP, 3 vasculitis, 8 SLE and 18 'CTD' including the 8 with JDM plus 3 jSSc, 4 jMCTD and 3 with overlap syndromes.	Video NFC, magnification 66x. All fingers except thumbs examined in children. Fourth fingers only in healthy adults. Single blinded observer.	Cross sectional, single centre study. Qualitative and quantitative methods including capillary density and morphology.	Definite nailfold capillary derangement present in 14/18 (78%) subjects with CTD (JDM, SSc, MCTD, or overlap syndromes) compared with 13% in SLE/JIA and none in HC/PR. Most abnormal findings in subjects with CTD - lower linear density/increased capillary loop width compared to other groups. Patients with JDM and SSc had the lowest density values. Significant difference between CTD & HCs, but no significant difference between primary RP and HCs.	Not applicable.	None	This studied confirmed significant difference between CTD and healthy controls. Patients with JDM and jSSc had the lowest NFC density.

(continued)

Table 1 (continued)

Reference	Number of subjects with IIM	Comparators if relevant—healthy controls/other disease	NFC technique used	Summary of methods	Summary of results	If longitudinal component, duration of follow up and key points	Associates	Key conclusions
Smith et al. 2004 [69]	60 JDM.	None.	Freeze-frame video microscopy, magnification not stated. 8 fingers examined. Single blinded observer.	Cross sectional, single centre study. Newly diagnosed patients seen between 1993–2002. NFC at diagnosis, performed by single investigator. Disease activity score (DAS) performed by a second investigator. Each investigator blinded to results of the other.	Two variables in NFC assessment—End row capillary number & terminal loop vascular bush formation were associated with severity of rash and duration of untreated disease (but not muscle symptoms) in children with JDM before administration of therapy.	Not applicable.	Greater symptom duration prior to therapy associates with worsening NFC structure as indicated by increased bushy & dilated loops, as well as end row capillary drop out. Disease activity score (DAS)-skin, but not DAS-muscle was associated with NFC and end row capillary loss.	This was one of the earliest studies to show that NFC associated with length of time of untreated disease and severity of skin disease associates with nailfold end row capillary loop drop out.

Ingegnoli et al. 2005 [70]	8 JDM; 6 with follow up data.	Between group comparisons:55 JIA, 6 PRP, 7 MCTD, 34 SLE, 8 jSSc, 70 HCs (50 children, 20 adults). With follow up data: 1 PRP, 10 SLE, 6 jSSc, 3 MCTD.	Video NFC using optic probe of 200 x magnification. Every finger of each hand examined.	Cross sectional single centre study with longitudinal component. NVC images coded and analysed by 2 observers. Qualitative and quantitative analysis. Evaluated capillary density, size, shape, arrangement and avascularity.	JIA and PRP similar to HCs. Percentage of major abnormalities significantly increased in MCTD, SLE and JDM. In JDM, a significant increase of major capillary abnormalities were seen ($p < 0.0001$), including elongated, enlarged, giant and bushy loops. During follow up, 8/26 (30.8%) of patients with major NFC pattern abnormalities, including 2 JDM, did not show any changes in their capillary findings. In 11/26 (42.3%) of children with major abnormalities, including 4 JDM, at the time of first examination, sequential examination showed modification in the morphology with progressive disorganisation of capillaries.	At least 12 months (range 12–168). In JDM, change over time in NFC morphology and density with increase in capillary loss and avascular areas seen in some but not all patients. In a proportion of patients, nailfold changes remained stable.	None.	This study confirmed that major NFC abnormality seen in JDM, SLE, MCTD and jSSc, but none of the JIA or SLE patients had scleroderma pattern. It also confirmed dynamic change in NFC over time in a proportion (but not all) JDM patients.

(continued)

Table 1 (continued)

Reference	Number of subjects with IIM	Comparators if relevant—healthy controls/other disease	NFC technique used	Summary of methods	Summary of results	If longitudinal component, duration of follow up and key points	Associates	Key conclusions
Nascif et al. 2006 [71]	13 JDM and 5 with overlap syndrome (myositis/SSc). 7/18 patients with JDM or JDM/SSc overlap had NFC more than twice.	None.	Optical microscope with magnification 10–16 times. Fingers examined (excluded thumbs) by same researcher, blinded to results of assessments for levels of disease activity.	Cross sectional single centre study with longitudinal component. 26 capillaroscopic examinations in total—13 during active phase and 13 in remission. Evaluated microhaemorrhages, capillary enlargement, morphological abnormalities, and level of dropout (recorded as 0–3; 0 = no drop out, 3 = extensive or confluent areas of dropout).	12/13 examinations during active disease phase showed significant abnormalities consistent with scleroderma pattern on NFC compared to 5/13 (38%) during inactive disease. Level of dropout was statistically higher in the active disease group ($p = 0.031$). 5/7 patients with NFC on ≥ 2 occasions progressed from active to inactive phase of disease. 2/5 had initial abnormal NFC findings that normalised, 1/5 had improved disease activity without change in NFC and in 2/5 patients, there were no alterations.	Duration of follow up not specifically stated. Patients were seen between May 1998–May 2003. Significant NFC abnormalities more frequent during active phase of disease. NFC can change (normalise) over time with inactive disease, but this was not seen in all patients.	NFC alterations (particularly capillary drop out) associate with active disease. NFC findings correlated with clinical and laboratory data in 20/26 (77%) examinations.	This study showed that capillary drop out offered the greatest statistical difference separating active and inactive disease. The study confirmed dynamic change in NFC over time in JDM related to disease activity in a proportion but not all patients.

Stringer et al. 2008 [72]	84 JDM.	None.	Methods for NFC not defined. Clinical examination of nailfold abnormalities documented as present/absent.	Inception cohort, single centre. Clinical laboratory and treatment data recorded at each study visit including normal/abnormal NFC changes.	At time point of 6 months post diagnosis, presence of Gottron's papules and abnormal nailfold capillaries predicted a longer time to remission. This relationship was stronger than that of Gottron's/abnormal NFC as individual predictors.	5 years (range 0.3–14 years).	Longer time to remission when NFC abnormalities present at 6 months post diagnosis, particularly when Gottron's papules also present.	This study found that the presence of NFC abnormalities plus Gottron's at 6 months post diagnosis associates with longer time to remission.
Christen-Zaech et al. 2008 [73]	61 JDM.	None.	Freeze-frame video microscopy, magnification not stated. 8 fingers examined. Single blinded observer.	Longitudinal single centre study including patients pre-treatment. Required at least 2 NFC or DAS assessments to be included. Values obtained at enrolment and follow up were analysed to determine association between the primary predictor (DAS) and NFC. NFC and DAS graded by individuals without knowledge of results of other measurement.	Over 36 months, end-row loop regeneration was associated with lower skin DAS ($p < 0.001$) but not muscle DAS ($p = 0.98$). In children with treated JDM, a unicyclic disease course was associated with increased end row loop regeneration and improvement in both skin DAS and muscle DAS at 36 months, which was maintained at 60 months in 81% of patients.	Mean follow up time of 29.6 +/− 10.2 months (range 3.2–38.6). The non-unicyclic disease course usually involved continuing skin manifestations with persistent NFC changes.	End row loop regeneration and decreased bushy loop numbers were associated with shorter duration of untreated disease. Over 36 months, end row loop regeneration associated with lower DAS-skin but not DAS-muscle. At 36 months, increased end row loop regeneration and improvement in DAS-skin and DAS-muscle were associated with unicyclic disease course.	This study confirmed that persistent NFC abnormalities can associate with a non-unicyclic disease course. It also found that NFC changes correlated with cutaneous but not musculoskeletal signs over a 36 month period.

(continued)

Table 1 (continued)

Reference	Number of subjects with IIM	Comparators if relevant—healthy controls/other disease	NFC technique used	Summary of methods	Summary of results	If longitudinal component, duration of follow up and key points	Associates	Key conclusions
Ostrowski et al. 2010 [74]	80 JDM.	12 children with normal nailfold end row loops at diagnosis were compared with the remaining 68 children.	Freeze-frame video microscopy, 8 fingers excluding thumbs (magnification not stated). The total number of end row loop per mm over 8 digits were divided to yield mean end row loop for each patient. An end row loop score of <7000 considered abnormal.	Longitudinal single centre study. All NFC studies were performed by one investigator at time of clinic visit. DAS determined by another independent investigator. Logistic regression used to look for potential predictors of abnormal nailfold end row loop at baseline, 24 months and 36 months.	At diagnosis, children with normal end row loop had a shorter duration of disease ($p = 0.03$) and lower skin DAS ($p = 0.045$). Over time, 7/12 with normal NFC at diagnosis developed abnormal end row loop by 24 months, and another had abnormal NFC at 47 months. 2 out of 3 with normal NFC at 24 months developed abnormal NFC at 36 months. Children with normal end row loop at baseline had significantly higher end row loop at 24 and 36 months, but differences between normal and abnormal decreased over time.	End row loop analysed as continuous variable, comparing 2 groups of children at 24 and 36 months follow up. Over time, increased likelihood of having abnormal nailfold end row loops associated with longer duration of untreated disease ($p = 0.02$) and higher skin DAS ($p = 0.004$).	Normal end row loop at diagnosis associated with shorter duration of untreated disease and lower skin DAS.	This study confirmed that NFC changes can associate with a longer duration of untreated disease, but also skin activity at time of diagnosis. It showed that a higher skin DAS at diagnosis associated with the presence or development of abnormal end row loop over time.

Schmeling et al. 2011 [52]	92 JDM, including an inception cohort of 28 with newly diagnosed JDM.	None.	Stereomicroscope, magnification not stated. right fourth digit (or left fourth digit if examination of right impractical). Nailfold capillary density determined. Nailfold capillary density of <6 capillary loops/mm was considered abnormal.	Single centre retrospective study capturing longitudinal follow up (1–26 visits per patient; median 9 visits). Total of 809 clinic visits with concurrent NFC collected over a time period of 5.5 years. In all patients, nailfold capillary density performed by a trained research assistant who did not have knowledge of disease activity status of patients. Disease activity measured by muscle scores (MMT, CMAS), muscle enzymes, quality of life measures and modified DAS (skin/muscle).	Disease activity (muscle and skin) significantly associated with loss of end row nailfold capillary over time. All patients in inception cohort (n = 28) with newly diagnosed JDM had a reduced baseline nailfold capillary density that improved as the disease improved, but this did not predict longer term outcome or disease course. Normalisation of NFC was seen in 6/23 (27.3%) at 6 months and a further 4/17 (further 23.5%) at 12 months.	28/92 JDM patients were newly diagnosed and had baseline NFC at diagnosis. All of these had reduced capillary density at baseline and showed notable improvement over time with treatment.	Loss of nailfold end row loop moderately associated with skin disease activity and more moderately associated with musculoskeletal involvement/function. For each capillary per millimetre increase in NFC density, the likelihood of having normal health-related quality of life increased by 24% [odds ratio (OR) = 1.24, P = 0.0009]. Likewise, overall quality of life, CHAQ, MMT, overall disease severity and pain were related to nailfold capillary density.	This study showed that reduced NFC density can be a sensitive diagnostic marker for JDM and a responsive measure of disease activity over time.

(continued)

Table 1 (continued)

Reference	Number of subjects with IIM	Comparators if relevant—healthy controls/other disease	NFC technique used	Summary of methods	Summary of results	If longitudinal component, duration of follow up and key points	Associates	Key conclusions
Piotto et al. 2012 [56]	30 JDM.	Between group comparisons:60 JIA, 30 SLE, 20 localised scleroderma, 4 SSc, 3 MCTD.	Optical microscope at 10- and 16x magnification, same observer.	Cross sectional single centre study. Clinical and laboratory tests as well as NFC performed in all patients.	Most patients (76.2%) had normal NFC. The major changes in NFC characterising scleroderma pattern were observed in patients with JDM, SSc and MCTD. No association with SLE/localised scleroderma. 26/30 with JDM (86.6%) had active disease. 22/26 NFC exams (84.6%) performed during the active phase of the disease showed scleroderma pattern, while the 4 exams performed during disease remission were normal ($P = 0.002$).	Not applicable.	NFC changes associated with active disease, and were normal in remission. NFC deletion score and number of dilated and bushy capillaries were statistically greater in the group with active disease.	This study confirmed that scleroderma pattern was seen in JDM, MCTD and SSc but not SLE, JIA and localised scleroderma. Disease activity associated with NFC in JDM and was normal in those patients in disease remission.

Barth et al. 2018 [75]	58 JDM	45 HC (age and sex matched).	Video microscope, 200x magnification. All fingers (not thumbs) examined. NFC analysis performed by assessor blinded to clinical data. Qualitative and quantitative data.	Cross sectional single centre study. Single assessor performed NFC and clinical examination in all patients with a median disease duration of 16.8 (range 2–38) years.	JDM patients had lower nailfold capillary density and more frequent neovascular pattern than controls. JDM patients with active disease had lower capillary density than HCs (mean difference of 1.19/mm). 50% of patients with active versus 21% of patients with inactive disease had low capillary density. Neovascular pattern observed in 60% of those with active disease versus 21% with inactive disease.	Not applicable.	Low nailfold capillary density and neovascular pattern associates with active disease. All disease activity scores were higher in patients with low nailfold capillary density compared to those with normal capillary density. Patients with neovascular pattern were also more likely to have higher disease activity and impaired muscle function.	This study confirmed that decreased nailfold capillary density and neovascular pattern associated with higher levels of disease activity and also impaired muscle function after median to long-term follow up.
Barth et al. 2019 [76]	58 JDM (same patient cohort as Barth et al. 2018)	None.	Video microscope, 200x magnification. NFC performed by single clinician and analysed by single researcher blinded to clinical information. Nailfold capillary density and neovascular pattern assessed. Cut off for low nailfold capillary density < 6 capillaries /mm.	Cross sectional single centre study. Clinical examination after a mean of 17 years disease duration, PFT measurements performed, HRCT in 56 patients, ECG and ECHO.	21/58 (36%) had low nailfold capillary density. Neovascular pattern observed in 24/58 (41%). Low nailfold capillary density was associated with low DLCO values, and signs of airway disease more prevalent on HRCT in the group with low nailfold capillary density. No significant associations between low nailfold capillary density and cardiac measures were observed after adjusting for age.	Not applicable.	Patients with low NFC density (n = 21) had lower forced vital capacity, total lung capacity and more often had low DLCO values compared to patients with normal NFC density (n = 37).	This study suggested that NFC density was associated with lung involvement but not cardiac involvement in JDM.

(continued)

Table 1 (continued)

Reference	Number of subjects with IIM	Comparators if relevant—healthy controls/other disease	NFC technique used	Summary of methods	Summary of results	If longitudinal component, duration of follow up and key points	Associates	Key conclusions
Khojah et al. 2022 [77]	96 JDM.	None.	NFC at diagnosis recorded for later analysis. Earlier images using freeze frame video microscopy, magnification 12x. Later digital images with dermatoscope (18x). 8 digits excluding thumbs. End row loop quantified by mean end row loop/mm of the number of fingers analysed for each patient.	Cross sectional, retrospective chart review, single centre study. Patients with JDM followed for ≥5 years, divided into 3 groups according to MSA status (anti-p155/140 / other MSA/MSA negative). Lipodystrophy as assessed by physician assessment and DXA fat distribution. Documentation of NFC end row loop obtained at diagnosis.	Patients with anti-p155/140 had significantly decreased end row loop counts at baseline, prolonged duration of untreated disease at diagnosis, and less frequent monophasic disease course.	Not applicable.	Anti-p155/140 myositis antibodies had significantly decreased end row loop counts at baseline compared to other MSA groups evaluated in this study.	Patients that were positive for anti-p155/140 (now typically classified as anti-TIF1) in this study had significantly worse end row loop counts compared to those with other MSA or MSA negative groups and were less likely to have a monophasic disease course. Authors suggest that this MSA may impact the vascular component of JDM.
Nozawa et al. 2022 [23]	172 JIIM, vast majority JDM.	None.	Stereoscopic microscope or handheld microscope. Data collected included NFC morphology and density to <6 loops/mm, but NFC changes grouped as overall normal or abnormal for the purpose of analysis.	Retrospective inception cohort, single centre study. Evaluated clinical and laboratory features, as well as disease activity and damage items to determine risk factors for calcinosis.	Calcinosis found in 44 patients (25.6%). In univariate analysis, the only risk factor significantly associated with the development of calcinosis was NFC abnormality at baseline (HR 4.86, $p = 0.03$). In multivariate analysis the only risk factor associated with development of calcinosis was the presence of NFC abnormality (HR 4.98, $p = 0.03$).	Median follow up 8.5 (range 0.1–28.3) years. Three distinct groups of disease activity—Class 1: Persistent high activity, class 2: Chronic moderate disease activity, class 3: High early disease activity but long-term low disease activity.	NFC abnormalities associated with risk of development of calcinosis.	In this inception cohort the only clinical or laboratory feature at baseline that predicted development of calcinosis was NFC abnormality.

Shenavandeh, Rashidi. 2022 [58]	150 IIM patients including 25 JDM, 81 DM, 25 CADM, 19 PM evaluated according to EULAR/ ACR criteria. Second analysis of 104 patients according to Troyanov and Senécal classification [78, 79] did not include JIIM.	Between group comparison of IIM.	Stereomicroscopy, 250x magnification. Qualitative and quantitative assessment. 8 fingers, excluding thumbs examined.	Cross sectional single centre study.	Scleroderma pattern dominant in JDM, seen in 18/25, (72%). Non-specific abnormalities seen in 7/25 (28%).	Not applicable.	Scleroderma pattern associates with high global and skin activity in DM. Associates for JDM not detailed in this study.	This study confirms that abnormal NFC, particularly scleroderma pattern, is common in JDM, similar to DM and CAMD but not PM.
Pachman et al. 2023 [66]	140 JDM.	46 HC.	Freeze frame video microscopy (18x).	Single centre retrospective cohort. association of NFC with clinical/laboratory data assessed.	JDM patients had fewer end row loops than HCs.	Not applicable.	More damage to end row loops with longer duration of untreated disease. Children with decreased end row loops had more skin disease than muscle disease. Anti-TIF1 associated with lower end row loops. Periungual haemorrhages at first assessment closely associated with dysphagia.	This study confirms an association of NFC changes (particularly capillary density) with duration of untreated disease, increased clinical symptoms (particularly skin disease), and anti-TIF1 in addition, nailfold haemorrhages were found to associate with dysphagia.

(continued)

Table 1 (continued)

Reference	Number of subjects with IIM	Comparators if relevant—healthy controls/other disease	NFC technique used	Summary of methods	Summary of results	If longitudinal component, duration of follow up and key points	Associates	Key conclusions
Khojah et al. 2023 [80]	68 JDM.	77 HC.	Freeze frame video microscopy (18x). 8 fingers examined. Analysis of NFC images performed by a single observer. Each patient's mean end row loop/mm was calculated by averaging the end row loop/mm of the 8 fingers and GraphPed prism used to calculate the area under the curve measuring end row loop cumulatively across the study duration.	Retrospective chart review, single centre study. Patients with at least 5 year follow up data and at least 4 NFC assessments at a prespecified time point (0, 6, 12, 24, 36, 48 and 60 months from initiation of medical therapy) were included. disease activity measured by standard assessments. Patients grouped according to disease course (monophasic, polycyclic or chronic).	Mean end row loop for treatment-naïve JDM was significantly lower than HCs and despite improvement in end row loop over time, it remained below the expected normal level of HCs. Rate of improvement varied according to disease course, with monocyclic course showing more improvement than chronic or polycyclic disease course. Significant correlation between the end row loop area under the curve for monocyclic short versus chronic, and monocyclic long versus chronic disease course. JDM patients with lipodystrophy exhibited a lower area under the curve than those without lipodystrophy. End row loop had no association with calcification.	Follow up for a minimum of 5 years. Despite improvement with treatment, end row loop count remained below normal even after 5 years. Patients requiring multiple immunosuppressants tended to have lower end row loop area under the curve.	Rate of improvement in end row loop quicker in monocyclic disease course compared to chronic or polycyclic. JDM patients with lipodystrophy exhibited a lower area under the curve than those without lipodystrophy. Negative association between duration of oral steroid use and end row loop area under the curve.	This study confirmed that persistently decreased nailfold capillary density reflected by low end row loop area under the curve associated with chronic disease course, and also with lipodystrophy.

Melsens et al. 2023 [53]	22 JDM.	Between group comparisons:204 HC, 20 primary RP, 20 jSLE, 13 jScl, 21 localised scleroderma 18 MCTD, 95 JIA.	Videocapillaroscopy, 200x magnification. All fingers except thumbs. Reading and reporting followed capillaroscopic protocol of the EULAR study group on microcirculation in rheumatic diseases. Qualitative & quantitative parameters.	Cross sectional, multi-centre study (13 centres worldwide), capturing patients with juvenile onset connective tissue disease and matched HCs.	Patients with JDM had a significantly lower nailfold capillary density compared to HCs. Nailfold capillary density in patients with primary RP was similar to that of HCs. Capillary dimension was significantly increased in JDM compared to HCs. Patients with JDM also exhibited significantly more abnormal shapes compared to HCs. Significantly more micro-haemorrhages were seen in JDM (85.3%) compared to HCs (39.2%). Odds to exhibit a scleroderma pattern higher in CTD (including JDM) compared to HC.	Not applicable.	None described.	This study confirms that JDM associated with significantly lower capillary density, increased capillary dimensions, more abnormal shapes and more haemorrhages than HCs.
Bogojevic et al. 2024 [81]	90 IIM: 5 JDM, 37 DM, 35 PM, 13 CADM.	35 PRP (control group) and between IIM group comparison.	Details of NFC equipment/ magnification not given. Quantitative and qualitative assessment for NFC.	Cross sectional single centre study.	Patients with JDM showed a high prevalence of scleroderma changes (4/5, 80%).		Not applicable –JDM excluded from comparison with control group.	This study confirmed a high prevalence of scleroderma pattern in JDM similar to DM and CADM.

APLS Anti phospholipid syndrome, *CADM* Clinically amyopathic dermatomyositis, *CHAQ* Childhood Health Assessment Questionnaire, *CMAS* Childhood Myositis Assessment Scale, *CTD/jCTD* Connective Tissue Disease/Juvenile onset Connective Tissue Disease, *DAS* Disease Activity Score, *DLCO* Diffusion capacity of the lungs for carbon monoxide, *DXA* Dual energy X ray absorptiometry (bone density scan), *ECG* Electrocardiogram, *ECHO* Echocardiogram, *HCs* healthy controls, *HRCT* High Resolution Computed Tomography, *JDM* Juvenile dermatomyositis, *JIA* Juvenile Idiopathic Arthritis, *MCTD* Mixed Connective Tissue Disease, *MMT* Manual Muscle Testing, *MRI* Magnetic resonance imaging, *MSA* Myositis Specific Antibody, *NFC* Nailfold Capillaroscopy, *PRP* Primary Raynaud's phenomenon, *PFT* Pulmonary Function Test, *RP* Raynaud's phenomenon, *SLE/jSLE* Systemic Lupus Erythematosus/juvenile onset Systemic Lupus Erythematosus, *SSc/jSSc* Systemic sclerosis/juvenile onset systemic sclerosis.

Table 2 Summary of some of the studies in adult patients examining nailfold capillaroscopic abnormalities in patients with idiopathic inflammatory myopathies

Reference	Number of subjects with IIM	Comparators if relevant—healthy controls/other disease	NFC technique used	Summary of methods	Summary of results	If longitudinal component, duration of follow up and key points	Associates	Key conclusions
Ganczarczyk et al. 1988 [63]	19 PM and 16 DM.	Between subgroup comparison.	Stereomicroscope. Magnification 20X. 8 fingers.	Cross-sectional.	Enlarged loops seen more frequently in DM than in PM, and more avascularity in DM.	Not applicable.	Capillary abnormalities more pronounced in patients with pulmonary involvement, arthritis and RP. Patients with disease duration <3 years had the more marked capillary abnormalities.	This was one of the earliest studies to show that patients with DM had more marked capillary changes (compared to PM) and to suggest associations with disease duration, RP and lung disease, although numbers were small.
Nagy & Czirják. 2004 [82]	26 DM/PM (out of 447 patients studied in total) 9 had DM.	Between group comparisons. 186 RP, 65 UCTD, 47 SLE, 14 RA, 9 primary SS, 102 SSc.	Stereomicroscope. Magnification 10-100X. Single observer.	Cross-sectional study. Single centre.	7/26 patients (26.9%) had a scleroderma pattern. 'Bizarre shaped loops' most commonly seen in patients with DM/PM.	Not applicable.	Not examined specifically for IIM.	One of the earlier studies to demonstrate abnormality in IIM.

Selva-O'Callaghan et al. 2010 [83]	53 IIM (34 DM, 17 PM, 2 IBM).	IIM vs HC, DM vs PM. Patients with high (abnormal) capillaroscopy scores (n = 15) vs those without (n = 38). 40 HC.	Stereomicroscope. Magnification 250x. One blinded observer.	Cross-sectional study. 8 fingers examined. Parameters assessed included capillary density (< 7 loops/mm = abnormal). Semiquantitative analysis.	Capillaroscopy abnormal as per authors' scoring system in 23 (43%) of patients. More abnormalities in patients with DM than with PM.	Not applicable.	Muscle disease activity/severity higher in those with the most abnormal capillary scores. RP and ILD more common in those with higher (abnormal) scores. Of the 6 patients with cancer associated IIM, 3 had 'severe' derangement (compared to 3/47 without cancer). No association with anti-synthetase or anti-PM-Scl antibodies.	Further confirmation that capillaroscopic abnormalities are more marked in DM than in PM.

(continued)

Table 2 (continued)

Reference	Number of subjects with IIM	Comparators if relevant—healthy controls/other disease	NFC technique used	Summary of methods	Summary of results	If longitudinal component, duration of follow up and key points	Associates	Key conclusions
Mercer et al. 2010 [84]	24 IIM (14 PM, 6 DM, 4 overlap).	IIM vs HC, DM vs PM. 35 HC.	Videocapillaroscopy (ring finger non-dominant hand). Magnification 300x. Quantitative analysis: Capillary density/mm. Apex and total loop width averaged across first 5 capillaries from right hand side of each nailfold.	Cross-sectional study with longitudinal component.	IIM vs HC: Capillary density lower, dimensions higher, in IIM. Arborised capillaries and avascular areas more frequent. DM vs PM: Capillaries more abnormal in DM than in PM (overlap group were the most abnormal).	16 patients' (and 27 HCs) nailfolds re-examined after 6–12 months (12 PM, 3 DM, 1 overlap).	No relation with RP. Lower capillary density in the 8 patients with anti-Jo-1 antibodies. Capillary density fell over time but not significantly in patients with IIM, no change in HCs. Some patients demonstrated marked changes in morphology over time.	This paper provided quantitative analysis and allowed tracking over time (but single nailfold only examined).
Mugii et al. 2011 [85]	50 DM.	DM vs HC. Patients with scleroderma pattern vs patients without. 20 HC	Videocapillaroscopy. Magnification 300x. Single observer. Semiquantitative assessments. Included RBC velocity. RBC velocity measured in 3 capillaries from each ring finger.	Cross-sectional study with longitudinal component.	37 (74%) patients with DM, but no HC, had scleroderma pattern. RBC velocity lower in patients with DM than HC but not significantly.	12 patients with DM re-examined after an average of 9.2 months). Scores for irregularly enlarged capillaries, haemorrhages and loss of capillaries decreased (i.e. improved) with stabilisation of disease. No change in RBC velocity.	Patients with scleroderma pattern had higher CK levels and higher muscle disease activity than those without. Scores for haemorrhages associated with skin disease.	Most patients with DM have abnormal capillaries, and degree of abnormality associated especially with muscle disease. Improved appearances after treatment.

Manfredi et al. 2015 [86]	52 patients with IIM (29 DM, 23 PM).	DM vs PRP, PM vs PRP, DM vs PM. DM short duration (≤ 6 months) vs longer duration (14 and 15 patients respectively). 52 patients with PRP.	Videocapillaroscopy. Magnification 200x. 8 fingers (at least 2 images per nailfold). Single blinded observer.	Cross-sectional study. Qualitative and semi-quantitative assessments.	Abnormalities (e.g. reduced capillary density) in DM vs PRP, and DM vs PM, but few abnormalities in PM vs PRP. Density reduced in DM vs PM. Density reduced short DM vs long DM. More giant capillaries short DM vs long DM. 69% DM had scleroderma pattern (0% PM) more common in shorter disease duration (non-significant).	Not applicable.	Capillary enlargement (giant capillaries) and loss were more marked in shorter duration disease. Ramified capillaries equally represented in short and longer duration disease.	The characteristic capillaroscopic abnormalities of DM are much less commonly seen in PM than in DM, and more marked in early disease.

(continued)

Table 2 (continued)

Reference	Number of subjects with IIM	Comparators if relevant—healthy controls/other disease	NFC technique used	Summary of methods	Summary of results	If longitudinal component, duration of follow up and key points	Associates	Key conclusions
Manfredi et al. 2016 [87]	29 DM.	DM vs 'all' SSc DM vs early SSc DM vs active SSc DM vs late SSc. 90 SSc (30 each of early, active, late capillaroscopic patterns).	Videocapillaroscopy. Magnification 200x. 8 fingers (at least 2 images per nailfold). Single blinded observer.	Cross-sectional study with longitudinal component. Qualitative and semi-quantitative assessments.	'Giant-ramified' capillaries (ramified capillaries with a diameter of >50 μm) almost exclusive to DM. Density lower in SSc vs DM (except in early SSc subgroup). Giant capillaries more common in SSc than in DM (except for late pattern SSc).	20 patients with DM and 90 with SSc re-assessed after 30 months. In DM: Reduction in giant capillaries. Increase in ramified capillaries. Increase in capillary density. In SSc: Increase in ramified capillaries early/active subgroups. Reduction in capillary density early/active, no change in late.	No association reported with RP.	'Giant-ramified' capillaries are specific for DM. Capillaroscopic appearances in DM improve over time (in contrast to in SSc, when abnormalities progress).
Pizzorni et al. 2018 [88]	24 DM	DM vs SSc. Anti-Jo-1 positive (n = 11) vs anti-Jo-1 negative (n = 13). 24 SSc.	Videocapillaroscopy. Magnification 200x. 8 fingers. Single observer.	Retrospective study. Cross-sectional with longitudinal component.	19/24 (79%) of patients with DM had scleroderma-pattern. Giant capillary and microhaemorrhage scores lower (i.e. less severe) in DM than in SSc, but ramification and disorganisation scores higher in DM, especially in early disease.	12 patients with DM re-examined after 3 years. Capillaroscopy 'scores' were unchanged over time (in this cohort with well-established disease), but the percentage of patients with ramified capillaries increased over time.	Capillaroscopy scores similar between anti-Jo-1 positive and negative patients.	The degree of different NFC abnormalities differed between DM and SSc, although numbers were small.

Kubo et al. 2019 [45]	70 IIM (52 DM, 18 PM)	IIM vs SSc, DM vs PM, IIM with scleroderma spectrum changes (n = 39) vs those without (n = 31). 60 SSc, 40 HC.	Videocapillaroscopy. Magnification 200x. 8 fingers. Single blinded observer.	IIM patients were treatment naïve at baseline. Cross-sectional study with 1 year follow-up after treatment in patients with IIM.	Scleroderma-spectrum pattern in 55.7% of patients with IIMs (65.4% DM, 27.8% PM) vs 80% of patients with SSc.	Patients re-examined after 1 year: Capillary abnormalities disappeared in more than half the patients with IIM after immunosuppressive therapy.	Among patients with IIM, those with scleroderma patterns were more likely to have skin disease than those without, but muscle enzymes and prevalence of RP were similar in those with and without scleroderma patterns. Anti-MDA5 and anti-TIF-1ɣ antibodies were more likely, and anti-ARS antibodies less likely to be present in those with scleroderma patterns than in those without. Patients with scleroderma pattern changes were more likely to have moderate or severe perivascular inflammation on skin biopsy.	This was one of the first studies to report autoantibody associations. A key finding was regression of capillaroscopic abnormalities in this cohort with early, previously untreated disease.

(continued)

Table 2 (continued)

Reference	Number of subjects with IIM	Comparators if relevant—healthy controls/other disease	NFC technique used	Summary of methods	Summary of results	If longitudinal component, duration of follow up and key points	Associates	Key conclusions
Sebastiani et al. 2019 [67]	190 ASynS,	ASynS vs PRP. Anti-Jo-1 positive (n = 133) vs anti-Jo-1 negative (n = 57). 75 PRP.	NFC images acquired using different systems. magnification 100-200x. Images transferred for central reading by a single blinded observer.	Retrospective, multicentre study.	Nailfold capillary abnormalities in 62.1% of patients with ASynS (vs 29.3% with PRP). Giant capillaries in 31.1% of patients, avascular areas in 20.5%, ramified capillaries in 49.5%, SSc-like pattern in 35.3% ($p < 0.005$ versus PRP).	Not applicable.	SSc-like pattern associated with anti-Jo-1 positivity, longer disease duration, and later onset ILD.	Most patients with ASynS had nailfold capillary abnormalities: Ramified capillaries were the commonest abnormality.
Soubrier et al. 2019 [89]	43 patients with IIM and interpretable images: 17 DM, 8 overlap myositis, 12 ASynS, 6 IMNM.	Between IIM subgroups. DM vs SSc, Overlap myositis vs SSc. 32 SSc and interpretable images.	Videocapillaroscopy. Magnification 100X. 8 fingers, 2 raters.	Cross-sectional, single centre.	Giant capillaries, substantial disorganisation, and avascular zones seen only in patients with DM and overlap myositis (never in ASynS or IMNM).	Not applicable.	Numbers were too small to identify associations with autoantibodies.	This study further confirmed that in patients with IIM, abnormalities are seen mainly in patients with DM and overlap syndromes.
Miossi et al. 2019 [90]	23 DM (early onset <12 months' symptoms).	Baseline vs follow-up (n = 15).	Stereomicroscope. Magnification 10-20x. 10 fingers (whole nailfold examined). Single observer.	Cross-sectional study with longitudinal component.	Capillaroscopic abnormalities were 'improved' at follow-up.	15 patients re-examined after a median of 3.21 years.	Capillary density and avascular areas correlated with serum angiogenin.	In this cohort of patients with early disease, capillary abnormalities regressed with treatment.

Wakura et al. 2020 [91]	27 DM-ILD.	Anti-MDA5 positive (n = 10) vs anti-ARS positive (n = 17).	USB microscopy (Dino-Lite). Magnification 200x. ,8 fingers. Two blinded observers.	Retrospective, cross-sectional study.	Patients who were anti-MDA5 positive had higher microhaemorrhage scores and higher capillary disorganisation scores than these who were anti-ARS positive.	Not applicable.	Degree of capillary loss correlated with total fibrosis scores on HRCT.	The degree of nailfold capillaroscopic abnormality may relate to severity of ILD.
Hamaguchi et al. 2021 [92]	11 DM, all anti-MDA5 positive	Baseline vs post-treatment	Videocapillaroscopy, both ring fingers.	Retrospective, observational, longitudinal study.	10/11 (91%) had irregularly enlarged capillaries and 11/11 (100%) had haemorrhages at baseline, reducing to 2/11 (18%) and 0/11 (0%) post-treatment.	Patients re-examined after treatment (duration not stated).	Not directly examined.	Capillaroscopic abnormalities regressed with treatment (no details of treatment given).
Chanprapaph et al. 2021 [93]	32 DM.	DM vs SLE, DM vs SSc. 54 SLE, 51 SSc, 108 HC.	USB microscopy (Dino-Lite). Magnification 200x. Ring and little fingers of both hands.	Cross-sectional study. Single centre.	Bushy capillaries found more often in DM than in SSc. Over 90% of patients with DM had 'scleroderma-type pattern' of capillary abnormality.	Not applicable.	No relationship between capillaroscopic abnormality and skin disease (as assessed by cutaneous assessment tool for myositis) in patients with DM.	Abnormalities characteristic of DM could be well visualised with USB microscope.

(continued)

Table 2 (continued)

Reference	Number of subjects with IIM	Comparators if relevant—healthy controls/other disease	NFC technique used	Summary of methods	Summary of results	If longitudinal component, duration of follow up and key points	Associates	Key conclusions
Johnson et al. 2021 [94]	15 DM.	Baseline vs post-treatment.	Videocapillaroscopy. Magnification 200x. 8 fingers.	Prospective cohort study.	With treatment, capillary density increased, mean apical diameter reduced.	13 patients restudied after treatment (mean interval duration 12 months, range 9–15 months).	Capillary density was associated with global disease activity, and with cutaneous, muscle and constitutional disease.	Nailfold capillary abnormalities regress with treatment, and capillary density was associated with disease activity.
Shenavandeh, Rashidi. 2022 [58]	150 IIM patients including 81 DM, 25 CADM, 19 PM, 25 JDM, evaluated according to EULAR/ ACR criteria with second analysis of 104 patients evaluated according to Troyanov and Senécal classification [78, 79]: 53 pure DM, 51 overlap myositis.	Comparative analysis of IIM subgroups.	Stereomicroscopy, magnification 250x. Qualitative and quantitative assessment. 8 fingers, excluding thumbs examined.	Cross sectional single centre study. Patients selected and evaluated using both the EULAR/ ACR and Troyanov and Senécal classification.	Scleroderma pattern dominant ($\geq$70%) in DM, CADM and overlap myositis, but less common in PM—Seen in 8/19 patients (42%) defined by EULAR/ ACR criteria. Using Troyanov and Senécal criteria, > 75% of patients with pure DM or overlap myositis had a scleroderma pattern.	Not applicable.	Scleroderma pattern associated with high skin disease activity and global disease activity in DM and overlap myositis.	This study confirms that abnormal NFC, particularly scleroderma pattern is common in DM and CADM but not PM. It also discusses differences depending on classification criteria used, due to inclusion of overlap myositis. In DM and overlap myositis, some associations were seen between NFC abnormalities and markers of disease activity.

Paudyal et al. 2023 [95]	62 DM (49 had CADM).	None.	Dermatoscope. Magnification 10x. 10 fingers. Single observer.	Cohort study with longitudinal component.	Most patients had abnormalities, including bushy capillaries in 47/54 (87.0%) and scleroderma-like pattern in 26/54 (48.1%).	54 patients re-examined at 12 and 24 weeks. 'Improvement' including in terms of avascular areas at 24 weeks.	Did not directly correlate capillaroscopy scores with disease activity, but examined changes in disease activity in relation to baseline capillaroscopy findings.	Results suggest that dermoscopy may be sufficiently sensitive to detect change over time in nailfold capillary abnormalities in patients with DM.
Hysa et al. 2023 [96]	30 DM.	Comparison with SSc (n = 601), MCTD (n = 70) and other CTDs.	Videocapillaroscopy. Magnification 200x. 8 fingers.	Retrospective, single site study of 1181 patients being assessed for RP.	Patients with DM had comparable numbers of giant capillaries, capillary dilations and microhaemorrhages (and similar capillary density) to patients with SSc.	Not applicable.	Not examined.	Capillary changes in patients with DM were similar to those in SSc, although fewer patients with DM were included than with SSc.

(continued)

Table 2 (continued)

Reference	Number of subjects with IIM	Comparators if relevant—healthy controls/other disease	NFC technique used	Summary of methods	Summary of results	If longitudinal component, duration of follow up and key points	Associates	Key conclusions
Torres-Ruiz et al. 2024 [51]	155 IIM (including 95 with DM, 26 with ASynS, 12 with IMNM, 2 with PM and 10 with overlap myositis).	Between group comparisons.	Videocapillaroscopy 8 fingers.	Cross-sectional study with longitudinal component, with a focus on autoantibodies. Three centres from 3 countries.	Only 14 (9%) patients reported to have normal capillaries. Scleroderma pattern in approximately half of patients with DM and overlap myositis, 81% of patients with ASynS had non-specific changes.	23 patients re-examined when disease controlled (duration not given). Abnormalities regressed as disease became inactive.	The key associates reported were with autoantibodies. SSc pattern most represented with anti-TIF-1ɣ (10/17), anti-Mi2 (6/9), and anti-SAE (4/4). Non-specific abnormalities found with anti-Jo-1 (14/18).	Abnormalities were most marked in patients with DM and overlap myositis: Findings in those with ASynS were 'between' those with DM and PM. Autoantibody associations were a key result of this study.
Bogojevic et al. 2024 [81]	90 IIM: 37 DM, 35 PM, 13 CADM, 5 JDM.	DM vs PRP, PM vs PRP, CADM vs PRP. 35 with PRP	Not stated.	Cross-sectional study.	A scleroderma pattern was reported in 81.9% of DM, 2.9% of PM, 76.9% pf CADM.	Not applicable.	Patients with a scleroderma pattern were those most likely to have cutaneous manifestations, RP and ILD.	This study further highlighted the increased prevalence of nailfold capillary abnormalities in patients with DM and CADM compared to in PM.

ARS aminoacyl-tRNA synthetase, *ASynS* anti-synthetase syndrome, *CK* creatine kinase, *DM* dermatomyositis, *CADM* clinically amyopathic dermatomyositis, *IIM* Idiopathic inflammatory myopathy, *IMNM* immune-mediated necrotising myopathy, *HC* healthy controls, *ILD* interstitial lung disease, *JDM* juvenile dermatomyositis, *MAA* myositis associated antibody, *MSA* myositis specific antibody, *NFC* nailfold capillaroscopy, *PM* polymyositis, *PRP* primary Raynaud's phenomenon, *RA* rheumatoid arthritis, *RBC* red blood cell, *RP* Raynaud's phenomenon, *SLE* systemic lupus erythematosus, *SS* Sjogren's syndrome, *SSc* systemic sclerosis, *UCTD* undifferentiated connective tissue disease patients within this study had JDM. Each child was examined using a standardized nailfold video capillaroscopy technique with a 200x magnification contact lens, capturing 8 fingers. NFC was assessed quantitively and qualitatively. Patients with JDM had a significantly lower nailfold capillary density with a mean of 6.3 capillaries/linear mm (S.D. 2.0) compared to healthy controls who had a mean nailfold capillary density of 8.5 capillaries /linear mm (S.D. 1.2). In contrast, nailfold capillary density in patients with primary Raynaud's phenomenon was similar to that of healthy controls. An increased number of dilated capillaries were seen in JDM with a mean of 1.5 dilated capillaries/linear mm (S.D 1.2) compared to healthy controls (mean 0.5 dilated capillaries/linear mm, S.D. 0.6). Patients with JDM also exhibited significantly more abnormal shapes compared to healthy controls, with 0.9/linear mm (S.D. 1.0) in JDM, and 0.3 (S.D 0.3) in healthy controls. Significantly more patients with JDM (85.3%) had micro-haemorrhages than healthy controls (39.2%) [53].

Studies in Adults

Maricq and LeRoy reported over 50 years ago that marked nailfold capillary abnormalities occur in patients with DM as well as in patients with SSc [62]. Several studies (Table 2) have demonstrated abnormalities in patients with IIM compared to healthy controls or to patients with primary Raynaud's phenomenon, especially in patients with DM [81, 83–86]. Manfredi et al., in their study of 52 adult patients with IIM (29 DM, 23 PM) and 52 with primary Raynaud's phenomenon reported abnormalities in most of the evaluated parameters (for example capillary loss, giant capillaries, ramified capillaries) in IIM compared to primary Raynaud's phenomenon [86]. As mentioned in the next section, these abnormalities were almost exclusively in patients with DM (as opposed to with PM). In a retrospective study of 190 patients with ASynS [67], NFC appearances were significantly different to those in 75 patients with primary Raynaud's phenomenon: for example 35.3% of patients with ASynS had an 'SSc-like' pattern compared to none of those with primary Raynaud's phenomenon, and 49.5% of patients had ramified capillaries compared to 6.7% of patients with primary Raynaud's phenomenon. Note that the term 'SSc-like' was used in this study [67] to describe a pattern similar to the scleroderma pattern. Some authors have used this term, or 'scleroderma-like' to describe a pattern which has the elements of a scleroderma pattern but which does not conform completely to any of the 'early', 'active' or 'late' patterns described by Cutolo et al. [98].

Comparing JIIM with SSc or Other Connective Tissue Disease

Studies in Children

Several studies have identified NFC abnormalities in JDM, jSSc, MCTD and jSLE, but scleroderma pattern, seen frequently in JDM and jSSc, is not apparent in jSLE [41, 56, 70]. Melsens et al. found a similarly lower nailfold capillary density in patients with JDM and SSc relative to healthy controls (6.3 capillaries/linear mm [S.D. 2.0] in JDM and 5.2 capillaries/linear mm, [S.D. 1.9] in SSc, compared to 8.5

capillaries/linear mm in healthy controls) [53]. Nailfold capillary density was also reduced relative to healthy controls in patients with MCTD (7.1 capillaries/linear mm, S.D. 1.3), localised scleroderma (7.7 capillaries/linear mm, S.D. 1.2) and jSLE (7.6 capillaries/linear mm, S.D. 1.3) but not in JIA. The decreased nailfold capillary density seen in patients with localised scleroderma in this study is surprising, and it is important to note the small numbers of patients within each connective tissue disease subgroup. Other studies including patients with localised scleroderma compared to JDM have noted lack of scleroderma pattern in patients with localised scleroderma [41, 56].

As mentioned above, Melsens et al. found that patients with JDM had an increased number of dilated capillaries compared to healthy controls. Differences were also seen in patients with MCTD and jSSc (mean of 1.8 capillary dilatations / linear mm in both MCTD and SSc, compared to mean of 1.5 capillary dilatations/ linear mm in JDM). Similarly more abnormal capillary shapes were seen in patients with JDM, MCTD and jSSc relative to healthy controls, whereas the number of abnormal shapes was found to be similar to healthy controls in patients with primary Raynaud's phenomenon, jSLE, localised scleroderma and JIA [53]. Microhaemorrhages were observed in patients from all CTD groups (JDM 85.3%, jSSc 84.6%, MCTD 77.8%, jSLE 80%), with the proportion of patients with microhaemorrhages significantly greater than those with primary Raynaud's phenomenon (55%) or healthy controls (39.2%) [53].

Studies in Adults

Manfredi et al. [87] examined 29 patients with DM and 90 patients with SSc who were selected on the basis of their capillaroscopic pattern (30 'early', 30 active' and 30 'late') (Table 2). They reported appearances in DM which tended to be 'between' the different subgroups of SSc (e.g. capillary loss in DM more marked than in 'early' SSc pattern but less than in active/late groups). 'Giant-ramified' capillaries (ramified capillaries with a diameter of >50 μm) were almost exclusive to DM, and occurred early on in the disease course. Change over time differed between 20 of the patients with DM who were studied longitudinally over 30 months compared to the 90 patients with SSc. There was a tendency for patients with DM (unlike those with SSc) to revert towards normal: in DM density increased over time and severity score for giant capillaries fell, although the score for ramified capillaries rose [87]. The authors highlighted that a key difference between DM and SSc was the finding of 'giant-ramified' capillaries early on in the disease course (ramified capillaries tend to occur later on in the SSc disease course and are not 'giant') and suggested that distinction should be made between a 'scleroderma-pattern' and a 'DM-pattern.' These findings were supported in a study of 24 patients with DM and 24 with SSc where the score for ramified capillaries was higher in those patients with disease duration less than one year (compared to more than one year) [88]. In this study, patients with DM had higher scores for ramified capillaries and capillary disorganisation than those with SSc, but lower scores for giant capillaries and microhaemorrhages [88].

Other studies have compared capillaroscopy findings between patients with IIM and SSc and have reported abnormalities in IIM although these tend to be less prevalent than in SSc [45, 89]. In a study of 1181 patients with Raynaud's phenomenon secondary to different connective tissue diseases referred to a single centre [96], 30 patients with DM displayed very similar degrees of capillary abnormality to 601 patients with SSc: comparable proportions of patients with DM had giant capillaries (73% of DM, 73% of SSc), capillary dilations i.e. diameter between 20 and 50 μm (96% DM, 99% SSc) and microhaemorrhages (70% DM, 70 SSc), and capillary density was similar (6.5 capillaries/mm ± 0.75 in patients with DM versus 7.04 ± 0.18 in patients with SSc) [96]. The fact that even studies from the same centre [88, 96] can report somewhat differing results may reflect the heterogeneity of the diseases in question and (perhaps) different disease durations.

That bushy capillaries are found more often in DM than in SSc has also been shown in a study from Thailand including comparison between 32 patients with DM and 51 with SSc [93]. This study was of interest because it demonstrated that these abnormalities can be well demonstrated using a USB microscope (magnification 200x).

Comparing JDM/DM with Other Subtypes of IIM

Studies in Children

Several studies have shown that DM is associated with the greatest degree of capillary abnormality compared to other IIM sub-types. This is less well determined in JIIM than in adults due to the rarity of non-JDM phenotypes sub-types in juvenile-onset disease. In an observational cross sectional study of 90 patients diagnosed with IIM according to EULAR/ACR classification criteria, 5 patients had JDM. Patients with JDM exhibited a high frequency of scleroderma pattern (4/5, 80%), similar to DM (30/37, 81.9%) and CADM (10/13, 76.9%) [81].

Studies in Adults

Several studies have highlighted how DM is the subtype of IIM associated with the greatest degree of capillary abnormality [45, 51, 63, 83, 84, 87] and this has been highlighted in a recent review article [98]. Over the years, conflicting results have been reported regarding scleroderma patterns in patients with PM. This may partly be explained by heterogeneity in the diagnostic or classification criteria used. In studies using the Bohan and Peter or equivalent criteria, patients described within PM groups may include individuals who would now be defined by the presence of anti-Jo-1 antibody as ASynS using the EULAR/ACR criteria. This may help to explain why Kubo et al., who distinguished patients as PM (n = 18) or DM (n = 52) using the Diagnostic Criteria of the Ministry of Health, Labour and Welfare in Japan 1995, which includes the presence of anti-aminoacyl-tRNA synthetase antibodies as one of the nine features of PM/DM, identified a scleroderma-like pattern in 22.2% of PM and 32.7% of DM patients [45]. Although Bohan and Peter, Sontheimer's criteria for CADM and EULAR/ACR criteria were also applied to this cohort, data for NFC patterns according to classification criteria were not shown. Manfredi et al., defining patients as PM (n = 23) or DM (n = 29) by the Bohan and Peter criteria, reported how all the abnormalities assessed were more prevalent in the 29 patients with DM compared to the 23 patients with PM. For example, ramified capillaries were noted in 58.6% of patients with DM but only 8.7% of patients with PM, and giant capillaries (noted in 65.5% of patients with DM), avascular areas (noted in 31% of patients with DM) and a 'scleroderma pattern' (noted in 69% of patients with DM) were not found in any patients with PM [86]. The authors also described a significant reduction in number of capillaries seen in 75.9% of DM patients compared to only 4.2% of PM patients and no control patients. The study did not distinguish ASynS from PM/DM. Later studies have included a broader range of IIM subtypes, reflecting the evolving classification of IIM and including the study by Torres-Ruiz et al. [51] described in the next paragraph. In the study of 90 patients with IIM (37 DM, 35 with PM, 13 with CADM and 5 with JDM) already mentioned under 'studies in children' Bogojevic et al. reported a scleroderma pattern in 81.9% of DM, and 76.9% of CADM, but only 2.9% of PM, confirming previous studies suggesting that capillary abnormalities are much less prevalent in the PM subgroup [81].

Patients with ASynS appear to have NFC alterations similar to DM as opposed to PM, perhaps reflecting the role of vasculopathy in the pathophysiology of ASynS [98]. Bernardino et al. found that all 17 patients with DM and all 4 patients with ASynS investigated in this study had a scleroderma pattern on nailfold videocapillaroscopy, in contrast to the 3 patients with PM, in whom none had a scleroderma pattern [99]. Torres-Ruiz et al. evaluated 155 patients from three centres in Mexico, Spain and the United States of America, investigating nailfold capillaroscopy abnormalities and their associations. In this study, DM (n = 95), PM (n = 2), ASynS (n = 26), IMNM (n = 12), IBM (n = 7), overlap myositis (n = 10) were defined by the EULAR/ACR 2017 classification criteria [51]. They reported how the 26 patients with ASynS had capillary abnormalities but these were less marked than in patients with DM [51]. They identified a scleroderma pattern in only 4 out of 26 (15.3%) of patients with ASynS compared to 51.5% in DM and none in PM. A non-specific pattern was found in 80.7% of patients with ASynS and only 1 patient (3.8%) with ASynS had normal NFC [51].

In a study including 43 patients with inflammatory myopathy, pronounced abnormalities in terms of avascular areas and vascular disorganisation were seen only in patients with DM and overlap syndromes and not in patients with ASynS or IMNM, although subgroup numbers were small [89]. The authors excluded 5 patients with uninterpretable images, reflecting the real-world situation when not all people have well visualised capillaries.

Role of NFC as a Potential Marker of Disease Activity and of Treatment Response in DM/JDM

A key aim in the treatment of IIM is to treat early and aggressively in order to optimise health related quality of life and prevent disease damage. Systemic immunosuppressive therapy is guided by clinical findings, with the help of serological and radiological investigations. Currently available serum biomarkers may not reflect disease activity. Muscle enzymes can fall to normal range, particularly in children with JDM despite active muscle and skin inflammation [100]. More sensitive markers of disease activity are needed to guide therapy. Vascular biomarkers such as circulating endothelial cells, microparticles, and galectin-9, among others, show promise, but require further validation and are not currently available in routine clinical practice [29].

Studies in Children

Studies suggest that capillary loss associates with disease activity and internal organ involvement, thus NFC can be a useful non-invasive biomarker in clinical practice [52, 56, 66, 71, 73]. NFC abnormalities have been found to associate with active disease but normalise, or at least improve, with disease remission in many patients with JDM [56, 64, 71]. In a proportion of patients, however, NFC changes have been found to remain stable over time despite improvement in disease activity [70, 71]. It is possible that failure to show normalisation of NFC may relate to subclinical or immunological activity in a patient that has clinically inactive disease. However, Khojah et al. in a study of 68 patients with JDM with follow up data for at least 5 years including at least 4 NFC assessments, found the mean end row loop for treatment naïve JDM patients was significantly lower than that of the healthy control group (n = 77), and despite improvement over time, it remained below expected for healthy controls, even after 5 years [80]. The authors suggest that perhaps current therapeutic strategies do not adequately target endothelial function adequately.

Several studies (Table 1) in children have documented change over time in NFC morphology and density [52, 64, 70, 71, 80]. The most common NFC finding in JDM is reduced nailfold capillary density, prominent at time of diagnosis, with a tendency to improve over time in response to treatment [52, 71, 73]. In a study of 92 JDM patients, including 28 patients within an inception cohort with NFC at diagnosis and follow up, normalisation of nailfold capillary density was found over 12 months in almost 50% of cases, thought to be due to treatment [52].

The degree of morphological changes in NFC appears to correlate with the clinical course of JDM and several studies (Table 1) have documented an association between nailfold capillary density and disease activity [23, 52, 71, 73, 75]. Ostrowski et al., in a study of 80 children with JDM captured at diagnosis, 24 and 36 months follow up, found that a longer duration of untreated disease at diagnosis and higher skin-Disease Activity score (skin-DAS) at diagnosis was associated with the development of abnormal nailfold end row loops over time [74]. Schmeling et al. found loss of end row loops was moderately associated with skin and muscle disease activity that was more pronounced at the beginning of the disease course [52]. This retrospective study captured longitudinal follow up of 92 patients (total of 809 clinic visits) with concurrent NFC over a time period of 5.5 years. They reported that for each capillary per millimetre increase in NFC density, the likelihood of having a normal health-related quality of life (which was transformed to a binary normal or abnormal for purposes of analysis) increased by 24% (OR = 1.24, p = 0.0009). Nailfold capillary density also associated with overall quality of life, functional assessment (measured by Childhood Health Assessment Questionnaire, CHAQ), muscle strength (measured by Manual Muscle Testing, MMT), overall disease severity and pain in this study [52].

A single centre study by Barth et al. of 58 patients with JDM with a median disease duration of 16.8 years had NFC evaluated along with disease activity and damage scores [75]. NFC was also compared to 45 healthy controls. Compared with controls, patients with JDM had more microvascular abnormalities in all NFC measures including decreased nailfold capillary density, dilated capillaries, haemorrhages, scleroderma and neovascular pattern. Patients with active disease presented more frequently with neovascular pattern compared to those with inactive disease. Decreased nailfold capillary density and neovascular pattern were associated with higher levels of disease activity and impaired muscle function. This suggests that there is role for NFC as a biomarker of disease activity in both skin and muscle [75]. Similarly, Christen-Zaech et al., in a single centre longitudinal study of 61 patients with JDM, captured pre-treatment and monitored over time, with a mean follow up time of 29.6 +/− 10.2 months (range 3.2–38.6), showed that over 36 months end row loop regeneration was associated with lower cutaneous disease measured by the skin-DAS [73]. However, in contrast to the study by Barth et al., an association was not seen with muscle-DAS. In the study by Christen-Zaech et al., those patients that had a chronic disease course typically had continuing skin manifestations with persistent NFC changes. A longer duration of untreated disease correlated with worsening of NFC abnormalities [73]. Although NFC at time of diagnosis could not predict disease course, the persistence of vascular abnormalities linked to skin disease activity in this study suggests that more aggressive treatment should be considered even in the absence of muscle disease to prevent complications such as calcinosis.

The majority of studies in juvenile onset disease relate to JDM, but a case report of a 4 year old child with CAJDM demonstrated improvement in NFC in response to treatment, leading the authors to suggest that NFC can be used as a convenient prognostic and monitoring parameter for skin involvement seen in these patients [101].

The course of JIIM can be broadly separated into monocyclic, polycyclic or chronic. Chronic continuous course is defined as persistent disease activity for more than 2 years post-diagnosis, whereas in monocyclic (also called unicyclic) disease there is full recovery within 2 years without relapse [102]. Numerous studies (Table 1) have shown that a chronic disease course is associated with persistent NFC abnormalities [64, 68, 80]. In contrast, NFC changes return to normal in individuals with a limited or monocyclic disease course [64, 68, 80]. A study by Khojah et al. investigating data from 68 initially treatment-naïve patients followed over 5 years found variation in the rate of improvement in end row loop count depending on disease course [80]. Patients with monocyclic disease demonstrated a faster rate of improvement in end row loop count than those with a chronic disease course [80].

Polycyclic disease course is defined as a recurrence of disease activity, with at least one flare, after a period of remission for more than 6 months [102]. Huber et al. questioned whether patients with polycyclic disease were truly in remission as opposed to having sub-clinical persistent inflammation, thus representing a chronic disease course [102]. This theory is backed up in a study by Papadopoulou et al., showing that circulating endothelial cells as a marker of endothelial injury were significantly elevated in patients with active disease relative to inactive disease, and that both circulating endothelial cell and galectin-9 as markers of vasculopathy, were higher in patients with abnormal NFCs compared to those with normal capillaries [19]. The fact that circulating endothelial cells were elevated in a proportion of patients who had abnormalities of NFC but were considered clinically to have inactive disease supports the notion of clinically quiescent but immunologically active disease. This raises the question of whether NFC can help determine those patients who need more careful monitoring for signs or symptoms of disease chronicity to prevent future disease-related damage.

Studies in Adults

That capillary abnormalities might change over time in adults with IIM, especially in those with DM, has been recognised for many years [98]. This was well demonstrated in a case report from 2010 when very abnormal nailfold capillaries in a 40 year old male with DM improved dramatically after 6 months treatment with corticosteroids and immunosuppression [103]. De Angelis et al. performed nailfold videocapillaroscopy in 6 patients with DM and in 9 with SSc at monthly intervals for 3 months [104]. The investigators were careful to ensure that the same sections of the nailfolds (one from each finger) were considered/compared over the four time points. Appearances changed over 3 months in patients with DM but not in patients with SSc [104].

Given the reports of capillary abnormalities being most marked in early disease, it is likely that the degree of change over time (if any) may depend at least in part on the stage of disease at which patients are examined. In 16 patients with well-established IIM (only 3 with DM) followed over 6–12 months reported by Mercer et al., capillary density fell over time, although not significantly, and in some patients nailfold architecture changed markedly (change in capillary density – 1.4 capillaries/mm in IIM, −0.4 in healthy controls) [84]. Mugii et al. suggested that in 12 patients with active DM followed over an average of 9.2 months, scores for irregularly enlarged capillaries, haemorrhages and loss of capillaries decreased (i.e. improved) with stabilisation of disease [85]. Manfredi et al. reported that in 20 patients with DM followed over 30 months, there was a reduction in giant capillaries and an increase in capillary density (i.e. improvement) whereas the number of ramified capillaries increased (perhaps reflecting an attempt at angiogenesis) [87]. In 40 previously untreated patients with IIM, reported by Kubo et al., there was substantial improvement/regression in capillary appearances after one year of treatment [45]. The authors suggested that the nailfold abnormalities in IIM might be driven by perivascular inflammation (which they demonstrated on skin biopsy) which could be suppressed with immunosuppressant treatment.

Pizzorni et al. reported no significant changes over 3 years in capillaroscopy scores in 12 patients with DM, although the proportion of patients with ramified capillaries increased from 84% at baseline to 100% at 3 years [88]. However, patients recruited into this study had well established disease. 'Improvement 'in capillary appearances after treatment, as assessed using a stereomicroscope was observed in a cohort of 23 patients with very early DM (median duration of symptom 3 months) [90]: in the 15 patients re-examined after approximately 3 years, median capillary density increased from 5.0/mm to 7.3/mm and there were reductions (improvements) in the number of giant capillaries, avascular areas, and haemorrhages [90]. The number of 'bushy capillaries' did not change. In another study of patients with short disease duration (median 1 year, range 0–6 years), in the 13 patients who were studied after a mean treatment duration of 12 months (range 9–15 months), mean capillary density increased (4.71/mm at baseline and 6.84/mm at follow-up [$p = 0.006$]), and mean apical diameter fell (56.1 μm at baseline and 27.8 μm at follow-up [$p = 0.003$]), indicating improvement [94].

In a retrospective study of 11 patients with anti-MDA5 positive adult DM, capillaroscopic abnormalities regressed after treatment: 10/11 (91%) had irregularly enlarged capillaries and 11/11 (100%) had haemorrhages at baseline, reducing to 2/11 (18%) and 0/11 (0%) respectively post-treatment [92]. Nailfold capillary abnormalities also regressed in the 23 patients followed over time by Torres-Ruiz et al.: specifically as disease became inactive, capillary density increased and avascularity reduced [51].

A study from China of 62 patients with DM was of interest because it suggested that abnormalities in nailfold capillaries could be readily seen with a dermatoscope (magnification 10x): most patients had abnormalities, including bushy capillaries in 47/54 (87.0%) and scleroderma-like pattern in 26/54 (48.1%) [95]. Also, changes in certain capillaroscopic features including avascular areas (present in 75.9% of patients at baseline and 47.1% at 24 weeks) were demonstrated, suggesting the dermatoscope may be sufficiently sensitive to monitor change over time [95]. This study therefore confirmed findings from an earlier study in 2003 suggesting that nailfold capillary changes in patients with DM can be identified using a dermatoscope [105]. If this is confirmed in larger studies this has important implications for disease monitoring because the relatively low-cost dermatoscope is likely to be easily accessible to most rheumatologists and dermatologists.

Associates of Capillary Abnormality

Several studies have examined for associations between nailfold capillaroscopic abnormalities and clinical and laboratory features. Conflicting results/conclusions have a number of possible explanations, including differences in the way capillary abnormalities have been reported and in the way in which internal organ involvement is defined, the heterogeneity of the populations studied, and (often) the small numbers of patients studied. The main associates will be discussed here. Some others are mentioned in Tables 1 and 2.

Association with Disease Duration

Studies in Children

Smith et al., in a study of 60 patients with JDM determined that NFC findings were associated with length of time of untreated disease [69]. The greater the symptom duration prior to therapy, the worse the NFC structure with increased bushy and dilated loops and end row loop capillary drop out [69]. This was confirmed by Pachman et al. in a study of 140 JDM patients that identified that there was more damage to end row loop with longer duration of untreated disease [66]. Other studies have also shown association with duration of untreated disease and over time, end row loop regeneration associated with shorter duration of untreated disease [73, 74, 77].

Studies in Adults

Several studies (Table 2) have shown that in patients with DM, abnormalities are more marked in early disease. For example, Manfredi et al. reported that patients with disease duration of 6 months or less had more marked capillary enlargement and capillary loss than those with longer duration disease, although ramified capillaries were equally represented (and seen in the majority of patients) irrespective of disease duration [86]. The 37/50 patients with DM and a 'scleroderma' pattern reported by Mugii et al. had a shorter disease duration (mean 37.0 months) than the 13/50 without a scleroderma pattern (mean 75.8 months) [85]. Conversely amongst 190 patients with ASynS, a SSc-like pattern was more likely to be seen in later disease [67].

Association with Muscle Disease Activity and Severity

Studies in Children

Abnormal muscle biopsy findings with extensive loss of capillary bed have been found to corelate with abnormal NFC patterns as described above [41]. Christen-Zaech et al. found that a monocylic disease course associated with increased end row loop regeneration and improvement in both muscle and skin DAS at 36 months [73]. However, with regards to evaluating disease activity over time, although correlation has been found between NFC and skin disease, musculoskeletal findings captured by DAS-muscle do not appear to correlate with NFC end row capillary loss [69, 73]. In a study of 140 patients with JDM, Pachman et al. identified that children with decreased end row loop had more skin disease than muscle disease [66]. Schmeling et al. in a study of 92 JDM patients found that loss of end row loop associated with musculoskeletal involvement or function, but association was modest relative to the association seen for skin disease. The relationship was more pronounced at the beginning of disease course [52].

Studies in Adults

Different studies have varied in their conclusions as to whether the degree of nailfold capillaroscopy change is related to muscle disease activity and severity. An early study from 1988 reported no significant differences in nailfold capillary appearances in the 23 patients with muscle weakness compared to the eight without [63].

A study of 53 patients with IIM reported in 2010 suggested that muscle disease activity and severity were greater in those with the more abnormal capillaries [83]. Association with muscle disease activity was also suggested in a study of 50 adult patients with DM by Mugii et al. [85], but not in the 70 patients described by Kubo *et al* [45]. In the prospective study (including 13 patients studied before and after treatment) reported by Johnson et al., capillary density was independently associated with global disease as measured by the Myositis Intention to Treat Index (MITAX) and decreased capillary density was associated with muscle disease [94].

Association with Skin Disease

Studies in Children

Smith et al. determined from a study of 60 untreated JDM patients that skin involvement, measured by skin-DAS was associated with loss of end row capillary number and terminal loop vascular bush formation on NFC [69]. Higher skin-DAS at diagnosis has been associated with increased likelihood of abnormal end row loop when evaluated over 36 months, and end row loop regeneration has been associated with lower skin-DAS [73, 74]. Improvement in end row loop regeneration and skin-DAS have been associated with a monocyclic disease course and in contrast, persistence of skin disease and NFC changes have been associated with a non-monocyclic disease course [73]. In a study by Stringer et al., investigating 84 patients with JDM with the aim of determining predictors of disease course, the presence of NFC abnormalities plus Gottron's papules at 6 months post diagnosis predicted a longer time to remission. This relationship was stronger than for NFC abnormalities or Gottron's as individual predictors [72].

Studies in Adults

Mugii et al. showed an association between skin disease activity and the severity score for haemorrhages [85]. In the 70 patients reported by Kubo et al., skin changes were more prevalent in those patients with scleroderma pattern abnormalities than in those without, and patients with scleroderma pattern changes were more likely to have moderate or severe perivascular inflammation on skin biopsy [45]. Johnson et al. reported that decreased capillary density was associated with cutaneous disease [94]. Torres-Ruiz et al. reported that of the 78 patients with cutaneous features, 41 (52.5%) had a scleroderma pattern and 33 (42.3%) had non-specific abnormalities [51]. In the study by Bogojevic et al., of 90 patients with IIM, skin manifestations (Gottron's sign, heliotrope rash and periungual erythema) were found especially in those with a scleroderma pattern of capillary abnormality [81].

Other studies have not shown an association with skin disease [93]. There are many reasons for the inconsistent findings, including the patient populations (disease heterogeneity and difference disease durations), different ways of classifying disease, different methods of assessing skin disease and different methods of acquiring nailfold images and of interpreting nailfold capillaroscopy.

Association with Raynaud's Phenomenon

If might seem intuitive that severity of capillaroscopic change might be associated with presence and/or severity of Raynaud's phenomenon as reported in a number of studies [63, 81, 83]. However, several studies have found no association between the capillary abnormality and Raynaud's phenomenon [45, 57, 84].

Association with Autoantibodies

Studies in Children

In JDM, the presence of anti-P155/140 (now typically classified as anti-TIF1) autoantibodies was found to have a lower end row loop count when compared to patients with other MSA sub-types or negative MSA, raising the suggestion that this MSA may impact the vascular component of JDM [77]. This association was confirmed in a more recent study by the same group, evaluating 140 JDM patients [66].

Studies in Adults

As testing for MSA and Myositis Associated Antibodies (MAA) has become more widespread and as (in parallel) the classification of IIMs has evolved, the number of reports of associations between nailfold capillaroscopic appearances and autoantibodies is increasing. Findings have been somewhat conflicting, again most likely reflecting the heterogeneity of the IIMs, often the small number of patients studied and different capillaroscopic methods.

Mercer et al. found that capillary density was lower (4.8/mm) in 8 patients who were anti-Jo-1-positive compared to the 16 who were anti-Jo-1 negative (6.8/mm) [84]. However, in a later study including 24 patients with DM, Pizzorni et al. reported similar capillaroscopy findings in 13 patients who were anti-Jo-1 negative compared to the 11 who were anti-Jo-1 positive [88].

Later studies included a wider range of autoantibodies. In the study reported by Sebastiani et al. of 190 patients with ASynS, the 133 patients who were anti-Jo-1 antibody positive had a higher prevalence of a SSc-like pattern of capillaries (44%) than those who were anti-Jo-1 negative (21.5%) [67]. In 70 Japanese patients, the 39 patients with scleroderma pattern changes were more likely than those without to be positive for anti-MDA5 and anti-TIF1γ antibodies, but less likely to be anti-aminoacyl tRNA synthetase antibody positive [45]. Perhaps consistent with this, in a study of 27 patients with DM-ILD, the 10 patients who were anti-MDA5 antibody positive had higher scores for microhaemorrhages and capillary disorganisation than the 17 patients who were anti-aminoacyl-tRNA synthetase positive [91]. Torres-Ruiz et al. reported a detailed comparison of nailfold capillary abnormalities in patients with different MSA and MAA. Key findings were that a scleroderma pattern was most commonly found in patients with anti-TIF-1ɣ (10/17), anti-Mi2 (6/9), and anti-SAE (4/4) autoantibodies [51]. Non-specific abnormalities were found in patients who were anti-Jo-1 antibody positive (14/18). Bogogevic et al. reported that patients who had a non-specific capillaroscopic pattern were those most likely to be anti-Jo-1 positive [81].

Flatley et al., in their review of 37 papers (346 patients) searched for associations between capillaroscopic findings and MSAs and MAAs and made the point that few studies have specifically examined this issue: they identified only 51 patients (from 6 different reports) in whom MSA/MAA status was known and numbers were too small to draw any firm conclusions, although abnormalities were reported in most of the patients (including 31 positive for anti-MDA-5, 10 positive for anti-TIF-1ɣ and 6 positive for anti-NXP2) [61]. In conclusion, there are some pointers towards anti-MDA5, and anti-TIF1ɣ antibodies being associated with more marked capillary changes than are associated with anti-Jo-1, but more detailed studies are required to explore this further.

Association with Malignancy

An association between the severity of nailfold capillary change and malignancy has been reported in some studies, although patients numbers were small [83]. De Angelis et al. demonstrated nailfold capillary changes over a very short time frame (1–2 months) in a case report of cancer associated CADM [106]. Sugimoto et al. identified NFC abnormalities associated with anti-TIF-1ɣ cancer-associated DM and reported improvement over time as the patient's general condition improved [107]. Interestingly, worsening of NFC abnormalities over time in this case associated temporarily with enlargement of the primary lesion (small cell lung cancer) on contrast enhanced computerised tomography and improvement in NFC was seen with tumour shrinkage in response to therapy [107].

Association with Organ Involvement or Disease Complications

Systemic vasculopathy and subsequent microvascular remodelling may play an important role in involvement of various organs such as the lungs and gut.

Lung Involvement NFC abnormalities have been associated with pulmonary disease in DM and JDM [76, 108]. This raises the possibility of NFC being used in clinical practice to determine risk of complications such as ILD and prompting investigations to allow early detection and treatment of ILD when present. This is important since pulmonary involvement is associated with a poor prognosis in JDM and DM [109, 110]. However, it is important to note that pulmonary involvement was seen in a proportion of patients with normal NFC suggesting that other factors aside from microvascular involvement are relevant [76].

In a single centre study of 58 patients with JDM examined after a mean disease duration of 17 years, low nailfold capillary density was identified in 21 patients (36%) and found to be associated with pulmonary involvement determined by HRCT or pulmonary function tests [76]. Specifically, an association was found between low nailfold capillary density and smaller lung volumes (FVC and TLC) and reduced gas diffusion (DLCO). HRCT-assessed airway disease was more prevalent in patients with low capillary density compared to those with normal capillary density. Pulmonary involvement was mostly subclinical, which raises the possibility that NFC can be used as a non-invasive method to predict risk of complications such as ILD and prompt investigation [76].

Wakura et al. in their study of 27 patients with DM-ILD, reported that the degree of nailfold capillary loss was associated with total fibrosis score on HRCT (Spearman's correlation coefficient 0.73) [91]. The 3 patients who died due to ILD had higher microhaemorrhage and neoangiogenesis scores than the 24 who were still alive [91]. In a retrospective single centre study of 95 patients with IIM (27 DM, 22 PM, 29 ASynS, 3 IMNM and 14 overlap myositis), comparing those with and without ILD, the presence of ILD associated with avascular zones, low capillary density and microhaemorrhages on NFC [108]. In multi-variate analysis the presence of avascular areas, loss of capillary density and 'active pattern' as defined by Cutolo's classification were identified as predictors of IIM-ILD [108]. In patients with ASynS, Sebastiani et al. reported that a SSc-like pattern on NVC was associated with late onset ILD [67].

Cardiac Involvement In the study by Barth et al., described above of 58 children with JDM, there was no significant association of nailfold capillary density with cardiac involvement as determined by electrocardiography (ECG), Holter monitoring and echocardiography (ECHO) [76].

Gastrointestinal Involvement A small single-centre study of 6 patients with JDM demonstrated that patients with active JDM had decreased bioavailability of oral prednisolone compared to the equivalent dose of steroids administered by the intravenous route. Difference in intravenous methylprednisolone versus oral prednisolone bioavailability was associated with NFC end row loop, suggesting that those patients with capillary obliteration had decreased absorption of oral prednisolone. The authors speculated that the decreased end row loops seen on NFC of patients with active disease may also possibly occur in the gastrointestinal tract leading to impaired absorption of oral medications [73]. However, this study has very small patient numbers and thus should be interpreted with caution.

Pachman et al. found in a retrospective study of 140 JDM patients that the presence of periungual haemorrhages at first assessment closely associated with dysphagia [66]. Sieiro Santos et al. identified an association between dysphagia and low capillary density, avascular zones and enlarged capillaries on nailfold videocapillaroscopy in a retrospective study of 95 patients with adult-onset IIM, mentioned above, but the purpose of this study was to evaluate the relationship between nailfold capillary abnormalities and pulmonary outcomes and details of how dysphagia was assessed were lacking [108].

Calcinosis In a retrospective single centre study evaluating an inception cohort of 172 patients with JDM to determine risk factors for calcinosis, nailfold capillaroscopy abnormality at baseline was the only risk factor reaching statistical significance in univariate analysis with a hazard ratio of 4.86 ($P = 0.03$) [23]. In multivariate analysis including nailfold capillary abnormality, age of diagnosis, sex and duration of disease from onset to diagnosis, the presence of NFC abnormality remained the only statistically significant risk factor for calcinosis (HR 4.98, $P = 0.03$). Calcinosis was seen in 44 (26%) patients in this cohort and was more likely to develop in those with a chronic disease course [23]. Previous studies have also documented risk of calcinosis to be increased by a longer duration of untreated disease, longer disease course and more severe disease [111, 112]. Tsaltskan et al. found that for each additional year of disease duration, odds of calcinosis increased by 12% [22]. The strongest predictors of calcinosis were disease duration, periungual nailfold capillary changes and younger age at onset. However, Khojah et al. did not find an association between calcinosis and end row loop count [80]. It is suggested that worsening vasculopathy over time results in more tissue damage and scarring, with resultant dystrophic calcium deposition. By using NFC as a marker of disease activity and vasculopathy and treating aggressively, it is possible that complications such as calcinosis could be prevented or minimised. Torres-Ruiz et al. reported lower capillary density in patients with adult-onset IIM who had calcinosis than in those without calcinosis [51]. Of the 20 patients they studied who had calcinosis, 10 had a scleroderma patterns and 10 had non-specific abnormalities [51].

Lipodystrophy Khojah et al. identified that patients with lipodystrophy had a lower end row loop capillary count when cumulatively evaluated using area under the curve compared to those without lipodystrophy [80].

Future Research Applications

Recent years have seen an expansion of interest in examining and studying nailfold capillaries in children and adults with IIM. This is an exciting time for NFC research in patients with IIM, because of parallel advances in our recognition and understanding of the different IIM subtypes (including their different autoantibody associations) and in nailfold capillary image acquisition and interpretation, including (as discussed in chapter "Image Interpretation") international efforts to standardise interpretation.

As discussed earlier in this chapter, several studies have shown that especially in patients with DM/JDM, nailfold capillary abnormalities provide a very visible window into current disease 'status' i.e. active or inactive, progressing or 'improving' (perhaps in response to treatment). However, these studies have often been hampered by small patient numbers and subjectivity of image analysis. As NFC becomes more widely available, so the opportunities for large multicentre studies increase. These multicentre studies will be facilitated by the growing interest in applying artificial intelligence approaches to nailfold capillary image analysis [113]. These approaches hold promise for objective, quantitative, rapid image analysis, as discussed in chapter "Quantitative Analysis".

Future large-scale studies should include longitudinal studies of treatment response, studies examining NFC appearances as predictors of disease trajectories, and association studies. These association studies (including studies of autoantibody associations) should increase our understanding of IIM pathophysiology. Future studies should also include consideration of the patient perspective: do patients feel that seeing their nailfold capillaries improves their understanding of their disease, a key step in optimising their management.

Conclusions

The presence of NFC abnormalities is not universal in IIM, but when present, can be helpful in aiding diagnosis of the condition, monitoring disease activity and predicting risk of organ complications or disease damage. Decreased capillary density in particular is recognised as associating with global and skin-disease activity, as well as risk of ILD and calcinosis. Whilst NFC changes seen in IIM can be similar to those seen in SSc and MCTD, the presence of 'bushy' capillaries has been reported to be characteristic of IIM. Scleroderma pattern is commonly seen in JDM/DM (including CADM), overlap myositis, and ASynS, but not in PM. Thus, the pattern of NFC abnormality may help in disease classification. The EULAR/ACR classification for IIM has been reported to be sub-optimal for recognising CADM, and NFC has been proposed as a potential item for inclusion in classification criteria for skin predominant IIM. The importance of NFC in diagnosis and monitoring of juvenile onset IIM, where vasculopathy is particularly apparent, is recognised by its inclusion in UK and European consensus guidelines.

It is important to note that there are a number of conflicting results and conclusions across studies relating to NFC in IIM. There are many reasons for the inconsistent findings, including disease heterogeneity and difference disease durations within populations studies, different diagnostic or classification criteria used for subtypes of IIM, different methods of assessing disease activity and the way in which internal organ involvement is defined, and different methods of acquiring nailfold images and interpreting or reporting nailfold capillary changes. Nonetheless, many studies show the utility of NFC in current clinical practice, and hand-held low-cost devices make this easily accessible as a tool. Research applications include the possibility of NFC to help determine treatment response in clinical trials, mainly in DM/JDM as well as examining pathogenesis and of looking for associates.

References

1. Khoo T, Lilleker JB, Yu-Hor Thong B, Leclair V, Lamb JA, Chinoy H. Epidemiology of the idiopathic inflammatory myopathies. Nat Rev Rheumatol. 2023;19(11):695–712.
2. Meyer A, Meyer N, Schaeffer M, Gottenberg J-E, Geny B, Sibilia J. Incidence and prevalence of inflammatory myopathies: a systematic review. Rheumatology. 2015;54(1):50–63.
3. Lundberg IE, Fujimoto M, Vencovsky J, Aggarwal R, Holmqvist M, Christopher-Stine L, et al. Idiopathic inflammatory myopathies. Nat Rev Dis Prim. 2021;7(1):1–22.
4. Halilu F, Christopher-Stine L. Myositis-specific antibodies: overview and clinical utilization. Rheumatol Immunol Res. 2022;3(1):1–10.
5. Martin N, Krol P, Smith S, Murray K, Pilkington CA, Davidson JE, et al. A national registry for juvenile dermatomyositis and other paediatric idiopathic inflammatory myopathies: 10 years' experience; the juvenile Dermatomyositis national (UK and Ireland) cohort biomarker study and repository for idiopathic inflammatory Myopat. Rheumatology. 2011;50(1):137–45.
6. Shah M, Mamyrova G, Targoff IN, Huber AM, Malley JD, Rice MM, et al. The clinical phenotypes of the juvenile idiopathic inflammatory myopathies. Medicine (Baltimore). 2013 Jan;92(1):25–41.
7. Martin N, Krol P, Smith S, Beard L, Pilkington CA, Davidson J, et al. Comparison of children with onset of juvenile dermatomyositis symptoms before or after their fifth birthday in a UK and Ireland juvenile dermatomyositis cohort study. Arthritis Care Res. 2012;64(11):1665–72.
8. Mamyrova G, Kishi T, Targoff IN, Ehrlich A, Curiel RV, Rider LG, et al. Features distinguishing clinically amyopathic juvenile dermatomyositis from juvenile dermatomyositis. Rheumatology (Oxford). 2018;157(11):1956–63.
9. Naveen R, Rathore U, Agarwal V, Gupta L. Characteristics and outcomes of overlap myositis: a comparative multigroup cohort study in adults from the MyoCite cohort. Rheumatol Int. 2021;41:551–63.
10. Rider LG, Shah M, Mamyrova G, Huber AM, Rice MM, Targoff IN, et al. The myositis autoantibody phenotypes of the juvenile idiopathic inflammatory myopathies. Medicine (Baltimore). 2013;92(4):223–43.
11. Pauling JD, Christopher-Stine L. The aetiopathogenic significance, clinical relevance and therapeutic implications of vasculopathy in idiopathic inflammatory myopathy. Rheumatology (Oxford). 2021;60(4):1593–607.
12. Kwiatkowska D, Reich A. The significance of autoantibodies in juvenile Dermatomyositis. Biomed Res Int. 2021;2021:5513544.
13. Pinal-Fernandez I, Casal-Dominguez M, Huapaya JA, Albayda J, Paik JJ, Johnson C, et al. A longitudinal cohort study of the anti-synthetase syndrome: increased severity of interstitial lung disease in black patients and patients with anti-PL7 and anti-PL12 autoantibodies rheumatology key messages. Rheumatology. 2017;56:999–1007.
14. Pinal-Fernandez I, Casal-Dominguez M, Mammen AL. Immune-mediated necrotizing myopathy. Curr Rheumatol Rep. 2018;20(4):21.
15. Shelly S, Mielke MM, Mandrekar J, Milone M, Ernste FC, Naddaf E, et al. Epidemiology and natural history of inclusion body myositis a 40-year population-based study criteria for rating therapeutic and diagnostic studies. Neurology. 2021;96(21):e2653–61.

16. Oldroyd AG, Callen JP, Chinoy H, Chung L, Fiorentino D, Gordon P, et al. Evidence-based guidelines international guideline for idiopathic inflammatory myopathy-associated cancer screening: an international myositis assessment and clinical studies group (IMACS) initiative. Nat Rev Rheumatol. 2024;20(5):315.
17. Stübgen JP. Juvenile dermatomyositis/polymyositis and lymphoma. J Neurol Sci. 2017;377:19–24.
18. Rider LG, Nistala K. The juvenile idiopathic inflammatory myopathies: pathogenesis, clinical and autoantibody phenotypes, and outcomes. J Intern Med. 2016;280(1):24–38.
19. Papadopoulou C, Hong Y, Krol P, Al Obaidi M, Pilkington C, Wedderburn LR, et al. The vasculopathy of juvenile Dermatomyositis: endothelial injury, hypercoagulability, and increased arterial stiffness. Arthritis Rheumatol. 2021;73(7):1253–66.
20. Lim D, Fiorentino D, Werth V. Current concepts and advances in dermatomyositis: a dermatological perspective. Clin Exp Rheumatol. 2023;41(2):359–69.
21. Valenzuela A, Chung L, Casciola-Rosen L, Fiorentino D. Identification of clinical features and autoantibodies associated with calcinosis in dermatomyositis. JAMA Dermatol. 2014;150(7):724–9.
22. Tsaltskan V, Aldous A, Serafi S, Yakovleva A, Sami H, Mamyrova G, et al. Long-term outcomes in juvenile myositis patients. Semin Arthritis Rheum. 2020;50(1):149–55.
23. Nozawa T, Bell-Peter A, Marcuz JA, Whitney K, Vinik O, Shupak R, et al. Early abnormal Nailfold capillary changes are predictive of calcinosis development in juvenile Dermatomyositis. J Rheumatol. 2022;49(11):1250–5.
24. Rothwell S, Chinoy H, Lamb JA, Miller FW, Rider LG, Wedderburn LR, et al. Focused HLA analysis in Caucasians with myositis identifies significant associations with autoantibody subgroups. Ann Rheum Dis. 2019;78(7):996–1002.
25. Deakin CT, Bowes J, Rider LG, Miller FW, Pachman LM, Sanner H, et al. Association with HLA-DRβ1 position 37 distinguishes juvenile dermatomyositis from adult-onset myositis. Hum Mol Genet. 2022;31(14):2471–81.
26. Wilkinson MGL, Radziszewska A, Wincup C, Ioannou Y, Isenberg DA, Manson JJ, et al. Using peripheral blood immune signatures to stratify patients with adult and juvenile inflammatory myopathies. Rheumatology (United Kingdom). 2020;59(1):194–204.
27. Shakshouk H, Deschaine MA, Wetter DA, Drage LA, Ernste FC, Gibson LE, et al. Do histopathological features correlate with systemic manifestations in dermatomyositis? Analysis of 42 skin biopsy specimens from 22 patients. J Cutan Pathol. 2022;49(5):442–7.
28. Allenbach Y, Uzunhan Y, Toquet S, Leroux G, Gallay L, Marquet A, et al. Different phenotypes in dermatomyositis associated with anti-MDA5 antibody: study of 121 cases. Neurology. 2020;95(1):70–8.
29. McLellan K, Papadopoulou C. Update on biomarkers of vasculopathy in juvenile and adult myositis. Curr Rheumatol Rep. 2022;24(7):227–37.
30. Wienke J, Deakin CT, Wedderburn LR, van Wijk F, van Royen-Kerkhof A. Systemic and tissue inflammation in juvenile Dermatomyositis: from pathogenesis to the quest for monitoring tools. Front Immunol. 2018;9:2951.
31. Kim H. Updates on interferon in juvenile dermatomyositis: pathogenesis and therapy. Curr Opin Rheumatol. 2021;33(5):371–7.
32. Ma X, Gao H-J, Zhang Q, Yang M-G, Bi Z-J, Ji S-Q, et al. Endoplasmic reticulum stress is involved in muscular pathogenesis in idiopathic inflammatory myopathies. Front Cell Dev Biol. 2022;10:791986.
33. Duvvuri B, Pachman LM, Morgan G, Khojah AM, Klein-Gitelman M, Curran ML, et al. Neutrophil extracellular traps in tissue and periphery in juvenile Dermatomyositis. Arthritis Rheumatol (Hoboken, NJ). 2020;72(2):348–58.
34. Seto N, Torres-Ruiz JJ, Carmona-Rivera C, Pinal-Fernandez I, Pak K, Purmalek MM, et al. Neutrophil dysregulation is pathogenic in idiopathic inflammatory myopathies. JCI Insight. 2020;5(3):e134189.

35. Wilkinson MGL, Moulding D, McDonnell TCR, Orford M, Wincup C, Ting JYJ, et al. Role of CD14+ monocyte-derived oxidised mitochondrial DNA in the inflammatory interferon type 1 signature in juvenile dermatomyositis. Ann Rheum Dis. 2022;82(5):658–69.
36. Pachman LM, Nolan BE, DeRanieri D, Khojah AM. Juvenile Dermatomyositis: new clues to diagnosis and therapy. Curr Treat Options Rheumatol. 2021;7(1):39–62.
37. Rider LG, Wu L, Mamyrova G, Targoff IN, Miller FW. Environmental factors preceding illness onset differ in phenotypes of the juvenile idiopathic inflammatory myopathies. Rheumatology (Oxford). 2010;49(12):2381–90.
38. Saud A, Naveen R, Aggarwal R, Gupta L. COVID-19 and myositis: what we know so far. Curr Rheumatol Rep. 2021;23(8):63.
39. Wang G, Wang Q, Wang Y, Liu C, Wang L, Chen H, et al. Presence of anti-MDA5 antibody and its value for the clinical assessment in patients with COVID-19: a retrospective cohort study. Front Immunol. 2021;12:791348.
40. Preuße C, Allenbach Y, Hoffmann O, Goebel HH, Pehl D, Radke J, et al. Differential roles of hypoxia and innate immunity in juvenile and adult dermatomyositis. Acta Neuropathol Commun. 2016;4(1):45.
41. Spencer-Green G, Schlesinger M, Bove KE, Levinson JE, Schaller JG, Hanson V, et al. Nailfold capillary abnormalities in childhood rheumatic diseases. J Pediatr. 1983;102(3):341–6.
42. Gitiaux C, De Antonio M, Aouizerate J, Gherardi RK, Guilbert T, Barnerias C, et al. Vasculopathy-related clinical and pathological features are associated with severe juvenile dermatomyositis rheumatology key messages. Rheumatology. 2016;55:470–9.
43. Wienke J, Enders FB, Lim J, Mertens JS, Van Den Hoogen LL, Wijngaarde CA, et al. Galectin-9 and CXCL10 as biomarkers for disease activity in juvenile Dermatomyositis: a longitudinal cohort study and multicohort validation. Arthritis Rheumatol. 2019;71(8):1377–90.
44. Lerkvaleekul B, Veldkamp SR, van der Wal MM, Schatorjé EJH, Kamphuis SSM, van den Berg JM, et al. Siglec-1 expression on monocytes is associated with the interferon signature in juvenile dermatomyositis and can predict treatment response. Rheumatology (Oxford). 2022;61(5):2144–55.
45. Kubo S, Todoroki Y, Nakayamada S, Nakano K, Satoh M, Nawata A, et al. Significance of nailfold videocapillaroscopy in patients with idiopathic inflammatory myopathies. Rheumatology (Oxford). 2019;58(1):120–30.
46. Bohan A, Peter JB. Polymyositis and Dermatomyositis. N Engl J Med. 1975;292(7):344–7.
47. Leclair V, Lundberg IE. New myositis classification criteria—what we have learned since Bohan and Peter. Curr Rheumatol Rep. 2018;20(4):18.
48. Lundberg IE, Tjärnlund A, Bottai M, Werth VP, Pilkington C, de Visser M, et al. 2017 European league against rheumatism/American College of Rheumatology classification criteria for adult and juvenile idiopathic inflammatory myopathies and their major subgroups. Ann Rheum Dis. 2017;76(12):1955–64.
49. Patel B, Khan N, Werth VP. Applicability of EULAR/ACR classification criteria for dermatomyositis to amyopathic disease. J Am Acad Dermatol. 2018;79(1):77–83.e1.
50. Concha JSS, Pena S, Gaffney RG, Patel B, Tarazi M, Kushner CJ, et al. Developing classification criteria for skin-predominant dermatomyositis: the Delphi process. Br J Dermatol. 2020;182(2):410–7.
51. Torres-Ruiz J, Pinal-Fernandez I, Selva-O'Callaghan A, Campbell B, Muñoz-Braceras S, Mejía-Domínguez NR, et al. Nailfold capillaroscopy findings of a multicentric multiethnic cohort of patients with idiopathic inflammatory myopathies. Clin Exp Rheumatol. 2024;42(2):367–76.
52. Schmeling H, Stephens S, Goia C, Manlhiot C, Schneider R, Luthra S, et al. Nailfold capillary density is importantly associated over time with muscle and skin disease activity in juvenile dermatomyositis. Rheumatology. 2011;50(5):885–93.
53. Melsens K, Cutolo M, Schonenberg-Meinem D, Foeldvari I, Leone MC, Mostmans Y, et al. Standardized nailfold capillaroscopy in children with rheumatic diseases: a worldwide study. Rheumatology (United Kingdom). 2023;62(4):1605–15.

54. Chong BF, Werth V. Cutaneous lupus erythematosus and Dermatomyositis: utilizing assessment tools for treatment efficacy. J Invest Dermatol. 2022;142(3):936–43.
55. Dolezalova P, Young SP, Bacon PA, Southwood TR. Nailfold capillary microscopy in healthy children and in childhood rheumatic diseases: a prospective single blind observational study. Ann Rheum Dis. 2003;62(5):444–9.
56. Piotto DGP, Len CA, Hilário MOE, Terreri MTRA. Nailfold capillaroscopy in children and adolescents with rheumatic diseases. Rev Bras Reumatol. 2012;52(5):722–32.
57. Torrente-Segarra V, Hernández-Baldizón S, Mosquera JM, Antón J. The importance of nailfold capillaroscopy in children with rheumatic diseases. Lin Exp Rheumatol. 2021;39(Suppl 1):35.
58. Shenavandeh S, Rashidi F. Nailfold capillaroscopy changes with disease activity in patients with inflammatory myositis including overlap myositis, pure dermatomyositis, and pure polymyositis. Reumatologia. 2022;60(1):42–52.
59. Enders FB, Bader-Meunier B, Baildam E, Constantin T, Dolezalova P, Feldman BM, et al. Consensus-based recommendations for the management of juvenile dermatomyositis. Ann Rheum Dis. 2016;76(2):329–40.
60. Oldroyd AGS, Lilleker JB, Amin T, Aragon O, Bechman K, Cuthbert V, et al. British Society for Rheumatology guideline on management of paediatric, adolescent and adult patients with idiopathic inflammatory myopathy. Rheumatology. 2022;61(5):1760–8.
61. Flatley EM, Collins D, Lukowiak TM, Miller JH. Nailfold microscopy in adult-onset dermatomyositis in association with myositis antibodies. Arch Dermatol Res. 2024;317(1):34.
62. Maricq HR, LeRoy EC. Patterns of finger capillary abnormalities in connective tissue disease by "wide-field" microscopy. Arthritis Rheum. 1973;16(5):619–28.
63. Ganczarczyk ML, Lee P, Armstrong SK. Nailfold capillary microscopy in polymyositis and dermatomyositis. Arthritis Rheum. 1988;31(1):116–9.
64. Silver RM, Maricq HR. Childhood dermatomyositis: serial microvascular studies. Pediatrics. 1989;83(2):278–83.
65. Bertolazzi C, Cutolo M, Smith V, Gutierrez M. State of the art on nailfold capillaroscopy in dermatomyositis and polymyositis. Semin Arthritis Rheum. 2017;47(3):432–44.
66. Pachman LM, Morgan G, Klein-Gitelman MS, Ahsan N, Khojah A. Nailfold capillary density in 140 untreated children with juvenile dermatomyositis: an indicator of disease activity. Pediatr Rheumatol. 2023;21(1):1–9.
67. Sebastiani M, Triantafyllias K, Manfredi A, González-Gay MA, Palmou-Fontana N, Cassone G, et al. Nailfold Capillaroscopy characteristics of Antisynthetase syndrome and possible clinical associations: results of a Multicenter international study. J Rheumatol. 2019;46(3):279–84.
68. Spencer-Green G, Crowe WE, Levinson JE. Nailfold capillary abnormalities and clinical outcome in childhood dermatomyositis. Arthritis Rheum. 1982;25(8):954–8.
69. Smith RL, Sundberg J, Shamiyah E, Dyer A, Pachman LM. Skin involvement in juvenile dermatomyositis is associated with loss of end row nailfold capillary loops. J Rheumatol. 2004;31(8):1644–9.
70. Ingegnoli F, Zeni S, Gerloni V, Fantini F. Capillaroscopic observations in childhood rheumatic diseases and healthy controls. Clin Exp Rheumatol. 2005;23(6):905–11.
71. Nascif AKS, Terreri MTRA, Len CA, Andrade LEC, Hilário MOE. Inflammatory myopathies in childhood: correlation between nailfold capillaroscopy findings and clinical and laboratory data. J Pediatr. 2006;82(1):40–5.
72. Stringer E, Singh-Grewal D, Feldman BM. Predicting the course of juvenile dermatomyositis: significance of early clinical and laboratory features. Arthritis Rheum. 2008;58(11):3585–92.
73. Christen-Zaech S, Seshadri R, Sundberg J, Paller AS, Pachman LM. Persistent association of nailfold capillaroscopy changes and skin involvement over thirty-six months with duration of untreated disease in patients with juvenile dermatomyositis. Arthritis Rheum. 2008;58(2):571–6.
74. Ostrowski RA, Sullivan CL, Seshadri R, Morgan GA, Pachman LM. Association of normal nailfold end row loop numbers with a shorter duration of untreated disease in children with juvenile dermatomyositis. Arthritis Rheum. 2010;62(5):1533–8.

75. Barth Z, Witczak BN, Flatø B, Koller A, Sjaastad I, Sanner H. Assessment of microvascular abnormalities by Nailfold Capillaroscopy in juvenile Dermatomyositis after medium- to long-term Followup. Arthritis Care Res. 2018;70(5):768–76.
76. Barth Z, Schwartz T, Flatø B, Aaløkken TM, Koller A, Lund MB, et al. Association between nailfold capillary density and pulmonary and cardiac involvement in medium to longstanding juvenile dermatomyositis. Arthritis Care Res. 2019;71(4):492–7.
77. Khojah A, Liu V, Savani SI, Morgan G, Shore R, Bellm J, et al. Association of p155/140 autoantibody with loss of Nailfold capillaries but not generalized lipodystrophy: a study of Ninety-Six children with juvenile Dermatomyositis. Arthritis Care Res. 2022;74(7):1065–9.
78. Troyanov Y, Targoff IN, Payette M-P, Raynauld J-P, Chartier S, Goulet J-R, et al. Redefining Dermatomyositis. Medicine (Baltimore). 2014;93(24):318–32.
79. Senécal J, Raynauld J, Troyanov Y. Editorial: a new classification of adult autoimmune myositis. Arthritis Rheumatol. 2017;69(5):878–84.
80. Khojah A, Morgan G, Klein-Gitelman MS, Pachman LM. Juvenile dermatomyositis: association between nail fold capillary end row loop– area under the curve– and disease damage indicators. Pediatr Rheumatol. 2023;21(1):1–8.
81. Bogojevic M, Markovic Vlaisavljevic M, Medjedovic R, Strujic E, Pravilovic Lutovac D, Pavlov-Dolijanovic S. Nailfold Capillaroscopy changes in patients with idiopathic inflammatory myopathies. J Clin Med. 2024;13(18):5550.
82. Nagy Z, Czirják L. Nailfold digital capillaroscopy in 447 patients with connective tissue disease and Raynaud's disease. J Eur Acad Dermatol Venereol. 2004;18(1):62–8.
83. Selva-O'Callaghan A, Fonollosa-Pla V, Trallero-Araguás E, Martínez-Gómez X, Simeon-Aznar CP, Labrador-Horrillo M, et al. Nailfold capillary microscopy in adults with inflammatory myopathy. Semin Arthritis Rheum. 2010 Apr;39(5):398–404.
84. Mercer LK, Moore TL, Chinoy H, Murray AK, Vail A, Cooper RG, et al. Quantitative nailfold video capillaroscopy in patients with idiopathic inflammatory myopathy. Rheumatology. 2010;49(9):1699–705.
85. Mugii N, Hasegawa M, Matsushita T, Hamaguchi Y, Horie S, Yahata T, et al. Association between nail-fold capillary findings and disease activity in dermatomyositis. Rheumatology. 2011;50(6):1091–8.
86. Manfredi A, Sebastiani M, Cassone G, Pipitone N, Giuggioli D, Colaci M, et al. Nailfold capillaroscopic changes in dermatomyositis and polymyositis. Clin Rheumatol. 2015;34(2):279–84.
87. Manfredi A, Sebastiani M, Campomori F, Pipitone N, Giuggioli D, Colaci M, et al. Nailfold Videocapillaroscopy alterations in Dermatomyositis and systemic sclerosis: toward identification of a specific pattern. J Rheumatol. 2016;43(8):1575–80.
88. Pizzorni C, Cutolo M, Sulli A, Ruaro B, Trombetta AC, Ferrari G, et al. Long-term follow-up of nailfold videocapillaroscopic changes in dermatomyositis versus systemic sclerosis patients. Clin Rheumatol. 2018;37(10):2723–9.
89. Soubrier C, Seguier J, Di Costanzo M-P, Ebbo M, Bernit E, Jean E, et al. Nailfold videocapillaroscopy alterations in dermatomyositis, antisynthetase syndrome, overlap myositis, and immune-mediated necrotizing myopathy. Clin Rheumatol. 2019;38(12):3451–8.
90. Miossi R, de Souza FHC, Shinjo SK. Nailfold capillary changes in adult new-onset dermatomyositis: a prospective cross-sectional study. Clin Rheumatol. 2019;38(9):2319–26.
91. Wakura R, Matsuda S, Kotani T, Shoda T, Takeuchi T. The comparison of nailfold videocapillaroscopy findings between anti-melanoma differentiation-associated gene 5 antibody and anti-aminoacyl tRNA synthetase antibody in patients with dermatomyositis complicated by interstitial lung disease. Sci Rep. 2020;10(1):15692.
92. Hamaguchi Y, Mugii N, Matsushita T, Takehara K. Long-term changes in nail fold capillary abnormalities and serum fibroblast growth factor 23 levels in dermatomyositis patients with anti-melanoma differentiating antigen 5 antibody. J Dermatol. 2021;48(1):106–9.
93. Chanprapaph K, Fakprapai W, Limtong P, Suchonwanit P. Nailfold Capillaroscopy with USB digital microscopy in connective tissue diseases: a comparative study of 245 patients and healthy controls. Front Med. 2021;8:683900.

94. Johnson D, van Eeden C, Moazab N, Redmond D, Phan C, Keeling S, et al. Nailfold Capillaroscopy abnormalities correlate with disease activity in adult Dermatomyositis. Front Med. 2021;8:708432.
95. Paudyal A, Yang Y, Zheng M, Zhang X, Wang H, Gong S, et al. Assessment of nail fold capillary changes by hand-held dermoscopy in adult dermatomyositis: a single-Centre prospective study. Australas J Dermatol. 2023 Nov;64(4):514–21.
96. Hysa E, Pizzorni C, Sammorì S, Gotelli E, Cere A, Schenone C, et al. Microvascular damage in autoimmune connective tissue diseases: a capillaroscopic analysis from 20 years of experience in a EULAR training and research referral Centre for imaging. RMD Open. 2023 Jul;9(3):e003071.
97. Ingegnoli F, Herrick AL. Nailfold capillaroscopy in pediatrics. Arthritis Care Res. 2013;65(9):1393–400.
98. Piette Y, Reynaert V, Vanhaecke A, Bonroy C, Gutermuth J, Sulli A, et al. Standardised interpretation of capillaroscopy in autoimmune idiopathic inflammatory myopathies: a structured review on behalf of the EULAR study group on microcirculation in rheumatic diseases. Autoimmun Rev. 2022 Jun;21(6):103087.
99. Bernardino V, Rodrigues A, Lladó A, Panarra A. Nailfold capillaroscopy and autoimmune connective tissue diseases in patients from a Portuguese nailfold capillaroscopy clinic. Rheumatol Int. 2020 Feb;40(2):295–301.
100. Pachman LM, Abbott K, Sinacore JM, Amoruso L, Dyer A, Lipton R, et al. Duration of illness is an important variable for untreated children with juvenile dermatomyositis. J Pediatr. 2006;148(2):247–53.
101. Campos LMA, Sallum AME, Camargo CZ, Andrade LEC, Kayser C. Improvement of nailfold capillary microangiopathy after immunosuppressant therapy in a child with clinically amyopathic juvenile dermatomyositis. Rev Bras Reumatol. 2017;57(5):487–90.
102. Huber AM, Lang B, LeBlanc CM, Birdi N, Bolaria RK, Malleson P, et al. Medium- and long-term functional outcomes in a multicenter cohort of children with juvenile dermatomyositis. Arthritis Rheum. 2000;43(3):541–9.
103. Riccieri V, Vasile M, Macri V, Sciarra I, Stefanantoni K, De Luca N, et al. Successful immunosuppressive treatment of dermatomyositis: a nailfold capillaroscopy survey. J Rheumatol. 2010 Feb;37(2):443–5.
104. De Angelis R, Cutolo M, Gutierrez M, Bertolazzi C, Salaffi F, Grassi W. Different microvascular involvement in dermatomyositis and systemic sclerosis. A preliminary study by a tight videocapillaroscopic assessment. Clin Exp Rheumatol. 2012;30(2 Suppl 71):S67–70.
105. Bergman R, Sharony L, Schapira D, Nahir MA, Balbir-Gurman A. The handheld dermatoscope as a nail-fold capillaroscopic instrument. Arch Dermatol. 2003 Aug;139(8):1027–30.
106. De Angelis R, Bertolazzi C, Filippucci E, Gutierrez M, Grassi W. Fast microvascular remodelling in a patient with cancer-associated dermatomyositis: capillaroscopic followup. Rheumatology. 2010;49(2):400. https://doi.org/10.1093/rheumatology/kep281.
107. Sugimoto T, Mokuda S, Yamaguchi K, Araki K, Kohno H, Yoshida Y, et al. Rapid changes of nailfold capillary abnormalities during treatment for a patient with dermatomyositis complicated by lung cancer: a case report. Mod Rheumatol Case Rep. 2021;5(1):95–100.
108. Sieiro Santos C, Tandaipan JL, Castillo D, Codes-Mendez H, Martínez-Martínez L, Magallares B, et al. Nailfold videocapillaroscopy findings correlate with lung outcomes in idiopathic inflammatory myopathies–related interstitial lung disease. Rheumatology (Oxford). 2024;10:keae669. https://doi.org/10.1093/rheumatology/keae669. Epub ahead of print. PMID: 39658251
109. Huber AM, Mamyrova G, Lachenbruch PA, Lee JA, Katz JD, Targoff IN, et al. Early illness features associated with mortality in the juvenile idiopathic inflammatory myopathies. Arthritis Care Res. 2014;66(1):732–40.
110. Hallowell RW, Paik JJ. Myositis-associated interstitial lung disease: a comprehensive approach to diagnosis and management. Clin Exp Rheumatol. 2022;40(2):373–83.
111. Saini I, Kalaivani M, Kabra SK. Calcinosis in juvenile dermatomyositis: frequency, risk factors and outcome. Rheumatol Int. 2016 Jul;36(7):961–5.

112. Hoeltzel MF, Oberle EJ, Robinson AB, Agarwal A, Rider LG. The presentation, assessment, pathogenesis, and treatment of calcinosis in juvenile Dermatomyositis. Curr Rheumatol Rep. 2014;16(12):467.
113. Kassani PH, Ehwerhemuepha L, Martin-King C, Kassab R, Gibbs E, Morgan G, et al. Artificial intelligence for nailfold capillaroscopy analyses—a proof of concept application in juvenile dermatomyositis. Pediatr Res. 2024;95(4):981–7.

Nailfold Capillaroscopy in Other Rheumatological Diseases

John D. Pauling

Key Points

- Nailfold capillaroscopic abnormalities are seen in many autoimmune rheumatic diseases other than SSc and IIM
- The presence of SSc-pattern nailfold capillary abnormalities in the context of lupus, mixed connective tissue disease and primary Sjogren's syndrome is often associated with SSc-associated clinical manifestations such as severe Raynaud's, interstitial lung disease (ILD) and pulmonary arterial hypertension (PAH)
- Other disease-specific nailfold capillary abnormalities have been proposed such as the 'lupus-pattern' but nailfold capillaroscopy has not established as important a role in the diagnosis of other rheumatological diseases compared to SSc and IIM
- The presence of nailfold capillary abnormalities in 'other' rheumatological diseases provides important mechanistic insight into the presence of vasculopathy across the autoimmune rheumatic diseases
- Evidence of regression of nailfold capillary abnormalities following effective treatment of lupus and vasculitis provides evidence for potential vascular repair in the autoimmune rheumatic diseases

Introduction

The aetiopathogenesis and clinical features of the autoimmune rheumatic diseases are characterised by vasculopathy, inflammation/autoimmunity and aberrant tissue remodelling/fibrosis. In many of these connective tissue diseases, vasculopathy is

J. D. Pauling (✉)
Department of Rheumatology, North Bristol NHS Trust, Translational Health Sciences, Bristol Medical School, University of Bristol, Bristol, UK
e-mail: John.Pauling@nbt.nhs.uk

A. L. Herrick et al. (eds.), *Nailfold Capillaroscopy in Rheumatological Diseases*,
https://doi.org/10.1007/978-3-032-03970-5_8

the result of immune-mediated endothelial injury that weakens the structural integrity of the vessel wall leading to haemorrhage and vascular leak, eventually progressing to an obliterative microangiopathy with permanent capillary loss and avascularity. The aetiopathogeneis of vasculopathy and the role of nailfold capillaroscopy (NC) as a tool for directly visualising the microvasculature is described fully in earlier chapters. Quite reasonably, individual chapters of the present book have also been devoted to the clinical utility of nailfold capillaroscopy in the assessment of systemic sclerosis (SSc) (chapters "Image Interpretation" and "Nailfold Capillaroscopy in Systemic Sclerosis (Including Associations)"). Much of the research into nailfold capillaroscopy has focussed on SSc in view of the virtual omnipresence of Raynaud's phenomenon (RP) and NC abnormalities in SSc. The next most extensively investigated group of disorders for NC has been the Idiopathic Inflammatory Myopathies (IIM), since Lépine identified features of vascular injury in IIM, proposing the term 'angiomyositis' [1]. RP is also a frequent (but not universal) symptom in IIM which can often clinically overlap with SSc. The role of NC in the assessment of IIM is the focus of chapter "Nailfold Capillaroscopy in Idiopathic Inflammatory Myopathies".

As the method of nailfold capillaroscopy has been developed and refined in terms of image acquisition and analysis, a growing body of literature has also emerged describing the prevalence and clinical significance of nailfold capillaroscopic abnormalities in other rheumatological diseases. Studies in rheumatological disease other than SSc and dermatomysositis (DM) were often smaller studies and sometimes enrolled mixed populations of patients, particularly those undertaken before 2000. Advances in serological disease sub-setting and updated classification criteria may also have led to the historical misclassification of included patients as having rheumatoid arthritis (RA), undifferentiated connective tissue disease (uCTD), systemic lupus erythematosus (SLE), or mixed connective tissue disease (MCTD); for whom modern diagnostic work up would suggest IIM or SSc-spectrum disease. An interesting observation is that much of the work undertaken in NC prior to 1980 took an agnostic view of underlying diagnosis. This likely reflects the heterogeneous patient mix in nascent CTD clinics from the era, but it is also evident that investigators remained unsure in which of the individual CTDs NC would prove most clinically useful. Some of the early positive smaller studies may have been subject to publication bias and additional biases may have occurred on account of the subjective nature of traditional qualitative methods for reporting NC changes. To date, in contrast to SSc, nailfold capillaroscopy is primarily a research tool in non-SSc disorders and has yet to establish a role in disease classification or routine clinical assessment of such diseases. Nonetheless, NC abnormalities do appear to be present in some patients with other rheumatological diseases and some of the NC abnormalities described (e.g. 'brush-like' microhaemorrhages, see later) appear distinct from those associated with SSc and IIM; potentially providing valuable additional mechanistic insight into contribution of vascular injury in the aetiopathogenesis of other rheumatological diseases. Indeed, it is over 40 years since investigators considered the diagnostic specificity of specific NC findings in connective tissue disease (CTD) [2]. In overlap disease, the presence of SSc-pattern NC changes may support better understanding the relative contribution of SSc-spectrum disease to the overall clinical phenotype, which could also have clinical utility in disease subsetting and personalised medicine approaches. NC can also help delineate CTD-features in organ-specific autoimmunity that can occur in overlap with SSc. For example, scleroderma NC changes are found in over half of patients with interstitial pneumonia with autoimmune features (IPAF) and may support better characterisation of such patients with therapeutic implications [3] (Fig. 1). NC can also predict the presence of SSc features in patients with primary biliary cirrhosis [4]. In the present chapter, I shall discuss the prevalence and clinical utility of NC abnormalities in rheumatological diseases other than SSc and IIM. I shall sub-categorise the chapter into the CTDs, inflammatory arthropathy, vasculitis and other diseases. Where applicable, I shall draw comparisons with the more extensively studied changes present in SSc and IIM, highlighting relevant areas of unmet research need.

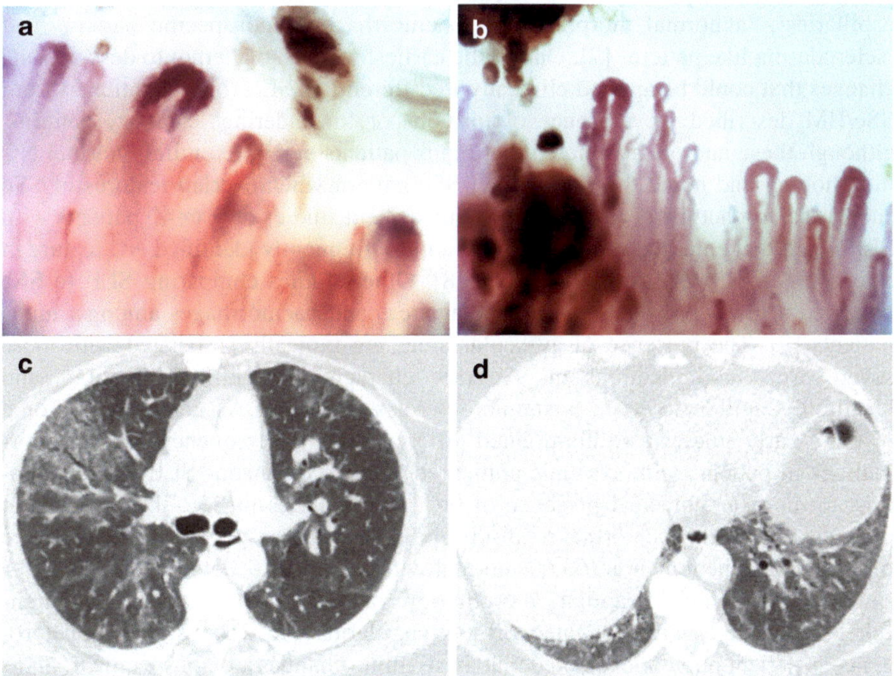

Fig. 1 Scleroderma-pattern nailfold capillary abnormalities (**a** and **b**) and bi-basal non-specific interstitial pneumonia (**c** and **d**) in a patient with idiopathic pneumonia with autoimmune features. There was a history of mild Raynaud's and identification of anti-Ro52 antibody but no other clinical features of systemic sclerosis

Connective Tissue Diseases

The term CTD is an umbrella term describing a heterogeneous group of multisystem diseases with shared aetiopathogeneic drivers and clinico-serological phenotypes; exemplified by the common presence of overlap features of two or more distinct clinical diseases in an individual patient. SSc and IIM important diseases making up the CTD spectrum alongside SLE, primary Sjogren's syndrome (pSS) and the archetypal overlap syndrome associated with anti-U1RNP antibodies referred to as MCTD.

Systemic Lupus Erythematosus

SLE is one of the commonest CTDs, affecting around 0.1% of the population and NC changes were first noted in this disease in the 1960s [5, 6]. An international systematic review, using the SCTC/EULAR consensus on standardised reporting of capillaroscopic findings, has synthesised the available evidence concerning the capillaroscopic abnormalities associated with SLE. A number of different capillaroscopic parameters appear to be significantly more prevalent in SLE patients compared to healthy controls. These can be summarised as the presence of 'tortuous capillaries', 'abnormal morphology', 'haemorrhages', 'nonspecific pattern' and 'scleroderma like pattern' [7]. One of the earliest studies to attempt to describe NC changes that could be applied clinically to differentiate SLE (only 5 patients) from SSc/IIM described the presence of tortuous or 'meandering' capillary patterns, although these authors also noted that lupus patients can have entirely normal NC morphology and noted the presence of SSc pattern when overlap features of SSc such as sclerodactyly were present [2]. Subsequent studies of over 40 patients with SLE noted that enlarged capillaries were a more frequently identified NC feature in SSc compared to SLE (86% vs 42%) [8]. Other studies comparing SLE to SSc observed a lower prevalence of avascular areas and haemorrhages amongst lupus patients [9]. The presence of avascular areas are typically associated with more severe organ complications of SSc (see chapters "Image Interpretation" and "Nailfold Capillaroscopy in Systemic Sclerosis (Including Associations)"). Some of these early studies also highlighted differences in the frequency of NC abnormalities in patients with systemic compared to more cutaneous SLE [10]. In contrast to the near universal presence of NC abnormalities in SSc, the majority of patients with SLE have normal nailfold capillaroscopy, irrespective of the presence of Raynaud's phenomenon (63.6% normal with RP vs. 82.9% without RP) [11]. A 'lupus pattern' nailfold capillary morphology was proposed (characterised by nailfold haemorrhages with elongated tortuous capillaries (Fig. 2) but studies of heterogeneous patient populations noted that these subtle changes are not specific to lupus and not uncommon in primary RP [12]. NC abnormalities are not uncommon in childhood-onset SLE and can evolve over time with SSc-like NC patterns found more commonly in patients with high disease activity and those with damage accrual (often exhibiting clinical features of SSc) [13]. Adult studies of SLE have

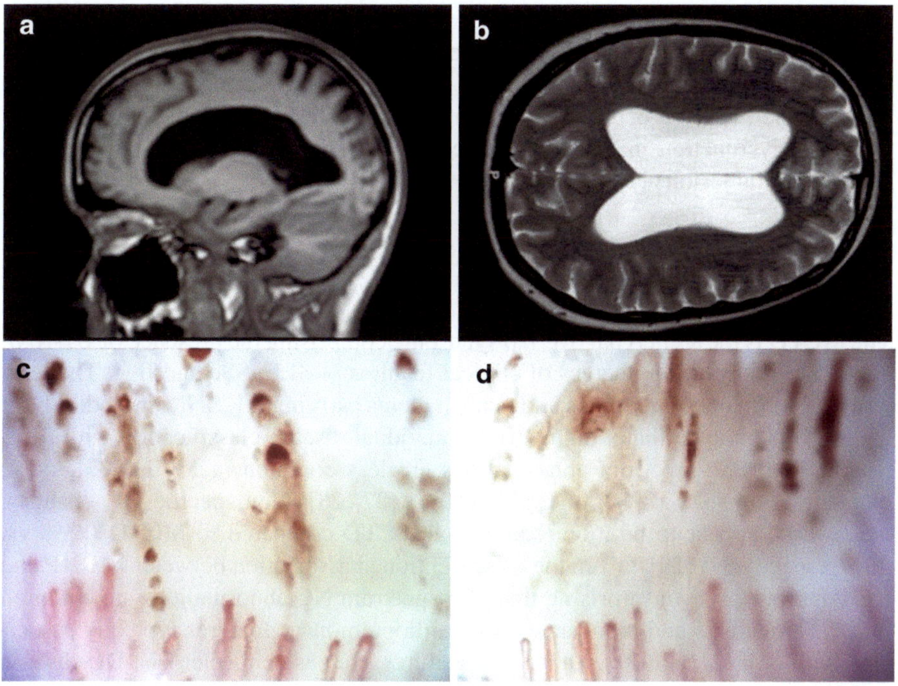

Fig. 2 Diagnostic value of NC in establishing a diagnosis in a 40 year old patient with unexplained myalgia and lower limb weakness (**a** and **b**) MRI brain revealed hydrocephalus and ventriculomegaly and; (**c** and **d**), 'Lupus pattern' nailfold capillary abnormalities with elongated nailfold capillaries with multiple associated brush-like microhaemorrhages. Other relevant clinical features included mild hair fall and new-onset Raynaud's phenomenon (positive Ro60, Ro52 and Ku antibodies)

also identified a range of NC morphological features, particularly when RP present, that appear to be associated with disease activity [14].

A number of studies have explored the relationship between NC abnormalities in SLE and the clinical phenotype, suggesting associations between SSc-like NC changes with the presence of RP (particularly in context of U1-RNP antibodies) [14–16], chilblains lupus [17], and ~ 30% of patients with cutaneous SLE *with* digital lesions present [18]. In contrast, others have reported that the association between U1RNP antibodies in SLE with abnormal NC (characterised by reduced capillary density) is independent of the presence of Raynaud's symptoms [19]. Raynaud's phenomenon (RP) is present in around half of people with SLE and appears to be associated with neurological involvement (and less common amongst patients with sicca symptoms) [11].

The presence of SSc-spectrum NC changes in SLE is also associated with traditional organ manifestations of SSc such as pulmonary arterial hypertension (PAH) [20, 21]. Indeed one study indicated a SSc-like NC pattern was associated with a 6.3-fold increased risk for PAH development in SLE patients [22]. Lupus nephritis meanwhile appears to be characterised by the presence of tortuous capillaries, higher capillary diameter/width (consistent with giant capillaries), capillary length and the presence of microhaemorrhages [15, 23]. There is no convincing association between the presence of NC changes in patients with SLE and the emergence of cognitive dysfunction in SLE [24], Jaccoud's arthopathy [25], or cutaneous SLE without digital lesions [18, 26].

Mixed Connective Tissue Disease

The MCTD is the archetypal overlap syndrome comprising the presence of U1-RNP antibodies and varying degrees of clinical features of SLE, SSc and IIM. The term remains, for many, contentious and many patients carrying U1-RNP antibodies have a clinical phenotype that would permit individual disease classification with SLE, SSc or IIM. SSc-spectrum abnormalities are less common in MCTD ~38–60%, compared with SSc (89%) and SLE (10%) [27, 28]. Non-specific NC changes, meanwhile, appear to be more common in uCTD compared to MCTD (83% vs. 46% respectively) [29]. Given the aforementioned association between U1RNP and RP symptoms, it is unsurprising that SSc-spectrum NC abnormalities are common in MCTD patients and associated with cardiopulmonary features typically associated with SSc [21, 30, 31]. Other SSc features such as skin sclerosis, DU disease and ILD are also more common in MCTD patients with scleroderma pattern NC changes, particularly in those with a severe reduction in capillary density and neoangiogensis [32]. The absence of scleroderma pattern NC changes is associated with a more inflammatory clinical phenotype (Fig. 3). A comparison of MCTD-ILD and SSc-ILD observed more frequent loss of capillaries in SSc-ILD group, while dilated capillaries were more characteristic of MCTD-ILD [31, 33]. The severity of restriction on lung function tests correlates with the severity of NC changes [33]. NC is not useful in MCTD at differentiating between patients with more inflammatory features such as skeletal muscle involvement [34].

Primary Sjogren's Syndrome

An assessment of the nailfold capillaries is not typically undertaken as part of the diagnostic work up in pSS, although RP occurs in around a third of people with pSS [35], whilst sicca symptoms have a similar prevalence in SSc. Given the considerable overlap that exists between individual CTDs, it is unsurprising that NC abnormalities are more prevalent in pSS compared with other forms of chronic inflammatory salivary gland disease [36, 37]. Within the CTDs, pSS most closely clinically resembles SLE and the 2 conditions share several clinical, serological, immunological and genetic features. These similarities extend to the frequency and nature of capillary morphological abnormalities identified on NC in pSS [38]. The presence of SSc features like RP and the presence of anticentromere antibodies are associated with a higher frequency of scleroderma-pattern NC changes [39–41]. In

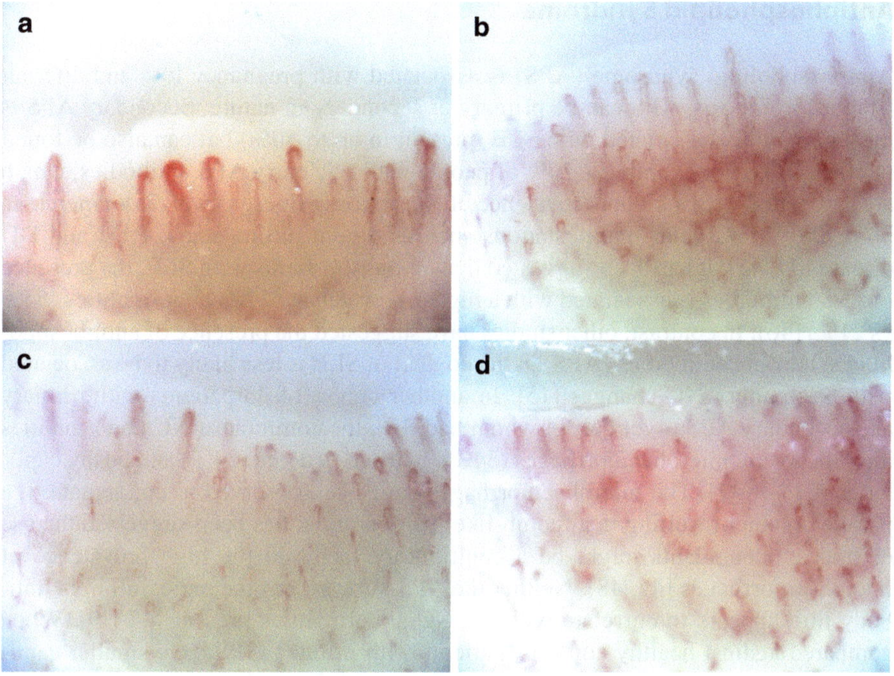

Fig. 3 Nailfold capillary abnormalities in a patient with inflammatory arthritis, Raynaud's phenomenon and mild puffy fingers carrying anti-U1RNP antibodies. There was subtle capillary dilation in the minority of digits (**a**) but capillary morphology and density was otherwise preserved (**b**–**d**). There were no other organ manifestations of scleroderma-spectrum disease

contrast, the more typical presence of anti-Ro and anti-La antibodies in pSS are not associated with distinct NC abnormalities [35, 41].

Undifferentiated CTD (uCTD)

The term uCTD is typically applied when insufficient clinical features are present to either classify or confidently make a clinical diagnosis of a specified CTD such as SLE, pSS, SSc or IIM. In this context, the application of NC has enormous utility in supporting clinicians to better classify disease. The identification of SSc-pattern changes may support classification of SSc (or VEDOSS) and identify patients at risk of SSc-associated clinical manifestations such as DU, PAH and ILD (Fig. 1) [42, 43]. In contrast, the presence of normal NC appearances might provide reassurance to both the clinician and the patient on the apparent absence of immune-mediated vascular injury.

Antiphospholipid Syndrome

Antiphospholipid syndrome (APS) is associated with pregnancy loss and arterial/venous thrombosis. APS can be primary or secondary in nature. Secondary APS is most commonly associated with SLE (present in up to 40%) but can also be found in other CTD. For example, ~20% of people with SSc carry APS antibodies, which are associated with a higher prevalence of NC abnormalities, as well as an increases propensity to vascular manifestations such as digital pitting scars, PAH and DU disease [44, 45]. It has been suggested that amongst patients with SLE, the presence of APS antibodies is associated with a higher prevalence of NC abnormalities (55% vs 21%) [46]. In contrast, other studies have suggested the presence of antiphospholipid syndrome antibodies (APS) in the context of SLE is less likely to be associated with SSc-pattern NC changes [15]. In another cohort of 33 patients with primary and secondary APS (over half of whom had RP), the commonest NC abnormalities identified were microhaemorrhages (54%), nailfold oedema (24%) and bushy capillaries (21%) [47]. The microhaemorrhages have been observed to congregate in a parallel manner resulting in a 'comb-like' pattern and it has been suggested the use of oral anticoagulants might be a contributory factor to the high prevalence of microhaemorrhages [47, 48]. Neither the APS-subtype nor the anticardiolipin antibody titre appears to correlate with the NC abnormalities present [47–49]. When compared against healthy controls, patients with primary APS have smaller capillary dimensions [50]. Microcirculatory damage on NC may be associated with prior thombotic events in primary APS. A comparison of primary APS and APS secondary to lupus suggested similar capillary morphology in both groups but microhaemorrhages were more common in SLE-APS [49].

Expert Opinion on the Role of NC in Other Connective Tissue Diseases

The NC abnormalities reported in SLE and APS are of interest and may be providing additional mechanistic aetiopathogenic insight. However, further large scale prospective studies, ideally with use of consensus description of capillaroscopic characteristics, such as the EULAR /SCTC consensus, are paramount [51]. Additional work would be valuable to explore the responsiveness of NC abnormalities to treatment in SLE and APS. It is unlikely NC will provide much additional diagnostic utility in these disease areas. In pSS, SLE and MCTD, the identification of SSc-like features on NC does provide additional diagnostic utility and may guide clinicians in identifying other SSc-like organ manifestations such as ILD and PAH, particularly in the absence of other clinicoserological features of SSc (Fig. 1).

Inflammatory Arthritis

Whilst considered distinct from the CTDs, the pathological hallmarks of inflammation/autoimmunity, vasculopathy and fibrosis are all present across the spectrum of non-CTD inflammatory arthritis and several studies have explored the NC changes associated with these conditions.

Rheumatoid Arthritis

RP occurs in around 20% of people with RA (varying according to definition applied) but ischaemic tissue damage is very rare. Irrespective of RP symptoms, a number of capillaroscopic features have been reported in RA. An early study that was agnostic to subsequently defined SSc-pattern NC changes proposed 3 patterns; the first characterised by small comma-shaped capillary loops; the second by long hair-pin loops spread in treillis form over the venular plexus in' slow, granular circulation'; and the third characterised by the presence of capillary haemorrhage and the irregular appearance of the loops, often of the "megacapillary" variety [52]. Other early studies observed a pronounced subpapillary plexus visibility with an increased number of elongated vessels in RA [53, 54].

Since SSc-pattern changes have been better categorised, it has been noted that non-specific NC changes can be found in nearly half of RA patients (higher in those with Raynaud's) but SSc-pattern changes are uncommon [55, 56].

Other studies have failed to identify differences in nailfold capillary morphology between RA and systemic vasculitis, but have noted increased capillary permeability amongst patients with vasculitis [57]. The NC appearances do not appear to differ between Rheumatoid Factor (RF) positive and RF-negative patients [54, 55, 58]. In contrast, the presence of extra-articular clinical manifestations appears to be associated with NC changes in RA [59]. Similarly, active RA is associated with reduced capillary density and appears to be improved by treatment with anti-TNF [60, 61]. In contrast, it has been suggested that JAK inhibition might worsen NC abnormalities in one small open-label study of RA [62].

Psoriatic Arthritis

The common identification of nail onycholysis in patients with psoriatic disease has resulted in a number of studies examining NC changes in psoriasis and psoriatic arthritis (PsA) (Fig. 4). In comparison to the elongated capillaries observed in RA, it has been suggested that patients with PsA are more likely to have shorter, fewer capillaries [53, 63]. All subsets of PsA patients have been reported to have lower capillary density and altered capillary dimensions as compared to patients with psoriasis alone [64]. Patients with psoriatic arthritis affecting the distal interphalangeal (DIP) joints and those with nail changes are more likely to have a reduction in arterial and venous capillary limb diameters [65]. Nailfold capillary abnormalities are

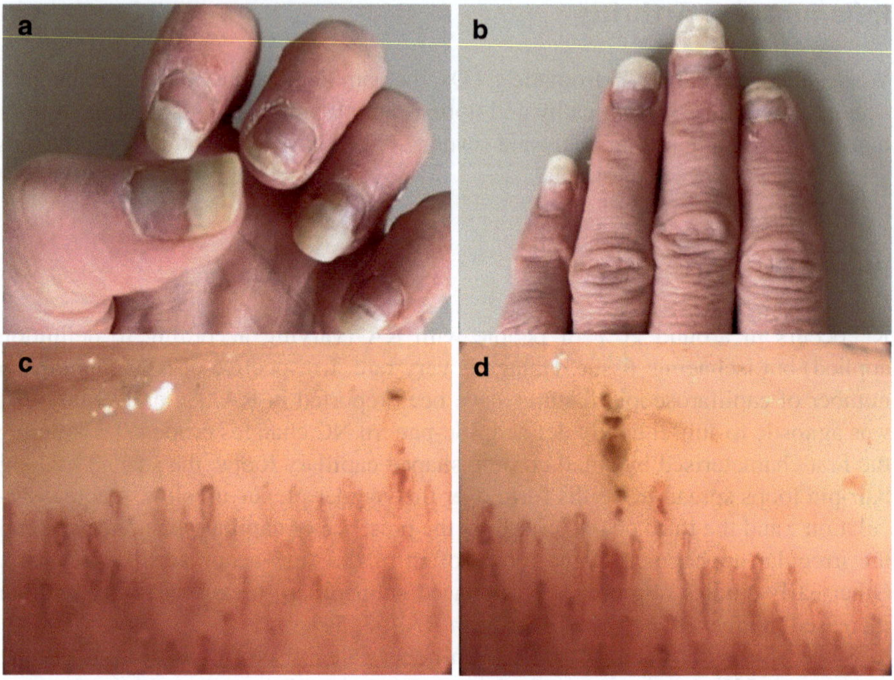

Fig. 4 Nailfold capillary abnormalities in a patient with psoriatic nail disease and Raynaud's phenomenon with (**a** and **b**), widespread onycholysis and nail pitting; and (**c** and **d**), subtle nailfold capillary abnormalities with occasional microhaemorrhages but preserved capillary density and capillary morphology

more common in psoriasis patients with anatomically adjacent periungual psoriatic plaque, nail pitting and onycholysis [66]. Others have noted a reduction in capillary loop density in patients with either psoriasis plus nail disease or psoriasis plus nail and DIP joint disease [65]. Intriguingly, given the occurrence of ischaemic acro-osteolysis in SSc, the presence of avascular areas and microaneurysm appear to be specific to the 'arthritis mutilans' subset of PsA in which severe bony destruction occurs [63]. NC tortuosities also appear to be more common in PsA [67]. Similar to RA, increased capillary permeability is not a feature of PsA [68].

Ankylosing Spondylitis

A limited number of studies have examined NC in ankylosing spondylitis (AS). Subtle changes such as nailfold peri-capillary oedema are common (~40%) but evidence of a true microangiopathy is rarer (~15%) and unrelated to disease severity [69]. The peri-capillary oedema may be immune-mediated and responsive to anti-TNF therapy [70]. Capillary morphological abnormalities meanwhile do not change after anti-TNF therapy [70].

Expert Opinion on the Role of NC in Inflammatory Arthritis

The identification of NC abnormalities in inflammatory arthritis is part of a broader body of work demonstrating immune-mediated vascular injury in inflammatory arthritis. Like in CTD, the presence of SSc-spectrum NC changes might indicate the presence of overlap disease and increased risk of SSc organ manifestations. It is unlikely that NC will ever have a diagnostic role in inflammatory arthritis, although the presence of NC abnormalities in inflammatory arthritis may have hitherto neglected clinical associations that could have practical implications for management.

Vasculitis

Given immune-mediated endothelial injury and altered vessel wall integrity are key aetiopathogenic drivers of SSc and IIM, there is a strong rationale for examining the role of NC in vasculitis and several studies have undertaken work in this field. As with CTD and inflammatory arthritis, many of the early studies applied loosely defined terms such as 'capillary loop dilatation' and 'immature morphology' to try and make sense of the capillary appearances visualised. As the NC changes of SSc were better described and classified, studies shifted their focus to look for these changes in other rheumatic diseases such as vasculitis. A number of studies have suggested that the presence of NC changes in vasculitis may correlate with high disease activity with resolution of changes following successful treatment [71, 72].

Large Vessel Vasculitis

A limited number of studies have considered the utility of NC in large vessel vasculitis. NC changes have been reported in ~40% of patients with Takaysau's vasculitis and appear to be associated with more severe disease [73]. Decreased capillary density with shortened, thin and tortuous capillaries have been noted in patients with subclavian artery involvement and may reflect generalised hypoperfusion of the digits [74, 75].

Medium Vessel Vasculitis

Kawasaki disease (KD) is a medium-sized vessel vasculitis of childhood that is notable for its propensity to affect the coronary arteries. Reduced capillary density (~40%) appears to be the commonest NC finding, particularly in the active phase of KD [76, 77]. Decreased capillary blood cell velocity has been noted in the active but afebrile phase of KD but resolves during convalescent phase [76]. Dilatation of the capillaries has also been reported in KD. There have been conflicting reports as to whether NC morphology and red cell velocity may be useful in predicting coronary artery involvement [76–78].

Small Vessel Vasculitis

One study of a heterogeneous population of patients with systemic autoimmune rheumatic disease noted a high proportion (92%) of 'avascular areas' in patients with Wegener's granulomatosis (now granulomatosis with polyangiitis, GPA) [12]. Other studies have suggested that, whilst retinal changes are highly prevalent and specific for GPA, non-specific NC changes are more typical in GPA (~80%) and no more prevalent than non-specific changes seen in healthy controls [79]. The prevalence and features of NC abnormalities in ANCA-associated vasculitis has formed the focus of a recent systematic review that suggested non-specific abnormalities including neoangiogenesis, capillary loss, microhaemorrhages, and bushy and enlarged capillaries are the more frequently observed NC changes and present in 70–80% of ANCA-vasculitis patients [80]. As with other forms of vasculitis, there appears to be differences in the NC pattern in the active and convalescent phases of the disease [80, 81].

Abnormalities at the nailfold are present in around half (54%) of children with Henoch-Schonlein purpura (HSP), typically characterised as capillary loop dilation and 'immature morphology' (horizontal distal plexuses and subpapillary plexuses) [82].

Behcet's Disease

Behcet's disease (BD) is a bespoke mixed-form of vasculitis characterised by significant large and smaller arterial and venous vascular features. A number of NC abnormalities have been observed in around 50–70% of people with Behcet's that include a variety of features including background pallor, microhaemorrhages, tortuous/branched capillaries, giant capillaries, avascular areas and abnormalities of venous plexus and irregularly arranged venules [83, 84]. Associations have been identified between NC abnormalities and active mucocutaneous disease, arthritis and superficial thrombophlebitis [83]. BD patients with a positive ANA are more likely to have non-specific NC abnormalities [85].

Expert Opinion on the Role of NC in Vasculitis

Whilst mechanistically interesting, it is unlikely NC will develop a role in the diagnostic assessment of vasculitis. NC abnormalities appear to be subtle and non-specific in nature. In large vessel vasculitis, such changes may simply be a consequence of reduced digital perfusion due to proximal stenoses. The lower prevalence of NC changes in the convalescent phase of small vessel vasculitis suggests reversibility with treatment and future longitudinal studies of vasculitis are needed to confirm and characterise this further.

Other Relevant Rheumatological Disease

A number of other conditions that might present to rheumatology clinics have been evaluated using NC. These include RP mimics such as thromboangiitis obliterans (Buerger's disease) in which elongated capillary length and even scleroderma-like NC patterns have been observed and may improve with smoking cessation, although larger studies are required to confirm this [86, 87]. Autoinflammatory diseases have also been assessed. Nailfold capillary abnormalities are uncommon in Familial Mediterranean fever but are characterised by capillary enlargement without micro-haemorrhages when identified [88, 89]. Presumed 'non-inflammatory' rheumatic diseases have been examined. For example, one study identified NC changes characteristic of PsA amongst patients with erosive osteoarthritis when compared to nodal osteoarthritis [90]. NC abnormalities with elongated capillaries and abnormal angiogenesis have also been noted in newer disease entities such as Middle Eastern Pain Syndrome and may be used to differentiate from fibromyalgia syndrome [91].

Conclusions

Over the last 50 years, the role of NC has been extensively studied in rheumatological diseases other than SSc and IIM. Indeed, many of the early studies of NC permitted a heterogeneous mix of patients owing to uncertainty over the clinical utility of NC in different diseases. The identification of NC changes across such a broad range of rheumatological disease highlights the importance of immune-mediated vascular injury across the spectrum of systemic autoimmune rheumatic disease. NC changes are less prevalent in 'other' rheumatological diseases but this may have considerable hitherto neglected clinical utility. The identification of SSc-pattern changes can be valuable in delineating the relative contribution of SSc features to disease pathogenesis. More work is needed to establish the role of NC in autoimmune rheumatic diseases in predicting treatment response which could guide more personalised treatment strategies for patients with autoimmune rheumatic disease.

References

1. Lépine R. Polymyosite (derinatomyosite; angiomyosite). Rev de Med. 1901;21:426–8.
2. Kenik JG, Maricq HR, Bole GG. Blind evaluation of the diagnostic specificity of nailfold capillary microscopy in the connective tissue diseases. Arthritis Rheum. 1981;24(7):885–91.
3. Romero-Bueno FI, Rodriguez-Nieto MJ, Palacios Miras C, Martinez Estupinan L, Martinez-Becerra MJ, Vegas Sanchez MC, et al. Fine-tuning characterization of patients with interstitial pneumonia and an underlying autoimmune disease in real-world practice: we get closer with Nailfold videocapillaroscopy. Front Med (Lausanne). 2023;10:1057643.

4. Fonollosa V, Simeon CP, Castells L, Garcia F, Castro A, Solans R, et al. Morphologic capillary changes and manifestations of connective tissue diseases in patients with primary biliary cirrhosis. Lupus. 2001;10(9):628–31.
5. Ross JB. Nail fold capillaroscopy—a useful aid in the diagnosis of collagen vascular diseases. J Invest Dermatol. 1966;47(4):282–5.
6. Lawler JC, Lumpkin LR. Cutaneous capillary changes in lupus erythematosus. Arch Dermatol. 1961;83:636–9.
7. Cutolo M, Melsens K, Wijnant S, Ingegnoli F, Thevissen K, De Keyser F, et al. Nailfold capillaroscopy in systemic lupus erythematosus: a systematic review and critical appraisal. Autoimmun Rev. 2018;17(4):344–52.
8. Lee P, Leung FY, Alderdice C, Armstrong SK. Nailfold capillary microscopy in the connective tissue diseases: a semiquantitative assessment. J Rheumatol. 1983;10(6):930–8.
9. Kabasakal Y, Elvins DM, Ring EF, McHugh NJ. Quantitative nailfold capillaroscopy findings in a population with connective tissue disease and in normal healthy controls. Ann Rheum Dis. 1996;55(8):507–12.
10. Studer A, Hunziker T, Lutolf O, Schmidli J, Chen D, Mahler F. Quantitative nailfold capillary microscopy in cutaneous and systemic lupus erythematosus and localized and systemic scleroderma. J Am Acad Dermatol. 1991;24(6 Pt 1):941–5.
11. Pavlov-Dolijanovic S, Damjanov NS, Vujasinovic Stupar NZ, Marcetic DR, Sefik-Bukilica MN, Petrovic RR. Is there a difference in systemic lupus erythematosus with and without Raynaud's phenomenon? Rheumatol Int. 2013;33(4):859–65.
12. Anders HJ, Haedecke C, Sigl T, Kruger K. Avascular areas on nailfold capillary microscopy of patients with Wegener's granulomatosis. Clin Rheumatol. 2000;19(2):86–8.
13. Schonenberg-Meinema D, Bergkamp SC, Nassar-Sheikh Rashid A, Gruppen MP, Middelkamp-Hup MA, Armbrust W, et al. Nailfold capillary scleroderma pattern may be associated with disease damage in childhood-onset systemic lupus erythematosus: important lessons from longitudinal follow-up. Lupus Sci Med. 2022;9(1):e000572.
14. Riccieri V, Spadaro A, Ceccarelli F, Scrivo R, Germano V, Valesini G. Nailfold capillaroscopy changes in systemic lupus erythematosus: correlations with disease activity and autoantibody profile. Lupus. 2005;14(7):521–5.
15. Furtado RN, Pucinelli ML, Cristo VV, Andrade LE, Sato EI. Scleroderma-like nailfold capillaroscopic abnormalities are associated with anti-U1-RNP antibodies and Raynaud's phenomenon in SLE patients. Lupus. 2002;11(1):35–41.
16. ter Borg EJ, Groen H, Horst G, Limburg PC, Wouda AA, Kallenberg CG. Clinical associations of antiribonucleoprotein antibodies in patients with systemic lupus erythematosus. Semin Arthritis Rheum. 1990;20(3):164–73.
17. Franceschini F, Calzavara-Pinton P, Quinzanini M, Cavazzana I, Bettoni L, Zane C, et al. Chilblain lupus erythematosus is associated with antibodies to SSA/Ro. Lupus. 1999;8(3):215–9.
18. Monfort JB, Chasset F, Barbaud A, Frances C, Senet P. Nailfold capillaroscopy findings in cutaneous lupus erythematosus patients with or without digital lesions and comparison with dermatomyositis patients: a prospective study. Lupus. 2021;30(8):1207–13.
19. Chebbi PP, Goel R, Ramya J, Gowri M, Herrick A, Danda D. Nailfold capillaroscopy changes associated with anti-RNP antibodies in systemic lupus erythematosus. Rheumatol Int. 2022;42(8):1355–61.
20. Atsumi T, Bae SC, Gu H, Huang WN, Li M, Nikpour M, et al. Risk factors for pulmonary arterial hypertension in patients with systemic lupus erythematosus: a systematic review and expert consensus. ACR Open Rheumatol. 2023;5(12):663–76.
21. Groen H, ter Borg EJ, Postma DS, Wouda AA, van der Mark TW, Kallenberg CG. Pulmonary function in systemic lupus erythematosus is related to distinct clinical, serologic, and nailfold capillary patterns. Am J Med. 1992;93(6):619–27.
22. Donnarumma JFS, Ferreira EVM, Ota-Arakaki J, Kayser C. Nailfold capillaroscopy as a risk factor for pulmonary arterial hypertension in systemic lupus erythematosus patients. Adv Rheumatol. 2019;59(1):1.

23. Adel H, Eldeeb AA, Hamdy F. Nailfold capillaroscopic changes in patients with glomerular diseases. Reumatol Clin (Engl Ed). 2025;21(1):101803.
24. Munguia-Realpozo P, Garcia-Carrasco M, Mendoza-Pinto C, Galaviz-Silva ML, Etchegaray-Morales I, Mendez-Martinez S, et al. Absence of association between nailfold capillary findings and mild cognitive dysfunction in systemic lupus erythematosus. Clin Rheumatol. 2022;41(9):2737–43.
25. Pimenta da Fonseca E, Lins CF, de Sa Ribeiro DL, Santos WGD, Rosa G, Machicado V, et al. Videocapillaroscopic findings in patients with systemic lupus erythematosus with or without Jaccoud Arthropathy. J Clin Rheumatol. 2021;27(6S):S198–203.
26. Ingegnoli F. Capillaroscopy abnormalities in relation to disease activity in juvenile systemic lupus erythematosus. Microvasc Res. 2013;87:92–4.
27. Felis-Giemza A, Ornowska S, Haladyj E, Czuszynska Z, Olesinska M. Relationship between type of skin lesions and nailfold capillaroscopy pattern in mixed connective tissue disease. Clin Rheumatol. 2022;41(1):281–8.
28. Todoroki Y, Kubo S, Nakano K, Miyazaki Y, Ueno M, Satoh-Kanda Y, et al. Nailfold microvascular abnormalities are associated with a higher prevalence of pulmonary arterial hypertension in patients with MCTD. Rheumatology (Oxford). 2022;61(12):4875–84.
29. Pizzorni C, Ferrari G, Schenone C, Hysa E, Carmisciano L, Gotelli E, et al. Capillaroscopic analysis of the microvascular status in mixed versus undifferentiated connective tissue disease. Microvasc Res. 2022;142:104367.
30. Sullivan WD, Hurst DJ, Harmon CE, Esther JH, Agia GA, Maltby JD, et al. A prospective evaluation emphasizing pulmonary involvement in patients with mixed connective tissue disease. Medicine (Baltimore). 1984;63(2):92–107.
31. Pallis M, Hopkinson N, Powell R. Nailfold capillary density as a possible indicator of pulmonary capillary loss in systemic lupus erythematosus but not in mixed connective tissue disease. J Rheumatol. 1991;18(10):1532–6.
32. Kasser C, Boleto G, Allanore Y, Avouac J. Nailfold videocapillaroscopy findings and associations with organ involvement in mixed connective tissue disease. Clin Exp Rheumatol. 2025;43(3):418–24.
33. Rajendran A, Maikap D, Padhan P, Misra R, Singh P. A comparison of Nailfold video Capillaroscopy findings in mixed connective tissue disease interstitial lung disease vs systemic sclerosis interstitial lung disease: a single-Centre study. Mediterr J Rheumatol. 2024;35(2):263–71.
34. Munteanu A, Kundnani NR, Caraba A. Nailfold capillaroscopy abnormalities and pulmonary hypertension in mixed connective tissue disease and systemic sclerosis patients. Eur Rev Med Pharmacol Sci. 2024;28(4):1314–26.
35. Corominas H, Ortiz-Santamaria V, Castellvi I, Moreno M, Morla R, Clavaguera T, et al. Nailfold capillaroscopic findings in primary Sjogren's syndrome with and without Raynaud's phenomenon and/or positive anti-SSA/Ro and anti-SSB/La antibodies. Rheumatol Int. 2016;36(3):365–9.
36. Bezuglov MF, Ivanova AV, Belikov ES, Tinigin PA. State of microcirculation and the system of hemostasis in Sjogren's disease, Sjogren's syndrome and chronic parenchymatous parotitis. Ter Arkh. 1985;57(8):88–90.
37. Melsens K, Leone MC, Paolino S, Elewaut D, Gerli R, Vanhaecke A, et al. Nailfold capillaroscopy in Sjogren's syndrome: a systematic literature review and standardised interpretation. Clin Exp Rheumatol. 2020;38 Suppl 126(4):150–7.
38. Ohtsuka T. Nailfold capillary abnormalities in patients with Sjogren's syndrome and systemic lupus erythematosus. Br J Dermatol. 1997;136(1):94–6.
39. Tektonidou M, Kaskani E, Skopouli FN, Moutsopoulos HM. Microvascular abnormalities in Sjogren's syndrome: nailfold capillaroscopy. Rheumatology (Oxford). 1999;38(9):826–30.
40. Vettori S, Irace R, Riccardi A, Iacono D, Pellecchia L, Vicedomini L, et al. Serum CXCL4 increase in primary Sjogren's syndrome characterizes patients with microvascular involvement and reduced salivary gland infiltration and lymph node involvement. Clin Rheumatol. 2016;35(10):2591–6.

41. Capobianco KG, Xavier RM, Bredemeier M, Restelli VG, Brenol JC. Nailfold capillaroscopic findings in primary Sjogren's syndrome: clinical and serological correlations. Clin Exp Rheumatol. 2005;23(6):789–94.
42. Vasile M, Avouac J, Sciarra I, Stefanantoni K, Iannace N, Cravotto E, et al. From VEDOSS to established systemic sclerosis diagnosis according to ACR/EULAR 2013 classification criteria: a French-Italian capillaroscopic survey. Clin Exp Rheumatol. 2018;36 Suppl 113(4):82–7.
43. van den Hoogen FKD, Fransen J, Johnson SR, Baron M, et al. 2013 classification criteria for systemic sclerosis: an American College of Rheumatology/European league against rheumatism collaborative initiative. Arthritis Rheum. 2013;65(11):2737–47.
44. Marie I, Jouen F, Hellot MF, Levesque H. Anticardiolipin and anti-beta2 glycoprotein I antibodies and lupus-like anticoagulant: prevalence and significance in systemic sclerosis. Br J Dermatol. 2008;158(1):141–4.
45. Chatterjee S, Pauling JD. Anti-phospholipid syndrome leading to digital ischaemia and rare organ complications in systemic sclerosis and related disorders. Clin Rheumatol. 2021;40(6):2457–65.
46. Bongard O, Bounameaux H, Miescher PA, De Moerloose P. Association of anticardiolipin antibodies and abnormal nailfold capillaroscopy in patients with systemic lupus erythematosus. Lupus. 1995;4(2):142–4.
47. Vayssairat M, Abuaf N, Deschamps A, Baudot N, Gaitz JP, Chakkour K, et al. Nailfold capillary microscopy in patients with anticardiolipin antibodies: a case-control study. Dermatology. 1997;194(1):36–40.
48. Ferrari G, Gotelli E, Paolino S, Pesce G, Nanni L, Colombo BM, et al. Antiphospholipid antibodies and anticoagulant therapy: capillaroscopic findings. Arthritis Res Ther. 2021;23(1):175.
49. Candela M, Pansoni A, De Carolis ST, Pomponio G, Corvetta A, Gabrielli A, et al. Nailfold capillary microscopy in patients with antiphospholipid syndrome. Recenti Prog Med. 1998;89(9):444–9.
50. Vaz JL, Dancour MA, Bottino DA, Bouskela E. Nailfold videocapillaroscopy in primary antiphospholipid syndrome (PAPS). Rheumatology (Oxford). 2004;43(8):1025–7.
51. Smith V, Herrick AL, Ingegnoli F, Damjanov N, De Angelis R, Denton CP, et al. Standardisation of nailfold capillaroscopy for the assessment of patients with Raynaud's phenomenon and systemic sclerosis. Autoimmun Rev. 2020;19(3):102458.
52. Merlen JF, Sarteel AM. Capillaroscopy in rheumatoid arthritis. Phlebologie. 1981;34(1):165–9.
53. Zaric D, Worm AM, Stahl D, Clemmensen OJ. Capillary microscopy of the nailfold in psoriatic and rheumatoid arthritis. Scand J Rheumatol. 1981;10(3):249–52.
54. Altomonte L, Zoli A, Galossi A, Mirone L, Tulli A, Martone FR, et al. Microvascular capillaroscopic abnormalities in rheumatoid arthritis patients. Clin Exp Rheumatol. 1995;13(1):83–6.
55. Sag S, Sag MS, Tekeoglu I, Kamanli A, Nas K, Aydin Y. Nailfold videocapillaroscopy results in patients with rheumatoid arthritis. Clin Rheumatol. 2017;36(9):1969–74.
56. Angeloudi E, Anyfanti P, Dara A, Pagkopoulou E, Bekiari E, Sgouropoulou V, et al. Peripheral nailfold capillary microscopic abnormalities in rheumatoid arthritis are associated with arterial stiffness: results from a cross-sectional study. Microvasc Res. 2023;150:104576.
57. Tan JH, Hoh SF, Win MT, Chan YH, Das L, Arkachaisri T. Childhood-onset systemic lupus erythematosus in Singapore: clinical phenotypes, disease activity, damage, and autoantibody profiles. Lupus. 2015;24(9):998–1005.
58. Hachulla E, Perez-Cousin M, Flipo RM, Houvenagel E, Cardon T, Catteau MH, et al. Increased capillary permeability in systemic rheumatoid vasculitis: detection by dynamic fluorescence nailfold videomicroscopy. J Rheumatol. 1994;21(7):1197–202.
59. Kuryliszyn-Moskal A. Cytokines and soluble CD4 and CD8 molecules in rheumatoid arthritis: relationship to systematic vasculitis and microvascular capillaroscopic abnormalities. Clin Rheumatol. 1998;17(6):489–95.
60. Caraba A, Stancu O, Crisan V, Georgescu D. Anti TNF-Alpha treatment improves microvascular endothelial dysfunction in rheumatoid arthritis patients. Int J Mol Sci. 2024;25(18):9925.

61. Anghel D, Sirbu CA, Petrache OG, Opris-Belinski D, Negru MM, Bojinca VC, et al. Nailfold Videocapillaroscopy in patients with rheumatoid arthritis and psoriatic Arthropathy on ANTI-TNF-ALPHA therapy. Diagnostics (Basel). 2023;13(12):2079.
62. Anyfanti P, Angeloudi E, Dara A, Pagkopoulou E, Moysidou GS, Deuteraiou K, et al. Non-invasive assessment of micro- and macrovascular function after initiation of JAK inhibitors in patients with rheumatoid arthritis. Diagnostics (Basel). 2024;14(8):834.
63. Salli L, Raimondi F, Pappalardo A. Periungual capillaroscopy in psoriatic arthritis. Clin Ter. 1999;150(6):409–12.
64. Elmesiry AM, Mahmoud SA, Mohamed MS, Aly H, Elmotaleb YA, Ghit MM, et al. Nailfold Capillaroscopy findings in patients with psoriasis vulgaris and different domains of psoriatic arthritis. J Psoriasis Psoriatic Arthritis. 2024;9(3):89–97.
65. Bhushan M, Moore T, Herrick AL, Griffiths CE. Nailfold video capillaroscopy in psoriasis. Br J Dermatol. 2000;142(6):1171–6.
66. Ohtsuka T, Yamakage A, Miyachi Y. Statistical definition of nailfold capillary pattern in patients with psoriasis. Int J Dermatol. 1994;33(11):779–82.
67. Cafaro G, Bursi R, Valentini V, Hansel K, Perricone C, Venerito V, et al. Combined semiquantitative nail-enthesis complex ultrasonography and capillaroscopy in psoriasis and psoriatic arthritis. Front Immunol. 2024;15:1505322.
68. Grassi W, Core P, Carlino G, Cervini C. Nailfold capillary permeability in psoriatic arthritis. Scand J Rheumatol. 1992;21(5):226–30.
69. Wendling D, Risold JC. Nailfold capillaroscopy and ankylosing spondylarthritis: incidence of anomalies, but absence of diagnostic and prognostic value. Rev Med Interne. 1994;15(7):448–51.
70. Batko B, Maga P, Urbanski K, Ryszawa-Mrozek N, Schramm-Luc A, Koziej M, et al. Microvascular dysfunction in ankylosing spondylitis is associated with disease activity and is improved by anti-TNF treatment. Sci Rep. 2018;8(1):13205.
71. Sendino Revuelta A, Barbado Hernandez FJ, Torrijos Eslava A, Gonzalez Anglada I, Sanchez P, de Rivera JM, Vazquez Rodriguez JJ. Capillaroscopy in vasculitis. An Med Interna. 1991;8(5):217–20.
72. Keret S, Mazzawi J, Slobodin G, Rimar O, Rosner I, Rozenbaum M, et al. Nailfold video capillaroscopy as a useful diagnostic tool in systemic vasculitis. Microvasc Res. 2022;143:104406.
73. Akdogan A, Erden A, Firat Senturk E, Kilic L, Sari A, Armagan B, et al. Capillaroscopic findings in Turkish Takayasu arteritis patients. Turk J Med Sci. 2019;49(5):1303–7.
74. Javinani A, Pournazari M, Jamshidi AR, Kavosi H. Nailfold videocapillaroscopy changes in Takayasu arteritis and their association with disease activity and subclavian artery involvement. Microvasc Res. 2019;122:1–5.
75. Wang L, Chen H, Ding Z, Ma L, Sun Y, Jiang L. Associations of microcirculation damage on nailfold capillaroscopy with supra-aortic severe ischemic events in patients with Takayasu arteritis. Clin Rheumatol. 2023;42(6):1625–34.
76. Huang MY, Huang JJ, Huang TY, Gupta-Malhotra M, Syu FK. Deterioration of cutaneous microcirculatory status of Kawasaki disease. Clin Rheumatol. 2012;31(5):847–52.
77. Reddy Konda VV, Jindal AK, Nadig PL, Banday AZ, Vinay K, Singh S. Microvascular changes on nailfold capillaroscopy in acute stage of Kawasaki disease: a new diagnostic paradigm for an enigmatic condition. Rheumatology (Oxford). 2024;63(2):392–8.
78. Sedaghat B, Raeeskarami SR, Tahghighi F, Assari R, Aghaei-Moghadam E, Razavi-Khorasani N, et al. The role of nailfold capillaroscopy in pediatric patients with Kawasaki disease. Reumatol Clin (Engl Ed). 2023;19(5):255–9.
79. Triggianese P, D'Antonio A, Nesi C, Kroegler B, Di Marino M, Conigliaro P, et al. Subclinical microvascular changes in ANCA-vasculitides: the role of optical coherence tomography angiography and nailfold capillaroscopy in the detection of disease-related damage. Orphanet J Rare Dis. 2023;18(1):184.
80. Screm G, Mondini L, Confalonieri P, Salton F, Trotta L, Barbieri M, et al. Nailfold Capillaroscopy analysis can add a new perspective to biomarker research in Antineutrophil cytoplasmic antibody-associated Vasculitis. Diagnostics (Basel). 2024;14(3):254.

81. Matsuda S, Kotani T, Wakura R, Suzuka T, Kuwabara H, Kiboshi T, et al. Examination of nailfold videocapillaroscopy findings in ANCA-associated vasculitis. Rheumatology (Oxford). 2023;62(2):747–57.
82. Greenberg LW. Nailfold capillary abnormalities in Henoch-Schonlein purpura. J Pediatr. 1983;103(4):665–6.
83. Wechsler B, Le TH, Mouthon JM, Cabane J, Godeau P. Periungual capillaroscopic aspects in Behcet's disease. Apropos of 30 cases. Annales de dermatologie et de venereologie. 1984;111(6–7):543–50.
84. Del Peral-Fanjul A, Atienza-Mateo B, Prieto-Pena D, Pulito-Cueto V, Blanco R. Vascular involvement in Behcet's disease: ultrasound assessment of femoral vein intima-media thickness, nailfold capillaroscopy and endothelial progenitor cells in a national referral Centre. Clin Exp Rheumatol. 2023;41(10):2008–16.
85. Mercade-Torras JM, Guillen-Del-Castillo A, Bujan S, Solans-Laque R. Nailfold videocapillaroscopy abnormalities and vascular manifestations in Behcet's syndrome. Clin Exp Rheumatol. 2024;42(10):2065–70.
86. Guidelli GM, Bardelli M, Fioravanti A, Selvi E. Nailfold capillaroscopy in Buerger's disease: a useful tool? Eur J Rheumatol. 2014;1(2):81–3.
87. Fahrig C, Heidrich H, Penninger C. Is the capillary microscopic determination of the visible capillary length a diagnostic criterion in thromboangiitis obliterans? Vasa. 1998;27(2):87–8.
88. Aytekin S, Aydin F, Akpolat T, Senturk N, Turanli AY. Evaluation of nailfold capillaries in familial Mediterranean fever patients. Clin Rheumatol. 2011;30(2):255–7.
89. Dinc A, Melikoglu M, Korkmaz C, Fresko I, Ozdogan H, Yazici H. Nailfold capillary abnormalities in patients with familial Mediterranean fever. Clin Exp Rheumatol. 2001;19(5 Suppl 24):S42–4.
90. Fioravanti A, Tofi C, Cerase A, Priolo F, Marcolongo R. Capillaroscopic findings in erosive and nodal osteoarthritis of the hands. Clin Rheumatol. 2001;20(3):174–6.
91. Elhamamy MH, Elbeialy AA, Mohamed MS, Abdelraheem SE, Elzomor HM. Is middle east pain syndrome (MEPS) a variant of fibromyalgia syndrome or a distinct disease? BMC Rheumatol. 2025;9(1):3.

Nailfold Capillaroscopy in Children

Clare E. Pain, Dieneke Schonenberg-Meinema, and Francesca Ingegnoli

Key Points

- Nailfold capillaroscopy is a non-invasive, safe and painless examination that is easy to perform on children using a variety of equipment. The capillaroscopy pattern in healthy children is similar to that in healthy adults, with a density of less than six capillaries per millimetre being pathological.
- ANA and capillaroscopy are recommended for the classification, evaluation and monitoring of RP. In pRP, capillaroscopy does not show a scleroderma pattern.
- Scleroderma patterns in jSSc, cSLE and JDM have been described, but longitudinal studies are lacking to understand whether these capillary changes are related to disease outcome and prognosis.
- In cSLE, capillary changes are predominantly abnormal capillary morphology and haemorrhages, with an overall pattern that can change over time.
- A scleroderma(-like) pattern with giant ramified capillaries and reduced density is often seen in JDM patients.

C. E. Pain (✉)
Department of Paediatric Rheumatology, Alder Hey Children's NHS Foundation Trust, Liverpool, UK
e-mail: clare.pain@alderhey.nhs.uk

D. Schonenberg-Meinema
Department of Pediatric Immunology, Rheumatology and Infectious Diseases, Emma Children's Hospital, Amsterdam University Medical Centers, University of Amsterdam, Amsterdam, The Netherlands
e-mail: d.schonenberg@amsterdamumc.nl

F. Ingegnoli
Rheumatology Unit, Department of Rheumatology and Medical Sciences, ASST Pini-CTO, Department of Clinical Sciences & Community Health, Dipartimento di Eccellenza 2023-2027, Università degli Studi di Milano, Milan, Italy
e-mail: francesca.ingegnoli@unimi.it

A. L. Herrick et al. (eds.), *Nailfold Capillaroscopy in Rheumatological Diseases*,
https://doi.org/10.1007/978-3-032-03970-5_9

Introduction

Nailfold capillaroscopy (NFC) is an important tool for specialists caring for children with Raynaud's phenomenon (RP) and with potential connective tissue diseases (CTDs). Not only does it play a central role in differentiating primary and secondary RP, it allows earlier diagnosis of CTDs in children and supports disease monitoring in juvenile dermatomyositis (JDM) with a growing interest in childhood onset SLE, juvenile systemic sclerosis (jSSc) and mixed/overlap CTD. However, confidence and use of NFC in children was reported as low in a UK study [1]. Formal training courses are now available for pediatric NFC which can provide hands-on training on video capillaroscopy.

As was already discussed in Chap. 3, different devices are available to perform NFC. Each device has its own (dis-)advantages concerning portability, user training, costs, magnification and possibility of storing of the images (Table 1). All of them can be used in adults and in children. Below are some considerations for the specific examination of NFC in the pediatric age.

In children no comparison studies have been performed yet (in any disease) for the different available capillaroscopy devices. Depending on their age the fingers are smaller and their ability to sit still might also be difficult in some children. In children for that reason, we advise the use of devices with a minimum of x200 magnification, if available.

Recent literature reviews provided an overview of the performance of different capillaroscopy devices in systemic sclerosis (SSc) when comparing them to the 'gold-standard' device nailfold videocapillaroscope [2, 4]. Dermatoscope images have a higher proportion of non-interpretable or non-classifiable images compared to images from videocapillaroscope. This means that the portable and affordable dermatoscope might function as a screening tool to identify a scleroderma pattern, but when in doubt or in case of non-interpretable results a second examination by videocapillaroscope should be performed for images with better visual quality and higher magnification. In a study of adult RP patients, approximately half required imaging with videocapillaroscope after (first try) examination with a dermatoscope [5]. USB

Table 1 Different types of devices for nailfold capillaroscopy

Type device	Magnification (max)	Portable device	Costs	Quality of images	Storage of images	User training
Opthalmoscope	15×	+	Low	+/–	–	–
Dermatoscope	10×	+	Low/ medium	+/–	–	–
Smartphone attachments	20×	+	Low/ variable	+	+	–
USB devices	300×	–	Low/ medium	+	+	+
Stereomicroscope	200×	–	Medium/ high	+	+	+
Videocapillaroscope	500×	–	High	++	+	+

Adapted from Ma et al. [2] and Schonenberg-Meinema et al. [3]

devices (cheap) and stereomicroscope (more expensive) are alternatives for video-capillaroscopy with good quality imaging but sensitivity and specificity have not yet been investigated for CTD's other than for adult SSc. Although these studies were performed in adults it is still important to consider these findings when examining children.

Standardised Approach of NFC in Children

The procedure of nailfold capillary examination by capillaroscopy is non-invasive and therefore easy to perform in children. Undergoing capillaroscopy examination is not painful and in many capillaroscopy devices the patient can look at the direct imaging on the screen which makes it easier for a child to be engaged and stay still during the examination.

The lowest age of reported capillaroscopy data is in 1–2 year old children [6]. Although RP often presents at teenager age, the indication to perform capillaroscopy can also be present in very young children. For instance, this is the case in patients with the suspicion of JDM, which can be seen in ages <4 years old. In JDM the nailfold capillary abnormalities are quite striking and helpful in diagnosis of this disease (discussed below in this chapter).

Before starting the procedure, it is recommended that the room temperature is a minimum of 20 degrees and that the pediatric patients are climatized for 15–30 min pre-examination, just as in adults [7]. The washing of their hands is also advised and preferably (if possible) a pre-instruction not to wear any nail polish. If they do have nail polish on their nails then the examination can be attempted to see if good images can be obtained, as long as the polish does not reflect the light in the camera.

In younger children below the age of 4 it is recommended to show how the device works on the fingers of their accompanying parent or teddy bear/doll that they have brought. After they are comfortable and at ease, the procedure can be performed while they are sitting on the lap of their parents. Some patience and experience of the examiner is needed for collecting good quality images because children have to stay still for some minutes. In most of the children this is possible by making jokes, pretending to be in a contest and with some minibreaks.

Children can have traumatic hemorrhages that should not be confused with pathological hemorrhages which can be seen in systemic autoimmune diseases. In all but especially in older children above 4 years old it is important to ask about recent hand trauma (including nail-biting and pulling of the folds), sports and hobbies that can induce traumatic lesions of the examination site. If trauma is reported, or noticed, then a note of that should be made in the patient chart with mentioning which finger it concerns to be able to correctly interpret the images. In teenagers, a manicure in the recent month should be asked about, as a cause for traumatic micro-hemorrhages. This group also has to be asked about use of caffeine, nicotine and vasoactive/-constrictive medication such as drugs for attention-deficit-hyperactivity disorder. The vasoconstrictive effects can influence visibility and suggest falsely low capillary density.

In a perfect world, just as in adults it would be ideal to examine eight fingers, excluding the thumbs. In practice, in the younger patient, examination of eight fingers with 4 images per finger is not always a realistic goal. In the youngest children it is advised to start with the non-dominant hand because that hand has less risk for trauma, thus the feasibility of high-quality imaging in those fingers (especially digits 3 and 4) might be the best. For younger patients two images per finger (centre of the nailfold) will be sufficient for diagnostic purposes. For purposes of follow-up and research (with storage of images) preferably four images per finger are advised, meaning that 32 images per patient are being collected. In adults, it has been shown that examination of less than eight fingers reduces the sensitivity to detect capillary changes [8]. Such studies have not yet been performed in the pediatric population.

Interpretation of the different variables from nailfold capillary images is performed according to the same European Alliance of Associations for Rheumatology Study Group on Microcirculation in Rheumatic Diseases (EULAR SG MC) criteria as in adults. The quantitative variables from nailfold capillaries in children are described by [3]:

1. Density per linear millimetre (counted at the distal row)
2. Dimension: apical diameter (in micrometre (μm))
3. (Ab)normal morphology
4. Haemorrhages

In earlier studies, different types of descriptions for capillary dimensions have been used, such as elongated limbs, diameter of afferent and efferent limbs, inter-capillary distances and apical diameter. Because of the inter-individual variability in all other variables for capillary dimension, currently only apical capillary diameter is suggested in the above standardized approach to describe capillary dimension.

To describe capillary morphology many different terms have been used in the past, such as 'tortuous', 'meandering', 'ramified', 'bushy' or 'bizarre' as capillary shapes [9–11]. To better harmonize the international terminology in reporting capillary variables there have been efforts to define what is 'normal' versus what is 'abnormal'. The definition for normal morphology has been discussed in earlier chapters. To summarize, normal capillary shapes have a stereotype hairpin shape with non-specific variations being crossing (once or twice) and tortuous (limbs bend but do not cross). Convexity of the tip is a requirement for interpretation as normal capillary morphology [12]. Subsequently, capillaries with other shapes than those described above have an *abnormal* morphology (see Fig. 1).

It is important to realize that the reliability to detect (ab)normal morphology has only been validated in capillaroscopy images from adults [13]. In recent years there have been more data describing the frequency of abnormal morphology in the healthy paediatric population [6].

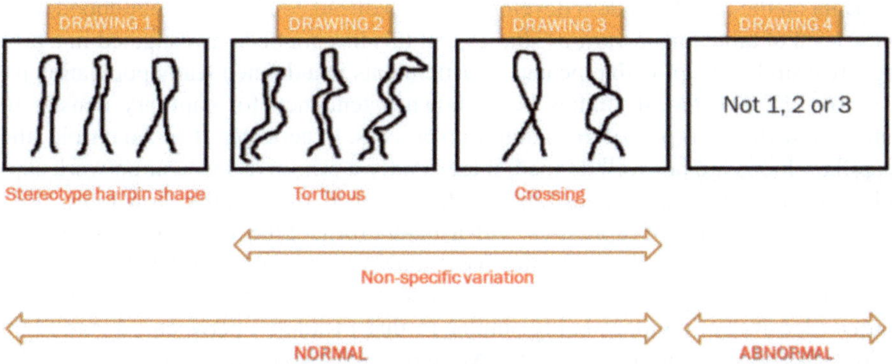

Fig. 1 Definitions for the interpretation of capillary shapes for normal and abnormal capillary morphology (copied image from Smith et al. 2016 [13])

Table 2 Capillaroscopic parameters and patterns in healthy adults and children according to EULAR definitions [6, 15]

Capillaroscopic characteristics	*Capillaroscopic patterns*				
	Non Scleroderma patterns		Scleroderma patterns		
	Normal	Non-specific abnormalities	Early	Active	Late
Density	≧ 7/mm (adults) ≧ 6–7/mm (children)	≧ 7/mm	≧ 7/mm	4–6 /mm	≦ 3 /mm
Dimension	< 20 μm	20–50 μm	> 50 μm	> 50 μm	≦ 50 μm
Abnormal morphology	Absent in adults May be seen in children	May be seen in adults and children	Absent in adults and children	Present in adults and children	Present in adults and children
Haemorrhages	Absent in adults May be seen in children	May be seen in adults and children	May be seen in adults and children	May be seen in adults and children	Absent in adults and children

Differences Between Healthy Adults Versus Healthy Children

An essential requirement in the assessment of microcirculatory abnormalities is knowledge of the normal nailfold capillary pattern in healthy adults and children. Until a few years ago, studies in healthy children aimed at defining normal capillary parameters were scarce, with some caveats [14]. They were performed with different equipment and magnifications, so the comparison with the normal adult model is only indirect, as shown in Table 2.

Data on the age-dependent development of nailfold capillaries in childhood have now been obtained from various studies, but this has not been investigated in a prospective study design with repeated measurements in a defined study population [6, 11, 16–22]. The oldest studies have shown a tendency for capillary density to increase with age as part of the maturation process. In neonates (1 or 2 days old) the capillary loops are not well defined, there is only a primitive vascular network supplied by arterioles and venules [20, 22]. Infants aged 1–6 months show rapid elongation and formation of capillaries, with a mature form of the microvascular network by 6 months [20, 22]. Some studies have shown a general age-related increase in capillary density in young children up to 6 years of age, with the number of capillaries (density) in children being similar to that of adults, between six and eight capillaries per millimetre [16–18, 21]. More recent data on capillaroscopy in healthy children has been published. An international multicentre study under the auspices of the EULAR SG MC described data from healthy children from 9 countries worldwide ($n = 204$) and, in general, found no significant correlation between capillary density and age [6]. There was a weak correlation ($R = 0.14$, $p = 0.046$) between density and age when the youngest age group (< 5 years of age) were excluded. Those healthy controls less than 5 years of age were found to have a significantly increased capillary density than other ages [6]. However, in a recent extensive study of 564 healthy children and adolescents by Dundar et al., capillary density was found to be significantly lower in the youngest age group (5–7 years of age) compared to other age groups, and a significant increase in density and capillary length was seen in teenage years compared to younger age groups [23]. In contrast, Melsens et al. used standardised quantitative and qualitative techniques for reporting and evaluated NFC in 8 fingers as opposed to only the fourth finger of the non-dominant hand. In general, a density of less than six capillaries per millimetre is pathological.

The number of non-specific capillary abnormalities is slightly associated with age, as are capillary dilations [6]. The same study reported a trend for the mean number of dilatations per mm to increase with age, as seen previously by Herrick et al. [6, 19].

It is worth mentioning some limitations in the interpretation of capillaroscopy, which remains an operator-dependent technique. Image quality is essential for correct analysis, but in children (as in adults) it can be compromised by local trauma leading to traumatic haemorrhages, which appear to be more common in childhood (Fig. 2) [6, 17].

A recent study has evaluated the impact of ethnicity or skin pigmentation on capillary density, investigating 145 healthy children with a mean age of 11.03 years. A significantly lower density was observed in subjects with an African / Afro-Caribbean and North African / Middle Eastern ethnicity compared to those with Caucasian ethnicity [24]. Previous studies including children and adolescents have not been as conclusive, but ethnic groups were less well defined as white and non-white and lower magnification methods were used for NFC [16, 25].

It is important to consider that a possible lower visibility in darker skin pigmentation may make capillary density look lower, and this should be considered with

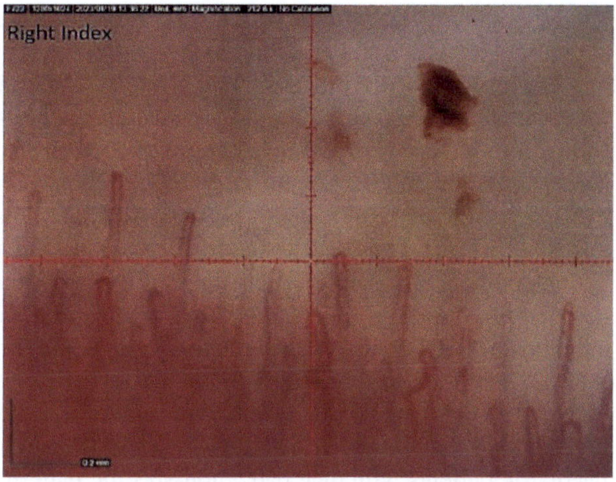

Fig. 2 NFC performed with Dinolite at Salford Royal rheumatology vascular service showing traumatic haemorrhages with haemosiderin deposition in a child with primary RP

the devices without extra light and lower magnification. The recent study from Bergkamp et al. used 200x magnification with good quality images from videocapillaroscope which makes these data reliable. In future studies on capillary density and age, skin colour should be considered and its influence taken into account. The association between subpapillary venular plexus visibility and growth and age is controversial [16, 18, 26]. Finally, the published data support the use of the same EULAR classification to define overall capillaroscopy patterns in adults and children [6]. The use of scleroderma- and scleroderma-like pattern terminology will be discussed in the sections of childhood onset SLE (cSLE) and JDM below in this chapter.

Paediatric Primary Raynaud's Phenomenon (pRP)

RP is defined as a vasospastic disorder, usually affecting the fingers and toes, characterised by episodic colour changes (blanching, cyanosis and hyperemia) in response to cold or emotional stress [27]. Although prevalence is influenced by gender and local environmental conditions (higher in females and colder climates), most population-based surveys estimate the prevalence of the disorder at 3–5% in the general population [28], and even higher in schoolchildren, where prevalence is estimated at 15%, with primary RP being most common in young females at up to 30% although this high number might also reflect those with acrocyanosis [29, 30].

Currently, the classification of RP identifies two main groups: primary RP (pRP) and secondary RP [27]. These two categories differ in their pathogenesis, course and outcome.

Specifically, pRP patients have a process related to a defect in thermoregulation that causes an exaggeration of the normal response to temperature, they have a favorable outcome because they have no underlying disease, and in this group approximately 30 to 50% of patients have a first-degree relative with the disease, supporting a genetic susceptibility [31].

Classification of RP into these two groups is important for early diagnosis, starting treatment and planning the timing of diagnostic tests, examinations and monitoring. The history is useful in differentiating RP from other conditions commonly seen in children and adolescents, such as acrocyanosis (i.e. persistent hypothermic cyanosis of the extremities) and primary pernio/chilblains, in which cold-induced vasospasm leads to a local inflammatory reaction of the skin tissue. As in adult patients with RP, in addition to a careful history, examination and investigations such as capillaroscopy and autoantibody profile are fundamental to the correct classification of RP. Currently, RP is the main indication for NFC, as it is a valuable tool in the differential diagnosis of RP in all age groups.

Nailfold capillaroscopic pattern is normal or non-specific with ANA negative in both adults and children with pRP. Cross-sectional studies have confirmed that most paediatric patients with pRP had a non-specific pattern [6, 11, 17, 32].

Longitudinally, 250 young patients with RP aged between 10 and 20 years were followed for 1–6 years after their first capillaroscopy in a prospective study to evaluate the role of capillaroscopy in predicting the development of connective tissue disease [33]. At the end of follow-up, 76% of the young patients were classified as having pRP, of whom 91% had normal capillaroscopic findings. The remaining 24% of patients developed undifferentiated connective tissue disease (10.8%) or specific CTD (12.8%). A normal capillaroscopic pattern was observed in most patients who developed undifferentiated connective tissue disease (81%), in 70% of patients with inflammatory arthritis, and in 67% of 9 patients with SLE [33]. Non-specific capillaries were found in both pRP and secondary RP. A small group of patients had a scleroderma pattern, and all developed a CTD within 6 months of undergoing capillaroscopy [33].

Based on the available evidence, recommendations for the assessment and monitoring of RP have been developed [34], as shown in Fig. 3. NFC should be performed at presentation in all young patients with RP, as should ANA testing. The combination of specific autoantibody positivity and NFC specific abnormalities identifies children at higher risk of conversion to systemic autoimmune CTD and careful evaluation of the patient at least every 3 months is mandatory [34]. Patients who were neither ANA positive nor had NFC changes were at lowest risk and at least annual assessment was recommended [34]. From paediatric clinicians, there have been questions about the necessity of this strict follow-up advice, especially for the groups without ANA or capillary abnormalities. We need more paediatric longitudinal data including all ages to better assess the risk of development of CTD in those that present with pRP.

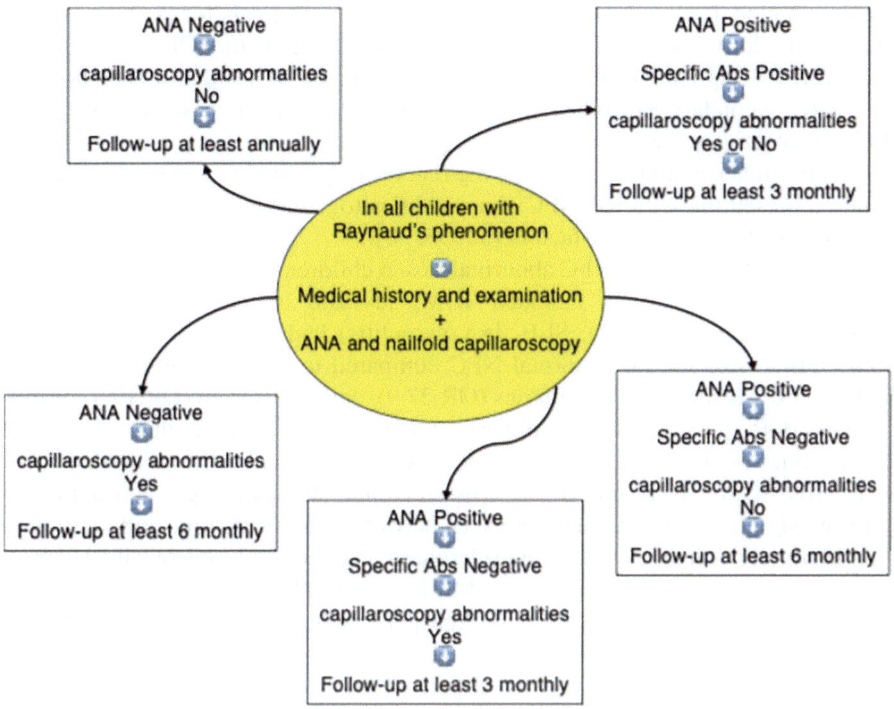

Fig. 3 Summary of recommendations for investigations and frequency of follow-up in children with RP [34]

Secondary Raynaud's Phenomenon in Children

RP is often the presenting feature of CTD in children. The CTDs associated with RP include jSSc, JDM, cSLE, jMCTD, juvenile Sjögren's syndrome (jSS) and overlap jCTDs. However, the risk factors for progression of a child presenting with RP to a definitive diagnosis of CTD are less well defined in children compared to adults [32, 33, 35, 36]. NFC is a key tool to differentiate primary RP from secondary RP in children as well as adults. As described above in section on pRP, NFC has been highlighted in several consensus guidelines as important to undertake together with a full blood count, inflammatory markers and ANA testing in all children presenting with RP [34, 37].

The largest prospective study on children and young adults with RP is described in detail in the section above on pRP [33]. A retrospective study showed that NFC was 'borderline' or 'abnormal' in 68% of those classified as secondary RP versus 23% of those classified with primary RP ($p < 0.001$) [32]. A further retrospective study of 83 patients classed as primary RP or secondary RP on whether a diagnosis of CTD was made, showed that of NCM parameters only capillary loss (defined as <6/mm) was associated with secondary RP ($p = 0.01$) [38]. In a multivariate logistic regression model including ANA, capillary loss was not a predictor of secondary RP but in a model without ANA it was an independent predictor (OR 3.98, CI 95% 1.22–12.99). Capillary loss alone had a sensitivity of 44.4% and a specificity of 84.4% for secondary RP. When combined with ANA this increased to 66.7% and 85.7% respectively [38].

Of the studies that have examined the risk of progression to a definitive CTD in children presenting with RP, NFC abnormalities together with positive ANA have been the most important risk factors [32, 33, 38].

A systematic review of NFC abnormalities in children showed that children with autoimmune disease (this included JDM, juvenile idiopathic arthritis (JIA), Kawasaki's disease, MCTD, SLE, IgA vasculitis) had an OR of 9.88 (95% CI 13.07–114.74) of having abnormal NFC compared to healthy controls [39]. The highest OR was for dilated capillaries (OR 27.9), density < 7/mm (OR 19.9), haemorrhages (OR 13.89) and giant capillaries (OR 12.87). Of the nine studies identified in this review, only four used videocapillaroscopy to visualise the nailfolds and all were cross-sectional. In one of the cross-sectional studies using videocapillaroscopy, no significant differences were seen between healthy children and those with JIA. Major abnormalities (including scleroderma pattern, reduced density, haemorrhages) were more frequent in jCTDs (MCTD, $p = 0.008$; cSLE, $p = 0.0002$; JDM, $p < 0.0001$) compared to healthy children [17]. A further study using NVC also showed significant changes (e.g., reduced density < 6, giants, haemorrhages) in secondary RP compared to healthy children [40]. However, their secondary RP included 9/32 with localised scleroderma and 4 with JIA which are not generally seen as CTD with systemic autoimmunity. Other studies suggest that neither of these conditions are associated with significant NFC capillary changes (except for possibly reduced density in localised scleroderma) compared with healthy controls [6, 17]. Notably, evaluation of 413 children worldwide with the EULAR/SCTC consensus standardized interpretation shows that the NFC assessment in juvenile rheumatic diseases differed significantly from healthy controls [6]. More specifically, the quantitative NFC characteristics were significantly lower or higher in the following subgroups compared with healthy controls: for density: lower in jSSc, JDM, MCTD, cSLE and localised scleroderma; for dilations: higher in jSSc, MCTD and JDM; for abnormal shapes: higher in JDM and MCTD; for haemorrhages: higher in jSSc, MCTD, JDM and cSLE. The qualitative NVC assessment of JIA, localised scleroderma and PRP did not differ from healthy controls, whereas the cSLE, jSSc, MCTD, JDM and cSLE subgroups showed more non-specific and scleroderma patterns, respectively.

These data confirm that the scleroderma patterns are associated with and predictive of secondary RP in children and adolescents, similar to adults. This occurs in almost all cases of jSSc and in most cases of jMCTD (>70%) [41, 42], and less frequently in cSLE (10–15%) [3].

One prospective study does report longitudinal data on NFC in 40 children who presented with isolated RP with no evidence of CTD [36]. The interval between repeat NFC was 6 months to 2 years with a mean of 1.6 years. This study showed that 4 children with non-specific findings had normal NFC on second evaluation and two children with normal NFC initially progressed to non-specific findings in one (not associated with a defined CTD diagnosis) and scleroderma pattern in another child who progressed to a diagnosis of MCTD.

Case 1

A 14-year-old girl presented with episodic colour change in her hands and feet associated with cold exposure. Attacks cause pain, numbness and impact on her function. She also reports her hands feeling stiff and she has puffy fingers not only with cold exposure. She has no digital ulcers and no other symptoms of note. Examination reveals puffy fingers, no digital pitting scars or digital ulcers. There is no sclerodactyly and no other skin involvement except for puffy fingers. NFC is shown in Fig. 4 and confirms a non-specific pattern. She has a normal full blood count, ESR and negative ANA, dsDNA and ENA screen and urinalysis.

On clinical review 6 months later, she has markedly improved with calcium channel blockers and no longer has puffy fingers. She has no new symptoms of note. NFC shows stable changes with no progression. One year later, she remains clinically well with negative autoantibodies, no skin or organ involvement of jSSc or other CTD. NFC still shows a non-specific pattern but with no new changes or progression. She remains under regular follow-up.

In a prospective study of 113 children and 2858 adults with RP without a previously known CTD, abnormal NVC (including reduced capillary density, dilations, giants, haemorrhages) were related to a positive ANA titre of ≥1:80 in adults but not in children [43]. As this study was not longitudinal, there is no data provided on risk of clinical progression to a defined CTD in this cohort.

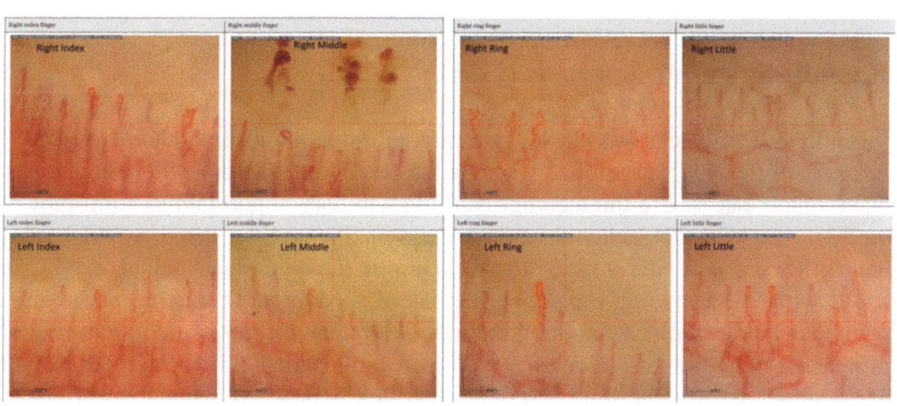

Fig. 4 NFC performed with Dinolite at Salford Royal rheumatology vascular service. Reduced capillary density (<7). 1–2 dilatations are seen in right index and left ring fingers. Abnormal shapes in right/left index and right ring, little finger. Multiple haemorrhages seen in right middle finger. Findings show a non-specific pattern

There is some suggestion from paediatric studies that secondary RP in children is due less frequently to SSc compared to in adults and more commonly to other CTDs, with frequency of jSSc being between 5.5–8.5% [33, 38]. We will come back to this topic in the other sections of this chapter.

Other non-rheumatological causes of secondary RP in children include drug therapies and in children, medications used to treat attention deficit hyperactivity disorder (e.g., central nervous system stimulants) are some of the most commonly associated [44, 45]. Whether secondary RP caused or exacerbated by CNS stimulants cause NFC abnormalities in children is yet to be determined but vasoconstrictive side effects seem to play a role (without pathological capillary changes).

At first assessment of a child with RP, children can be frequently classified into primary RP or secondary RP where a definite diagnosis of CTD can be made. Some children will fall into a grey area in between, neither having primary RP nor fulfilling a definite diagnosis and these children require careful monitoring including repeating NFC (see Case 1). Evidence is lacking as to how frequently NFC should be repeated in such cases but 6–12 monthly is often our approach.

Paediatric studies do suggest that the risk of development of CTD in a child with RP reduces over time with a retrospective cohort with a mean follow-up of 6.4 years showing the mean time between development of RP and diagnosis of a CTD was 2.1 years which was similar to the 2.4 years shown in the prospective study by Pavlov et al. [33, 38]. Of note, the secondary RP group who presented with RP as their cardinal symptom, all had other symptoms at presentation, commonly musculoskeletal [38]. This might mean that after 2 years of observation, and without any other symptoms, the risk for development of a CTD in a child with RP seems low. However, further longitudinal studies of children with RP with repeat NFC are required to better define the risk of development of CTD in children presenting with isolated RP and those that have some features to suggest a secondary RP without a definitive diagnosis.

Juvenile Systemic Sclerosis (jSSc)

Juvenile systemic sclerosis (jSSc) is a rare autoimmune disease characterised by sclerosis of the skin, vasculopathy (including RP, digital ulcers) and organ involvement which can be life-threatening. Nailfold capillary abnormalities form part of the EULAR/ACR 2013 classification criteria of SSc and the PReS/ACR/EULAR Padua Provisional Criteria jSSc [46, 47]. Despite the numerous studies on NFC in adults with SSc including predicting the risk of severity and future organ involvement, paediatric studies examining the role of NFC in diagnosis and monitoring of jSSc are lacking [48–50]. However, NFC is recommended to be performed as part of the initial assessment of a child or adult with SSc or when a diagnosis of SSc is suspected [51].

An international study is currently ongoing to validate the EULAR/ACR 2013 classification criteria in jSSc and will help increase the understanding of the role of NFC in diagnosis of these paediatric patients.

A comparison of NFC patterns in adults with juvenile (n = 30) and adult-onset (n = 2108) SSc showed that juvenile onset SSc more frequently showed scleroderma pattern compared to adult-onset SSc (93.3% versus 88%) with OR 2.44 (95% CI 0.57–10.41). Active scleroderma pattern was present in 58% of juvenile and 61% adult onset SSc and late scleroderma pattern in 61% and 55.5% respectively [52].

In a large international cohort of jSSc, nailfold capillary changes were reported in 120/161 (75%) but nailfold examination and definition of capillary abnormality were not standardised [53]. A large single-centre jSSc cohort identified nailfold capillary changes in 48/54 (89%) but did also not use the current standardised approach to categorise abnormalities [54]. Other studies have observed variable prevalences of abnormal nailfold capillaries in jSSc ranging from 40–100%, with differing definitions of abnormality and variable tools used to examine nailfolds [55–59].

In a French cohort, NFC abnormalities were noted in all patients who had capillaroscopy done (n = 15) with 11/15 described as scleroderma pattern and 4 with non-specific pattern [60]. Of those where findings were described as per Cutolo, early pattern was seen in 1 patient, active in 3 and late scleroderma pattern in 4 [60, 61]. Another cohort showed that 16/27 (60%) had early, 10/27 (37%) had active and 1(3%) had late pattern [59].

In the standardised NFC cross-sectional study in children, capillary density was the lowest in jSSc (mean capillary density 5.2/linear mm (SD 1.9) compared to other paediatric rheumatic diseases and to primary RP and was significantly lower than in healthy children (8.5 (SD 1.2)), albeit only 13 children with jSSc were included [6]. Additionally, jSSc patients had statistically more dilatations and more presence of haemorrhages than healthy children. Giants were seen in 11/13 (84.6%) compared to 3 (1.5%) of healthy children (OR 283.7 (CI 99.3% 33.2–5229.1). Scleroderma pattern was seen in 12/13 (99.3%) of the jSSc patients compared to 3/204 (1.5%) of healthy children (OR 465.9 (CI 99.3% 45.3–18,977); $p < 0.001$).

In a small longitudinal study with only 7 jSSc patients, all had scleroderma pattern but the number of affected fingers reduced at follow-up, suggesting the possibility of treatment modifying vasculopathy [62]. A previous study however, showed progressive changes in a small number of jSSc patients [17]. Improvement with treatment has been recorded in adults with SSc, particularly after autologous stem cell transplant [63, 64]. Further studies are needed in children.

Data is needed on longitudinal capillary changes in jSSc and whether changes map to disease outcomes and difference in prognosis. This is currently being investigated by an international study.

Childhood-Onset SLE (cSLE)

cSLE is a rare, but lifelong systemic autoimmune disease. It can be severe and possibly life-threatening. Capillaroscopy data are not part of any of the current SLE classification criteria, but in the last decade there has been a growing interest in the capillaroscopic abnormalities that are seen in SLE patients, not only in adult patients but also in cSLE. A systematic review showed that in adults with SLE abnormal capillary morphology and capillary hemorrhages are significantly more prevalent when compared to healthy controls [65]. A review in cSLE from 2020 showed that the literature on capillaroscopy data in cSLE was very scarce [66]. At that moment in time, capillary abnormalities (from only six studies) were not comparable due to different used definitions, especially for capillary morphology.

Since the international consensus on abnormal capillary morphology has been published in 2016 and 2018 [12, 13], it is possible to compare data between different studies. More recent studies, with use of these new standardized definitions from EULAR SG MC, have shown that the majority of cSLE patients show capillary changes when compared to age-matched healthy controls, although this still should be confirmed in larger cohorts [6, 67]. Just as in adults with SLE, these capillary changes are predominantly abnormal capillary morphology and small hemorrhages or 'extravasations' (often combined), seen in this cross-sectional study in up to 88% of cSLE patients (Figs. 5 and 6) [67]. Combined extravasations and abnormal shapes in the same finger were observed in 78% (n = 32/41) of SLE patients and in 60% of those patients this combination was detected in >4 fingers, making it a finding which deserves further study.

As in adults with SLE, cSLE patients also showed a higher number of capillary haemorrhages when compared to healthy children with comparable ages. The number of capillary haemorrhages per mm was correlated with disease activity (by

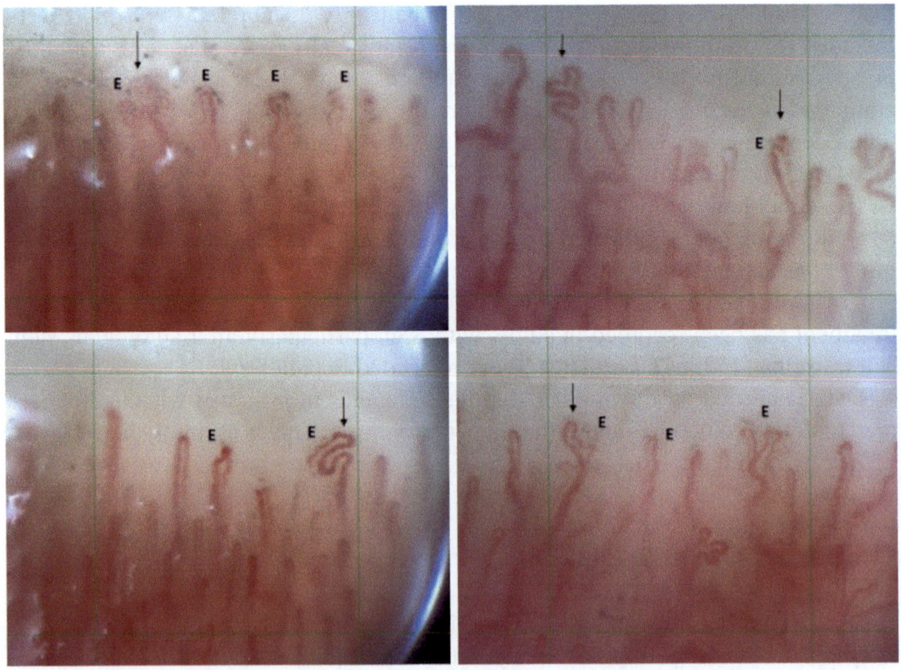

Fig. 5 NFC performed by videocapillaroscopy, green line 1 mm grid. Pericapillary extravasations (E) and abnormal shapes (arrows)

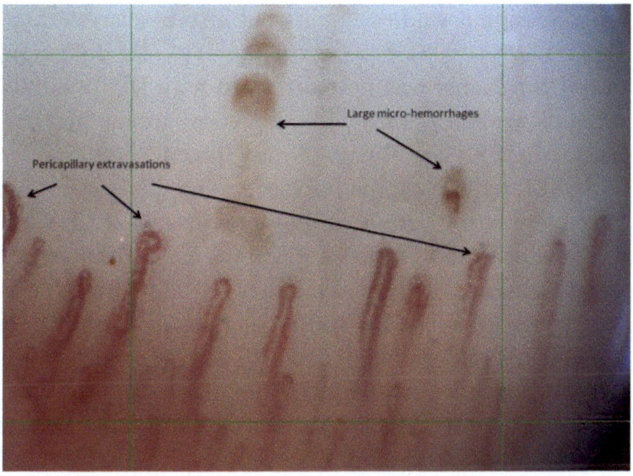

Fig. 6 NFC performed by videocapillaroscopy, green line 1 mm grid. Different subtypes of capillary hemorrhages in cSLE: Large hemorrhages and pericapillary extravasations

SLEDAI) [67]. The significant finding of more capillary haemorrhages in cSLE compared to healthy children was confirmed by the multicentre study from Melsens [6], although there was a little overlap in patient cohorts from both publications and cohort size was small (n = 20) [67].

A new subtype of capillary haemorrhage (called 'pericapillary extravasation') was described in the cross-sectional case-control study from Schonenberg-Meinema [67] (Fig. 5). This observation of a new subtype of capillary haemorrhage was in a later study validated by a good intra- and interrater agreement [68]. It was hypothesized that it might be capillary leakage that can be visually detected by the high-quality imaging from video-capillaroscopy with 200x magnification. Studies have not yet examined if these smaller capillary extravasations can also be detected by other devices or lower magnifications than video-capillaroscopy.

According to the standardized EULAR SG MC definitions, the main NVC pattern (by qualitative analysis) that has been observed in cSLE is called a 'nonspecific abnormalities' pattern. This means that the capillaries are not normal but also do not qualify to be classified as a scleroderma pattern. In the earlier mentioned cSLE study, these non-specific abnormalities were called 'microangiopathy' with the combination of capillary haemorrhages and abnormal morphology in the same capillaries [67]. These findings seem to correspond with the 'minor and major capillary abnormalities' from earlier studies [17, 69, 70]. Other recent studies show very similar observations calling them major abnormalities or non-specific abnormal capillary patterns in SLE [71–73]. Hypothetically these detailed observations may be more easily visualized by means of better quality imaging from the improved technology of the capillaroscopy devices. This non-specific NFC pattern, or microangiopathy, in cSLE should be further studied for its meaning of (long-term) vascular health in these patients.

Already in earlier studies a scleroderma NFC pattern was reported in cSLE, which has been debated as a possible sign for clinical overlap syndromes with jSSc [69, 74]. Ingegnoli reported in 2013 that some of those patients developed lung fibrosis, although these concerned adults with SLE [69]. In the more recent cross-sectional studies, giants but also a scleroderma(-like) pattern was seen in a subset (15%) of cSLE patients (Fig. 7) [6, 75]. Interestingly this scleroderma pattern in cSLE patients was not correlated with RP. In adults with SLE, capillary abnormalities were also seen without a correlation with RP [65]. In SSc capillary abnormalities and RP are always closely linked. Another difference between jSSc patients and cSLE patients is the presence of capillary abnormalities from early, active and late scleroderma pattern at the same time in cSLE [76]. In a longitudinal follow-up study, it was shown that a scleroderma pattern in cSLE was not correlated with overlap disease or clinical features of jSSc. However, a NFC scleroderma pattern in cSLE was associated with higher risk for specific *lupus-related* damage, as measured by SLICC damage index [62].

These recent findings raise the question as to whether the pathophysiology of these capillary abnormalities is quite different in these two systemic autoimmune diseases and if so should if we should name it differently. This phenomenon should be studied further to explore if capillary scleroderma(-like) patterns have prognostic meaning in cSLE and maybe should *not* be seen as a sign of overlap disease, or at least not in children [77]. In the meantime, for the clinician there should be awareness that all patients should regularly be screened for all organ systems in order to detect overlap disease, including the lungs in cSLE (lung function tests) and kidney in jSSc (urine sampling).

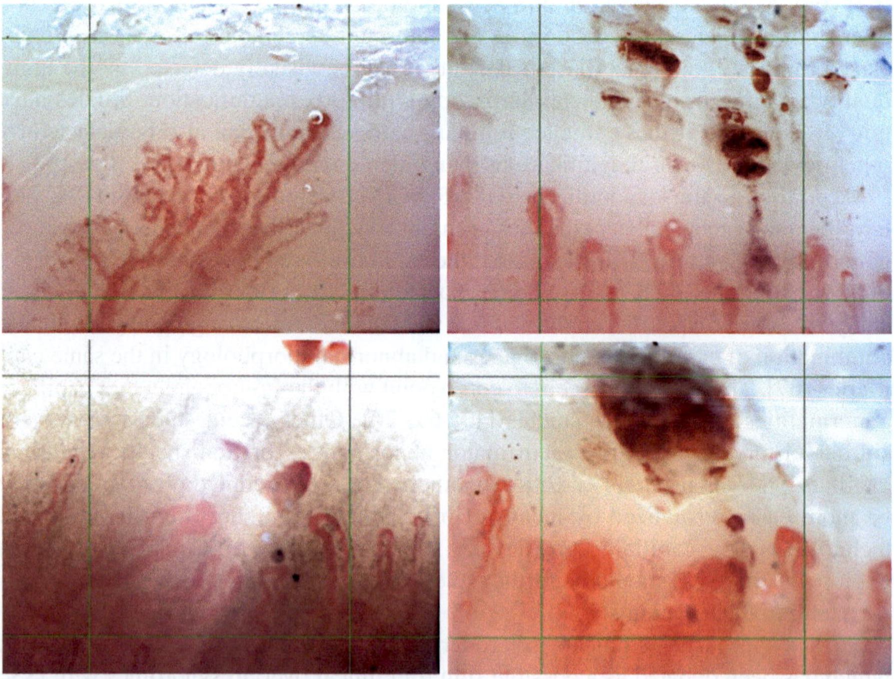

Fig. 7 NFC performed by videocapillaroscopy, green line 1 mm grid. NFC scleroderma(-like) patterns in cSLE patients

There have been some descriptions of capillary changes in cSLE over time. Both improvement and worsening of capillary abnormalities have been observed [17, 62, 69]. There is ongoing research on this topic. Until we have clarity about the meaning of these positive and negative changes it is recommended to repeat NFC on a regular basis in all CTD's, including cSLE.

Juvenile Dermatomyositis (JDM)

Just as cSLE, JDM is a rare disease often with a monocyclic course. There are not many studies published on the details of capillary abnormalities in JDM but we do know that 80–90% of JDM patients show capillary abnormalities [78]. In one cross-sectional study (n = 58) capillary changes in JDM patients were compared between active and inactive patients with a mean disease duration of 16.8 years [79]. In this study capillary density in JDM was significantly lower than in healthy controls. A low capillary density (mean 5.9 capillaries/mm) and a scleroderma-late pattern, both more prevalent in active JDM patients, were associated with higher disease activity. In both active (90%) and inactive (78%) patients a NVC scleroderma pattern was seen, with a high percentage of late scleroderma pattern (n = 11/30, 37%) in the active JDM patients. In other studies, a scleroderma(-like) pattern was also seen in the majority of JDM patients [6, 62]. Even more so than in SLE, capillary abnormalities in JDM seem to have a characteristic pattern where features from 'early-', 'active-' and 'late stage' scleroderma pattern can occur at the same time (Fig. 8). The capillary pattern in JDM is therefore often called a 'scleroderma-like' pattern. Of note, variable definitions have been used throughout literature for scleroderma like pattern, one of them stating it as a capillary pattern showing mixed microvascular markers of the scleroderma capillary patterns, but not fully fitting the definition for the single 'early', 'active' or 'late' scleroderma pattern [76]. Notably, this terminology had not been integrated in the EULAR/SCTC consensus on standardised description of capillaroscopic finding nor in the first multicentre study comparing with standardised capillaroscopic description children with connective tissue diseases versus healthy controls [6]. This nomenclature may be somewhat confusing for the paediatric clinician because scleroderma is a different disease with different treatments and prognosis when compared to JDM. This term is also difficult to explain to the patient itself because if they are diagnosed with JDM and they search on scleroderma they find information about this severe lifelong disease which they do not have.

One study in adults with DM explicitly describes giant-ramified capillaries as a finding that seems to occur mainly in DM patients, rarely seen in SSc [80]. This observation needs to be studied in JDM as well to further distinguish scleroderma from scleroderma-like patterns. It has been suggested that a lower capillary density in JDM can be associated with subclinical lung involvement but these patients had longstanding disease [81]. Skin colour was not considered in this study which might be a confounding factor for capillary density (see above in this chapter).

We need longitudinal follow-up studies in JDM, starting at diagnosis, to know if the severity of capillary changes can serve as a biomarker for risk of more severe organ involvement. JDM is discussed in more detail in Chap. 7.

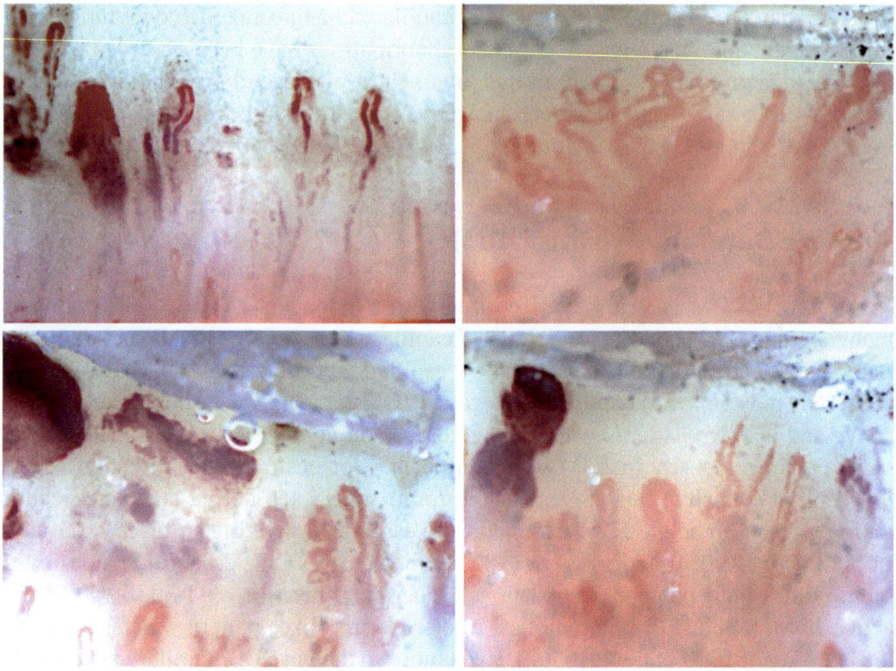

Fig. 8 NFC performed by videocapillaroscopy, green line 1 mm grid. NVC scleroderma-like patterns in JDM with in the right upper corner different stages of the capillary scleroderma pattern at the same time in one image

Juvenile Mixed Connective Tissue Disease (jMCTD) and Overlap Conditions

MCTD is characterised by anti-U1 RNP antibody and frequently has features of arthritis, RP, and can have overlapping features with SLE, SSc and myositis [82]. There are several diagnostic criteria with varying clinical features but all featuring the need for positive anti-U1 RNP to fulfil criteria. None of the items within the criteria (Sharp, Kasukawa, Alarcón-Segovia, Khan) include nailfold capillary abnormalities and none of these criteria have been validated in jMCTD [83–86].

A small number of studies have examined the role of NFC in jMCTD. In the standardised NFC cross-sectional study which included 18 children with MCTD, capillary density was significantly lower, number of dilatations higher with more abnormal shapes and haemorrhages compared to healthy children [6]. Scleroderma pattern was seen in 11/18 (61.1%) of the jMCTD patients which was similar to JDM and less common than in jSSc (92.3%). Giants were seen in 10/18 (55.6%) of jMCTD compared with 84.6% of jSSc.

In jMCTD there were significantly higher rates of abnormalities (such as avascularity, giant loops, hemorrhage) compared to healthy children ($p = 0.008$). This longitudinal study including 7 with jMCTD also showed progression of NFC changes towards more frequent scleroderma pattern [17].

Undifferentiated CTD

In a small cohort of children with undifferentiated CTD (uCTD) defined as RP and ANA autoantibodies, scleroderma pattern in NVC was seen in 9/13 (69.2%) which was less than in those with jSSc where 100% had scleroderma pattern [62].

Miscellaneous

There are very few reports in the literature of NFC in other childhood rheumatic diseases, which are briefly reviewed below.

In paediatrics, juvenile Sjögren's syndrome (JSS) is a rare autoimmune disease. Only one capillaroscopy study has recently been published [87]. The authors reported in JSS reduced capillary density associated with capillary haemorrhages and low C3 [87]. A hypothesis around these findings is that some of those patients studied could have had overlapping symptoms with SLE, because a low C3 is not matching with the diagnosis of SS and it is known that capillary haemorrhages are frequently seen in SLE.

NFC has also been performed in patients with JIA [11, 17, 74]. Capillary density, dimensions and morphology did not differ from those in healthy children; some non-specific variations in nailfold capillaries have been reported in JIA. Furthermore, the capillaroscopic appearance did not differ between the different JIA disease subgroups [11, 17]. This is as expected because JIA is not a systemic vascular disease.

The most common vasculitis in children is IgA vasculitis (previously known as Henoch-Schönlein purpura). Reported capillaroscopy abnormalities include increased non-specific capillary variations (i.e. tortuosity), pericapillary oedema and microvascular network disruption, which are abnormalities that did not completely resolve during clinical remission [88, 89].

Kawasaki disease (KD) is a systemic vasculitis affecting children. Studies in children with KD have reported capillary morphological abnormalities, reduced density and enlarged capillaries in both active and remission phases of the disease [90, 91]. The capillaroscopic pattern shows dynamic features [90]. During the remission phase, the number of enlarged capillaries decreased, and capillary density was significantly improved. In one study there was no correlation between coronary artery involvement and capillary density [91], in the other study a correlation was suggested with morphological abnormalities but EULAR criteria were not used [90–92].

NFC has also been performed in children with Turner syndrome, a chromosomal disorder caused by a complete or partial X monosomy, where hairpin capillaries and non-specific morphologic variations without a specific pattern have been reported [93].

Conclusion

Children are not little adults. This is an important message although capillaroscopic findings in adults and children with the same CTD's show comparable pathologic changes. There is still debate about normal values for different ages and skin colours. For other changes, such as capillary haemorrhages in cSLE, it is still unclear what these mean clinically. Large efforts for prospective studies in children with standardized consensus interpretation (e.g., EULAR/SCTC consensus) are highly needed. Box 1 highlights the research agenda for NFC in children.

In the last decade it has been shown that cSLE, jDM and jMCTD can also show scleroderma(−"like") capillary patterns. The nomenclature of the scleroderma-"like" pattern should be on the research agenda, especially in describing the capillary changes in diseases other than jSSc, certainly as this terminology had not been included in the EULAR/SCTC consensus.

Larger longitudinal studies examining clinical features, autoantibodies and NFC findings in children with CTDs will hopefully help us understand the role of NFC in defining disease phenotypes and risks of organ involvement (and thus screening recommendations). Until risks of organ involvement are better defined in jCTDs, it is important given the frequency of overlap features in the paediatric population and the possibility for phenotypes to change over time (e.g., from a more SLE to SSc phenotype) to fully assess the patient for evidence of vasculopathy (NFC, digital pits/ulcers, sclerodactyly, Raynaud's), skin, musculoskeletal, heart, lung, gastrointestinal and kidney involvement.

Box 1: Research Agenda for NFC in Children

- Further large-scale multi-ethnic cohort studies are needed to confirm whether age and skin colour influence normal values for density, abnormal morphology and apical diameter in healthy children.
- Examination of sensitivity of different capillaroscopy devices to detect capillary changes in children particularly those with small and narrow nailbeds.
- In children who present with RP without a clear diagnosis of CTD, there is a need to evaluate the current recommendations of screening with NFC and autoantibody testing including follow-up frequency and when to repeat NFC. This requires long-term data examining risk of progression to a CTD in paediatric RP patients.
- Perform longitudinal cohort studies in paediatric CTD's to analyse if NFC changes mirror the severity of vascular inflammation and have a prognostic value as a biomarker for disease activity, damage and/or development of future organ involvement.
- Increase our understanding of the role of scleroderma(-like) patterns in cSLE, JDM and MCTD/overlap CTD to predict (future) disease phenotype and to elucidate pathogenesis.

References

1. Anderson C, Leone V, Pain C. Comment on: Nailfold capillaroscopy: a survey of current UK practice and 'next steps' to increase uptake among rheumatologists. Rheumatology (Oxford). 2023;62(10):e303–e4.
2. Ma Z, Mulder DJ, Gniadecki R, Cohen Tervaert JW, Osman M. Methods of assessing Nailfold Capillaroscopy compared to video Capillaroscopy in patients with systemic sclerosis-a critical review of the literature. Diagnostics (Basel). 2023;13(13):2204.
3. Schonenberg-Meinema D, Cutolo M, Smith V. Capillaroscopy in the daily clinic of the pediatric rheumatologist. Best Pract Res Clin Rheumatol. 2024;38(3):101978.
4. Cutolo M, Smith V. Detection of microvascular changes in systemic sclerosis and other rheumatic diseases. Nat Rev Rheumatol. 2021;17(11):665–77.
5. Radic M, Snow M, Frech TM, Saketkoo LA, Cutolo M, Smith V. Consensus-based evaluation of dermatoscopy versus nailfold videocapillaroscopy in Raynaud's phenomenon linking USA and Europe: a European league against rheumatism study group on microcirculation in rheumatic diseases project. Clin Exp Rheumatol. 2020;38 Suppl 125(3):132–6.
6. Melsens K, Cutolo M, Schonenberg-Meinema D, Foeldvari I, Leone MC, Mostmans Y, et al. Standardized nailfold capillaroscopy in children with rheumatic diseases: a worldwide study. Rheumatology (Oxford). 2023;62(4):1605–15.
7. Ingegnoli F, Herrick AL, Schioppo T, Bartoli F, Ughi N, Pauling JD, et al. Reporting items for capillaroscopy in clinical research on musculoskeletal diseases: a systematic review and international Delphi consensus. Rheumatology (Oxford). 2021;60(3):1410–8.
8. Dinsdale G, Roberts C, Moore T, Manning J, Berks M, Allen J, et al. Nailfold capillaroscopy-how many fingers should be examined to detect abnormality? Rheumatology (Oxford). 2019;58(2):284–8.
9. Piotto DG, Len CA, Hilario MO, Terreri MT. Nailfold capillaroscopy in children and adolescents with rheumatic diseases. Rev Bras Reumatol. 2012;52(5):722–32.
10. Piotto DP, Sekiyama J, Kayser C, Yamada M, Len CA, Terreri MT. Nailfold videocapillaroscopy in healthy children and adolescents: description of normal patterns. Clin Exp Rheumatol. 2016;34 Suppl 100(5):193–9.
11. Dolezalova P, Young SP, Bacon PA, Southwood TR. Nailfold capillary microscopy in healthy children and in childhood rheumatic diseases: a prospective single blind observational study. Ann Rheum Dis. 2003;62(5):444–9.
12. Cutolo M, Melsens K, Herrick AL, Foeldvari I, Deschepper E, De Keyser F, et al. Reliability of simple capillaroscopic definitions in describing capillary morphology in rheumatic diseases. Rheumatology (Oxford). 2018;57(4):757–9.
13. Smith V, Beeckman S, Herrick AL, Decuman S, Deschepper E, De Keyser F, et al. An EULAR study group pilot study on reliability of simple capillaroscopic definitions to describe capillary morphology in rheumatic diseases. Rheumatology (Oxford). 2016;55(5):883–90.
14. Ingegnoli F, Herrick AL. Nailfold capillaroscopy in paediatrics. Arthritis Care Res. 2013;65(9):1393–400.
15. Smith V, Herrick AL, Ingegnoli F, Damjanov N, De Angelis R, Denton CP, et al. Standardisation of nailfold capillaroscopy for the assessment of patients with Raynaud's phenomenon and systemic sclerosis. Autoimmun Rev. 2020;19(3):102458.
16. Terreri MT, Andrade LE, Puccinelli ML, Hilario MO, Goldenberg J. Nail fold capillaroscopy: normal findings in children and adolescents. Semin Arthritis Rheum. 1999;29(1):36–42.
17. Ingegnoli F, Zeni S, Gerloni V, Fantini F. Capillaroscopic observations in childhood rheumatic diseases and healthy controls. Clin Exp Rheumatol. 2005;23(6):905–11.
18. Cony M, Klene-Boudard C, Fontan I, Sanciaume C, Sarrat P, Taieb A, et al. Periungual capillaroscopy patterns in normal children. Arch Fr Pediatr. 1992;49(3):171–4.
19. Herrick AL, Moore T, Hollis S, Jayson MI. The influence of age on nailfold capillary dimensions in childhood. J Rheumatol. 2000;27(3):797–800.
20. Leader S. Capillary microscopy in children. Am J Dis Child. 1932;44:403–16.

21. Maricq HR. Nailfold capillaries in normal children. J Nerv Ment Dis. 1965;141(2):197–203.
22. Mayer K. Observations on the capillaries of the normal infant. Am J Dis Child. 1921;22:381–7.
23. Dundar HA, Adrovic A, Demir S, Demir F, Cakmak F, Ayaz NA, et al. Description of the characteristics of the nailfold capillary structure in healthy children: a multi-centric study. Rheumatology (Oxford). 2024;63(SI2):SI152–9.
24. Bergkamp SC, Smith V, Kuijpers TW, Cutolo M, van den Berg JM, Schonenberg-Meinema D. Correlations between capillary density and degree of skin pigmentation in healthy children analysed by nailfold video capillaroscopy. Quant Imaging Med Surg. 2023;13(6):3938–47.
25. Andrade LE, Gabriel Junior A, Assad RL, Ferrari AJ, Atra E. Panoramic nailfold capillaroscopy: a new reading method and normal range. Semin Arthritis Rheum. 1990;20(1):21–31.
26. Whitson DW, Jones MB. Visibility of the nailfold capillaries in normal adolescents. Biol Psychiatry. 1971;3(3):281–7.
27. Herrick AL, Wigley FM. Raynaud's phenomenon. Best Pract Res Clin Rheumatol. 2020;34(1):101474.
28. Garner R, Kumari R, Lanyon P, Doherty M, Zhang W. Prevalence, risk factors and associations of primary Raynaud's phenomenon: systematic review and meta-analysis of observational studies. BMJ Open. 2015;5(3):e006389.
29. Jones GT, Herrick AL, Woodham SE, Baildam EM, Macfarlane GJ, Silman AJ. Occurrence of Raynaud's phenomenon in children ages 12-15 years: prevalence and association with other common symptoms. Arthritis Rheum. 2003;48(12):3518–21.
30. Fraenkel L. Raynaud's phenomenon: epidemiology and risk factors. Curr Rheumatol Rep. 2002;4(2):123–8.
31. Tervi A, Ramste M, Abner E, Cheng P, Lane JM, Maher M, et al. Genetic and functional analysis of Raynaud's syndrome implicates loci in vasculature and immunity. Cell Genom. 2024;4(9):100630.
32. Nigrovic PA, Fuhlbrigge RC, Sundel RP. Raynaud's phenomenon in children: a retrospective review of 123 patients. Pediatrics. 2003;111(4 Pt 1):715–21.
33. Pavlov-Dolijanovic S, Damjanov N, Ostojic P, Susic G, Stojanovic R, Gacic D, et al. The prognostic value of nailfold capillary changes for the development of connective tissue disease in children and adolescents with primary raynaud phenomenon: a follow-up study of 250 patients. Pediatr Dermatol. 2006;23(5):437–42.
34. Pain CE, Constantin T, Toplak N, Moll M, Iking-Konert C, Piotto DP, et al. Raynaud's syndrome in children: systematic review and development of recommendations for assessment and monitoring. Clin Exp Rheumatol. 2016;34(Suppl 100):200–6.
35. Koenig M, Joyal F, Fritzler MJ, Roussin A, Abrahamowicz M, Boire G, et al. Autoantibodies and microvascular damage are independent predictive factors for the progression of Raynaud's phenomenon to systemic sclerosis: a twenty-year prospective study of 586 patients, with validation of proposed criteria for early systemic sclerosis. Arthritis Rheum. 2008;58(12):3902–12.
36. Piotto DG, Hilario MO, Carvalho NS, Len CA, Andrade LE, Terreri MT. Prospective nailfold capillaroscopy evaluation of Raynaud's phenomenon in children and adolescents. Acta Reumatol Port. 2013;38(2):114–21.
37. Foeldvari I, Culpo R, Sperotto F, Anton J, Avcin T, Baildam E, et al. Consensus-based recommendations for the management of juvenile systemic sclerosis. Rheumatology (Oxford). 2021;60(4):1651–8.
38. Farenhorst CA, Roon AM, Gessel AI, Stel AJ, Bootsma H, Armbrust W, et al. Capillary microscopy is a potential screening method for connective tissue disease in children with Raynaud's phenomenon. Pediatr Rheumatol Online J. 2022;20(1):11.
39. Li AR, Burke CD, Purvis CS, Lee LW. Association between nailfold capillaroscopy abnormalities and autoimmune disease in pediatric populations. Pediatr Dermatol. 2022;39(2):197–204.
40. Gorski S, Bartnicka M, Citko A, Zelazowska-Rutkowska B, Jablonski K, Gorska A. Microangiopathy in Naifold Videocapillaroscopy and its relations to sE- selectin, Endothelin-1, and hsCRP as putative endothelium dysfunction markers among adolescents with Raynaud's phenomenon. J Clin Med. 2019;8(5):567.

41. Foeldvari I, Zhavania M, Birdi N, Cuttica RJ, de Oliveira SH, Dent PB, et al. Favourable outcome in 135 children with juvenile systemic sclerosis: results of a multi-national survey. Rheumatology (Oxford). 2000;39(5):556–9.
42. Mier R, Ansell B, Hall MA, Hasson N, Levinson J, Lovell D, et al. Long term follow-up of children with mixed connective tissue disease. Lupus. 1996;5(3):221–6.
43. Mueller M, Gschwandtner ME, Emminger W, Kiener H, Schnaubelt S, Giurgea GA, et al. Associations between nailfold capillary aberrations and autoantibodies in children and adults with Raynaud's phenomenon. RMD Open. 2023;9(1):e003077.
44. Goldman W, Seltzer R, Reuman P. Association between treatment with central nervous system stimulants and Raynaud's syndrome in children: a retrospective case-control study of rheumatology patients. Arthritis Rheum. 2008;58(2):563–6.
45. Umair HM, Sandler RD, Alunno A, Matucci-Cerinic M, Hughes M. Association between central nervous system stimulants used to treat attention deficit hyperactivity disorder (ADHD) and Raynaud's phenomenon: a scoping review. Semin Arthritis Rheum. 2021;51(6):1200–4.
46. van den Hoogen F, Khanna D, Fransen J, Johnson SR, Baron M, Tyndall A, et al. 2013 classification criteria for systemic sclerosis: an American college of rheumatology/European league against rheumatism collaborative initiative. Ann Rheum Dis. 2013;72(11):1747–55.
47. Zulian F, Woo P, Athreya BH, Laxer RM, Medsger TA Jr, Lehman TJ, et al. The Pediatric rheumatology European society/American College of Rheumatology/European league against rheumatism provisional classification criteria for juvenile systemic sclerosis. Arthritis Rheum. 2007;57(2):203–12.
48. Smith V, Riccieri V, Pizzorni C, Decuman S, Deschepper E, Bonroy C, et al. Nailfold capillaroscopy for prediction of novel future severe organ involvement in systemic sclerosis. J Rheumatol. 2013;40(12):2023–8.
49. Medsger TA Jr, Bombardieri S, Czirjak L, Scorza R, Della Rossa A, Bencivelli W. Assessment of disease severity and prognosis. Clin Exp Rheumatol. 2003;21(3 Suppl 29):S42–6.
50. Avouac J, Lepri G, Smith V, Toniolo E, Hurabielle C, Vallet A, et al. Sequential nailfold videocapillaroscopy examinations have responsiveness to detect organ progression in systemic sclerosis. Semin Arthritis Rheum. 2017;47(1):86–94.
51. Denton CP, De Lorenzis E, Roblin E, Goldman N, Alcacer-Pitarch B, Blamont E, et al. The 2024 British Society for Rheumatology guideline for management of systemic sclerosis. Rheumatology (Oxford). 2024;63(11):2956–75.
52. Ingegnoli F, Boracchi P, Gualtierotti R, Smith V, Cutolo M, Foeldvari I, et al. A comparison between nailfold capillaroscopy patterns in adulthood in juvenile and adult-onset systemic sclerosis: a EUSTAR exploratory study. Microvasc Res. 2015;102:19–24.
53. Foeldvari I, Klotsche J, Kasapcopur O, Adrovic A, Terreri MT, Sakamoto AP, et al. Gender differences in juvenile systemic sclerosis patients: results from the international juvenile scleroderma inception cohort. J Scleroderma Relat Disord. 2023;8(2):120–30.
54. Li JC, Tadros S, Rosser F, Torok KS. Pulmonary nodules in juvenile systemic sclerosis: a case-series from the National Registry for childhood onset scleroderma (NRCOS). Diagnostics (Basel). 2023;13(12):2103.
55. Martini G, Foeldvari I, Russo R, Cuttica R, Eberhard A, Ravelli A, et al. Systemic sclerosis in childhood: clinical and immunologic features of 153 patients in an international database. Arthritis Rheum. 2006;54(12):3971–8.
56. Borowiec A, Dabrowski R, Wozniak J, Jasek S, Chwyczko T, Kowalik I, et al. Cardiovascular assessment of asymptomatic patients with juvenile-onset localized and systemic scleroderma: 10 years prospective observation. Scand J Rheumatol. 2012;41(1):33–8.
57. Stevens BE, Torok KS, Li SC, Hershey N, Curran M, Higgins GC, et al. Clinical characteristics and factors associated with disability and impaired quality of life in children with juvenile systemic sclerosis: results from the childhood arthritis and rheumatology research Alliance legacy registry. Arthritis Care Res (Hoboken). 2018;70(12):1806–13.
58. Jindal AK, Patra P, Guleria S, Gupta A, Bhattad S, Rawat A, et al. Clinical profile, long-term follow-up and outcome of juvenile systemic scleroderma: 25 years of clinical experience from north-West India. Clin Exp Rheumatol. 2021;39 Suppl 131(4):149–56.

59. Adrovic A, Sahin S, Barut K, Kasapcopur O. Juvenile Scleroderma: A Referral Center Experience. Arch Rheumatol. 2018;33(3):344–51.
60. Jacquel L, Bechara R, Terzic J, Rameau AC, Chatelus E, Rossi-Semerano L, et al. An updated overview of juvenile systemic sclerosis in a French cohort. Pediatr Rheumatol Online J. 2025;23(1):13.
61. Cutolo M, Sulli A, Pizzorni C, Accardo S. Nailfold videocapillaroscopy assessment of microvascular damage in systemic sclerosis. J Rheumatol. 2000;27(1):155–60.
62. Schonenberg-Meinema D, Bergkamp SC, Nassar-Sheikh Rashid A, Gruppen MP, Middelkamp-Hup MA, Armbrust W, et al. Nailfold capillary scleroderma pattern may be associated with disease damage in childhood-onset systemic lupus erythematosus: important lessons from longitudinal follow-up. Lupus Sci Med. 2022;9(1):e000572.
63. Boonstra M, Ciaffi J, Noordhoek DC, Liem SIE, Beaart-van de Voorde LJJ, van Bijnen STA, et al. Improvement of microangiopathy after haematopoietic stem cell transplantation in systemic sclerosis. Clin Exp Rheumatol. 2022;40(10):1993–8.
64. Wildt M, Andreasson K, Hamberg V, Hesselstrand R, Wuttge DM. Treatment with mycophenolate mofetil is associated with improved nailfold vasculature in systemic sclerosis. Rheumatology (Oxford). 2024;63(2):385–91.
65. Cutolo M, Melsens K, Wijnant S, Ingegnoli F, Thevissen K, De Keyser F, et al. Nailfold capillaroscopy in systemic lupus erythematosus: a systematic review and critical appraisal. Autoimmun Rev. 2018;17(4):344–52.
66. Schonenberg-Meinema D, Melsens K, Nassar-Sheikh Rashid A, Cutolo M, Kuijpers TW, van den Berg JM, et al. Capillaroscopy in childhood-onset systemic lupus erythematosus: a first systematic review. Clin Exp Rheumatol. 2020;38(2):350–4.
67. Schonenberg-Meinema D, Bergkamp SC, Nassar-Sheikh Rashid A, van der Aa LB, de Bree GJ, Ten Cate R, et al. Nailfold capillary abnormalities in childhood-onset systemic lupus erythematosus: a cross-sectional study compared with healthy controls. Lupus. 2021;30(5):818–27.
68. Bergkamp SC, Schonenberg-Meinema D, Nassar-Sheikh Rashid A, Melsens K, Vanhaecke A, Boumans MJH, et al. Reliable detection of subtypes of nailfold capillary haemorrhages in childhood-onset systemic lupus erythematosus. Clin Exp Rheumatol. 2021;39(5):1126–31.
69. Ingegnoli F. Capillaroscopy abnormalities in relation to disease activity in juvenile systemic lupus erythematosus. Microvasc Res. 2013;87:92–4.
70. Ingegnoli F, Zeni S, Meani L, Soldi A, Lurati AF, Fantini F. Evaluation of nailfold videocapillaroscopic abnormalities in patients with systemic lupus erythematosus. JCR-J Clin Rheumatol. 2005;11(6):295–8.
71. Zhao T, Lin FA, Chen HP. Pattern of Nailfold Capillaroscopy in patients with systemic lupus erythematosus. Arch Rheumatol. 2020;35(4):568–74.
72. Shenavandeh S, Habibi S. Nailfold capillaroscopic changes in patients with systemic lupus erythematosus: correlations with disease activity, skin manifestation and nephritis. Lupus. 2017;26(9):959–66.
73. Raeeskarami SR, Namazi N, Assari R, Najafizadeh SR, Hassannejad Z, Ziaee V. The comparison of Nailfold Capillaroscopy between juvenile systemic lupus erythematosus and healthy controls: correlation with laboratory and clinical parameters. Int J Vasc Med. 2020;2020:7631958.
74. Piotto DG, Len CA, Hilario MO, Terreri MT. Nailfold capillaroscopy in children and adolescents with rheumatic diseases. Rev Bras Reumatol. 2012;52(5):727–32.
75. Schonenberg-Meinema D, Bergkamp SC, Rashid ANS, Gruppen MP, Middelkamp-Hup MA, Armbrust W, et al. Nailfold capillary scleroderma pattern may be associated with disease damage in childhood-onset systemic lupus erythematosus: important lessons from longitudinal follow-up. Lupus Sci Med. 2022;9(1):e000572.
76. Smith V, Pizzorni C, De Keyser F, Decuman S, Van Praet JT, Deschepper E, et al. Reliability of the qualitative and semiquantitative nailfold videocapillaroscopy assessment in a systemic sclerosis cohort: a two-Centre study. Ann Rheum Dis. 2010;69(6):1092–6.
77. Lambova SN. Scleroderma-like capillaroscopic pattern in SLE is not a sign of overlap syndrome in both adults and children. Lupus Sci Med. 2022;9(1):e000749.

78. Cancarini P, Nozawa T, Whitney K, Bell-Peter A, Marcuz JA, Taddio A, et al. The clinical features of juvenile dermatomyositis: a single-centre inception cohort. Semin Arthritis Rheum. 2022;57:152104.
79. Barth Z, Witczak BN, Flato B, Koller A, Sjaastad I, Sanner H. Assessment of microvascular abnormalities by Nailfold Capillaroscopy in juvenile Dermatomyositis after medium- to long-term Followup. Arthritis Care Res. 2018;70(5):768–76.
80. Manfredi A, Sebastiani M, Campomori F, Pipitone N, Giuggioli D, Colaci M, et al. Nailfold Videocapillaroscopy alterations in Dermatomyositis and systemic sclerosis: toward identification of a specific pattern. J Rheumatol. 2016;43(8):1575–80.
81. Barth Z, Schwartz T, Flato B, Aalokken TM, Koller A, Lund MB, et al. Association between Nailfold capillary density and pulmonary and cardiac involvement in medium to longstanding juvenile Dermatomyositis. Arthritis Care Res. 2019;71(4):492–7.
82. John KJ, Sadiq M, George T, Gunasekaran K, Francis N, Rajadurai E, et al. Clinical and immunological profile of mixed connective tissue disease and a comparison of four diagnostic criteria. Int J Rheumatol. 2020;2020:9692030.
83. Alarcon-Segovia D, Cardiel MH. Comparison between 3 diagnostic criteria for mixed connective tissue disease. Study of 593 patients. J Rheumatol. 1989;16(3):328–34.
84. Kahn M-F. Syndrome de sharp. La Revue du praticien (Paris). 1990;40(21):1944–5.
85. Kasukawa R. Mixed connective tissue disease. Intern Med. 1999;38(5):386–93.
86. Sharp GC, Irvin WS, Tan EM, Gould RG, Holman HR. Mixed connective tissue disease—an apparently distinct rheumatic disease syndrome associated with a specific antibody to an extractable nuclear antigen (ENA). Am J Med. 1972;52(2):148–59.
87. Lercara A, Malattia C, Hysa E, Gattorno M, Cere A, Lavarello C, et al. Microvascular status in juvenile Sjogren's disease: the first nailfold videocapillaroscopy investigation. Clin Rheumatol. 2024;43(2):733–41.
88. Zampetti A, Rigante D, Bersani G, Rendeli C, Feliciani C, Stabile A. Longitudinal study of microvascular involvement by nailfold capillaroscopy in children with Henoch-Schonlein purpura. Clin Rheumatol. 2009;28(9):1101–5.
89. Martino F, Agolini D, Tsalikova E, Bederti O, Principessa L, Martino E, et al. Nailfold capillaroscopy in Henoch-Schonlein purpura: a follow-up study of 31 cases. J Pediatr. 2002;141(1):145.
90. Huang MY, Huang JJ, Huang TY, Gupta-Malhotra M, Syu FK. Deterioration of cutaneous microcirculatory status of Kawasaki disease. Clin Rheumatol. 2012;31(5):847–52.
91. Reddy Konda VV, Jindal AK, Nadig PL, Banday AZ, Vinay K, Singh S. Microvascular changes on nailfold capillaroscopy in acute stage of Kawasaki disease: a new diagnostic paradigm for an enigmatic condition. Rheumatology (Oxford). 2024;63(2):392–8.
92. Sedaghat B, Raeeskarami SR, Tahghighi F, Assari R, Aghaei-Moghadam E, Razavi-Khorasani N, et al. The role of nailfold capillaroscopy in pediatric patients with Kawasaki disease. Reumatol Clin (Engl Ed). 2023;19(5):255–9.
93. Coelho SCSRA, Pinheiro VS, Solberg PFC, de Faria JP, Naliato ECO, Fernandes TJ, Guimarães MM. Nailfold video capillaroscopy in turner syndrome: a descriptive study. J Vasc Bras. 2007;6(4):325–31.

Research Methods; Functional Measures of Nailfold Capillaroscopy Including Permeability, Perfusion and Oxygenation

Andrea Murray and John Allen

Key Points

- Permeability of nailfold capillaries offers a potential imaging technique to elucidate pathogenesis, particularly relating to adaptive vs protective mechanisms and to understanding of the role of oedema in disease.
- Capillary blood flow (perfusion) can be measured by several different techniques. Capillary perfusion has been shown to differentiate between healthy controls and patients with systemic sclerosis (SSc) and to be a sensitive measure of response to pharmacological treatment. However, achieving accurate measures of flow remains challenging.
- Measuring oxygenation in nailfold capillaries is a novel technique, remaining firmly within the research arena and requiring validation; however, it offers exciting possibilities for assessing early disease and treatment response in clinical trials.

A. Murray (✉)
Centre for Musculoskeletal Research, Division of Musculoskeletal and Dermatological Sciences, The University of Manchester, Manchester Academic Health Science Centre, Manchester, UK

Northern Care Alliance NHS Foundation Trust, Salford, UK

National Institute for Health and Care Research (NIHR) Manchester Biomedical Research Centre, Manchester, UK
e-mail: andrea.murray@manchester.ac.uk

J. Allen
Vascular Optics and Microvascular Sensing, Centre for Intelligent Healthcare, Coventry University, Coventry, UK
e-mail: ad5325@coventry.ac.uk

A. L. Herrick et al. (eds.), *Nailfold Capillaroscopy in Rheumatological Diseases*,
https://doi.org/10.1007/978-3-032-03970-5_10

Introduction

With the advent of the 2013 systemic sclerosis (SSc) classification criteria [1] the structural assessment of nailfold capillaries is now well established into clinical practice both in SSc-spectrum disorders and also for other connective tissue diseases. Structural measures facilitate clinical diagnosis and discrimination of primary from secondary Raynaud's phenomenon. The incorporation of capillaroscopy into the clinical pathway for clinical diagnosis has led to other advancements which remain on the periphery between research and clinical fields, including standardization of protocols, handheld low-cost systems and machine learning software to enhance automated quantitative capillary measurement (see chapter "Quantitative Analysis" [2–5]). Other developments are still firmly within the remit of research. These include functional measurements such as permeability, perfusion and oxygenation. The limitations on such developments, in terms of translation from the laboratory to the outpatient clinic are mainly due to complexities of techniques (e.g. high-speed cameras to measure velocity) or their invasiveness (e.g. intravenous delivery of fluorophores): these limitations have impeded full validation. Functional capillary measures still need to prove their usefulness both for understanding pathophysiology and for determining real added value. Advantages include potentially aiding early detection particularly with the relatively new VEDOSS (Very Early Diagnosis of Systemic Sclerosis) proposal, when structural vascular changes are present but may not yet be conclusive and clinical symptoms are nonspecific [6]. Changes in function prior to, or in parallel to, structural changes potentially add sensitivity. Functional changes can be induced (e.g. by heat, cold or occlusion) and, whilst they are likely influenced by structural changes (which in a disease modifying process, take place over years), take place over much shorter time frames of minutes-hours. Functional changes may improve nailfold capillaroscopy's sensitivity to change, for example further reinforcing reported changes in capillary structure in trials of a vasodilators or disease modifying drugs [7, 8] and detecting subtle differences in flow or oxygenation with disease and/or intervention.

In this chapter we focus on research into measurement of functional aspects of the capillaries in three areas, at varying levels of progress: permeability, blood flow (perfusion) and oxygenation.

Permeability Assessments Using Capillaroscopy

Fluorescent Dye Perfusion in Nailfold Capillaries Relating to Local Skin Physiology

The relevance and role of nailfold capillary permeability relates to the surrounding physiology. At the dermal-epidermal junction the dermal papillae form an 'egg box' like structure tessellating with the epidermal ridges. Capillaries are embedded within these papillae (concentric collagen lamellae, layers of collagen fibrils) and, at the nailfold, where the capillaries are pushed beneath the nail and lie flat these

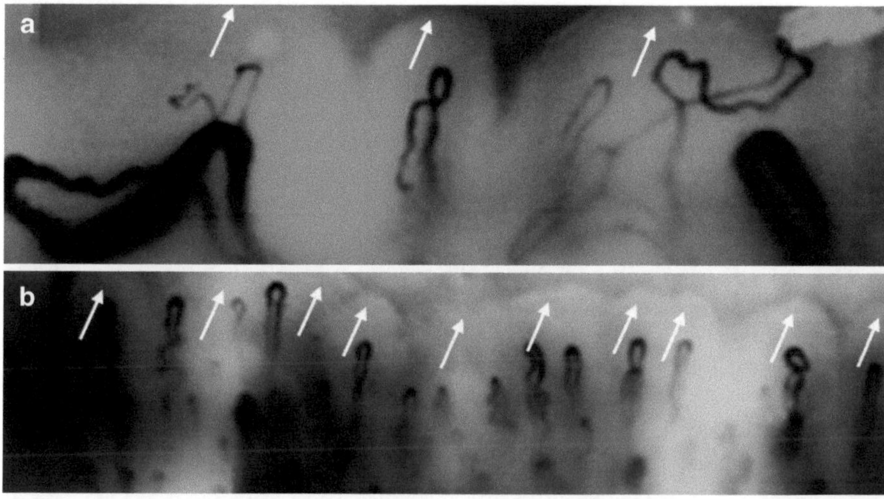

Fig. 1 Examples of cropped, nailfold capillary images, showing the 'halo' or dermal papillae (white arrows); (**a**) patient with SSc and (**b**) healthy control. Images have been contrast-enhanced (post-processed digitally) to show the halo clearly

papillae (sometimes referred to as the perivascular zone) can be observed as a 'halo' [9]. The halo is paler than the epidermis layer thus showing a contrasting region which has clearly defined boundaries (Fig. 1). Shirshin et al. confirmed that the perivascular zone corresponded to the border of 'viable epidermis' using the technique of two-photon tomography with fluorescence lifetime imaging. This technique excites endogenous fluorophores in the tissue to fluoresce and measures the lifetime it takes to decay. Since the nailfold tissue components (e.g. collagen or erythrocytes) have different properties then the boundaries between them can be identified. The authors hypothesized that increased halo size related to increased accumulation of interstitial fluid and identified that halo size was directly linked to clinically significant oedema observed in patients with heart failure [10].

Nailfold Transcapillary Diffusion (Permeability) Studies

At the nailfold, the assessment of transcapillary diffusion (dynamic fluorescence videomicroscopy), also referred to as permeability or leakiness, is carried out using a protocol of fluorescent dye intravenous injection into the antecubital vein. The bolus of sodium fluorescein [NaF]) travels to the hands and nailfolds over a measured period of time. The dye fluoresces when illuminated by light of a certain wavelength and the fluorescence itself is emitted at a different (lower energy) wavelength. Hence, the progress of the dye is monitored by nailfold capillaroscopy using a light source at the specific wavelength necessary to excite the fluorescent dyes (Fig. 2). The camera chosen then captures the image at the emission wavelength of the dye. For NaF ultraviolet (UV)/blue illumination is used (either a UV/blue light

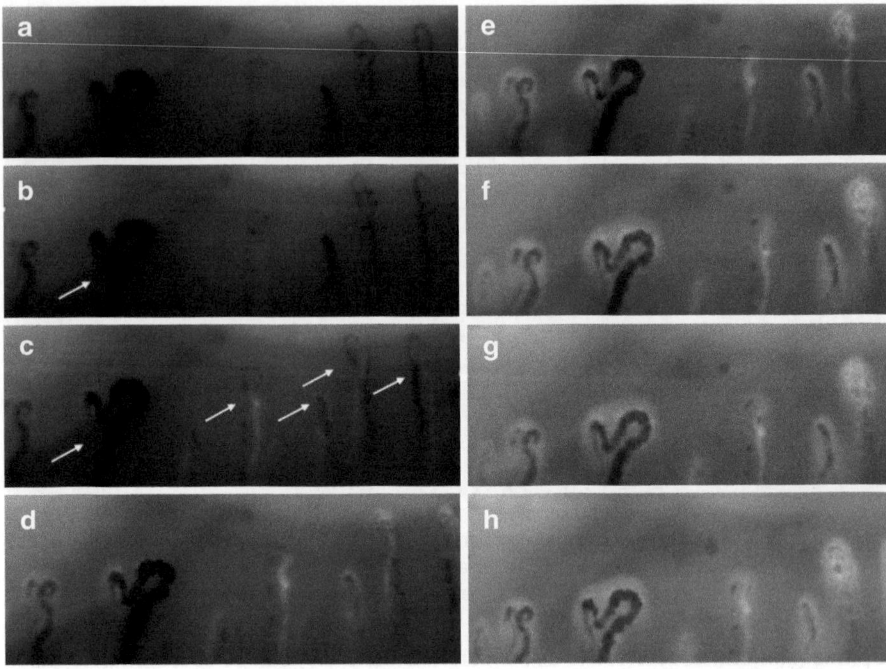

Fig. 2 Sequential images (**a**–**h**) taken from a fluoroscopy video of sodium fluorescein entering the capillaries and diffusing into the dermal papillae. White arrows highlight initial dye entering the capillaries

source or a broadband white light source with a filter, excitation in the blue 465–490 nm, emission in the green at 510–530 nm). Upon reaching the capillaries, the dye diffuses through the permeable capillary walls into the halo and beyond to the interstitial space, utilizing the intrinsic capillary properties essential for nutritional flow exchange. The dynamics of the dye permeating across the capillary wall and into the halo provides useful information on the condition of both the microvascular walls and the surrounding skin structure.

The technique was initially pioneered by Bollinger et al. in the late 1970s. NaF had long been used as a fluorescent marker for retinal angiography [11] and thus was an obvious choice for adaption to assess the microvasculature at the nailfold. Limitations include the invasive approach of the technique, requiring an intravenous bolus and with risk of anaphylactic reaction to the bolus.

In their seminal study in 1979, Bollinger et al. imaged 12 healthy controls, describing the appearance and evolution of dye through capillaries at the nailfold. It was observed that post injection, the dye could be seen initially in the capillaries, then in the 'halo' and then in the pericapillary interstitial space [12]. These early techniques were analogue, requiring significant effort to extract data from consecutive video frames displayed on TV screens. Therefore, permeability was only assessed in a small subset of capillaries manually. The studies that followed all used similar protocols: accounting for acclimatization (of approximately 20 min) at set room temperatures (approximately 24 ± 1 °C) to ensure homogeneity of conditions for all participants. Oil (often paraffin oil) was used on the nailfold to aid visualization and the hand was held at heart level with patients sometimes reclining. The bolus (varying concentrations, adjusted for estimated total blood volume) was then delivered. Outcomes included time from dye delivery to nailfold arrival and a measure of fluorescence dynamics with time. Imaging continued regularly for up to an hour, recording the spread of fluorescent dye across the nailfold area. Relative fluorescence curves were then plotted, e.g. frame intensity as a percentage of the maximum with time, from first observation of the dye to the end of the observation period.

Several more studies were carried out by Bollinger's group, including a study of 13 patients with SSc and 12 controls that identified increased permeability both at the capillary wall and the papillary border in the SSc group as compared to the controls, indicating abnormalities in the interstitial space. The time to dye arrival was not significantly different between the groups; however, the time from filling the first to the last capillary was less than 12 s for the control group but in 5 of the patients with SSc the dye arrival was markedly delayed to between 25 s to 5 min. For the healthy controls the halo filled relatively quickly and remained well defined for 10 min with some perfusion to more distant tissue (indicating an 'intact' boundary at the dermal-epidermal junction). In contrast for the patients with SSc the halo, often irregularly shaped, could not be observed in some capillaries due to blurring of the boundaries. The NaF dye preferentially permeated from the venular side of the capillary in patients but was symmetric for the control group. In capillaries with blurred boundaries, the dye diffused into the wider interstitial space quickly and easily, implying damage to boundaries where epithelial cell linings begin. The authors concluded that in patients with SSc there was faster transcapillary and interstitial transfusion from enlarged vessels. Whilst this could be due to increased capillary surface area, there was no correlation between the estimated surface area and the diffusion rate. They also reasoned that since blood flow in the fingers is lower in patients with SSc (also implied by finger temperature measurement being lower in the patients than controls) then faster or more perfusion cannot account for the increase in fluorescence intensity in patients. Thus, increased permeability is the most likely cause [9].

Grassi et al. debated whether increased permeability in SSc might be adaptive and protective rather than vasculopathy due to wall damage and oedema. They noted that increased permeability had been identified in capillaries under critical hypoxia, suggesting that despite a decreased perfusion due to cold fingers undergoing vasospasm, increased permeability over longer periods, may provide 'nutritional protection'. Additionally, they reported increased permeability with a heat stimulus in SSc. Thus, the increased permeability observed may be a compensatory mechanism to ensure that the tissue receives the nutrients it requires to function [13].

Permeability in Response to Medication

Grassi et al. [14] assessed the effect of nifedipine (a calcium-channel blocker) in 11 patients with SSc and 7 controls using NaF capillaroscopy alongside a cold challenge, before and after dosing. The study consisted of three visits: visit 1, baseline nailfold imaging following a 7 day washout period. At visit 2 (day 2), participants underwent (gloved) hand submersion into 5 °C water for 3 min. Capillary imaging was performed 2 min after removal from water. Visit 3 (day 4) participants took 10 mg of nifedipine orally and underwent the same cold challenge protocol 5 min later. There was no significant difference between any visit in terms of time for dye appearance for the control group (mean time 26.6–29.6 s for all visits). For the patients there was a significant delay in the time for dye appearance after cold challenge (mean time 27.5 [baseline] to 224.1 [visit 2] s). This was ameliorated by nifedipine to 112.7 s (but was still significantly delayed as compared to the baseline), indicating that nifedipine did not restore time to dye arrival back to baseline measures or to a time equivalent to healthy controls). The shape of the fluorescence intensity curves was also altered from baseline, with dye diffusion significantly decreased at visit 2, after cold challenge in patients. Post nifedipine and cold challenge (visit 3), the fluorescence levels in the patient cohort had increased to similar levels to the control group at baseline. This suggests that whilst the time to arrival was not restored to control levels, the overall diffusion of dye was 'normalised' by the administration of nifedipine. In the control group there was an unexpected increase in capillary permeability on cooling (proposed to be due to reactive hyperaemia). In contrast to the patient group, no significant difference in fluorescence levels was measured after nifedipine in healthy controls. The conclusion was that if vasomotor tone was already 'normal', as in the control group, then nifedipine had no effect on flow or permeability.

In a study of bosentan, 15 patients with limited cutaneous SSc were imaged in a single centre study and followed longitudinally. Patients were administered 16 weeks bosentan (62.5 mg for 4 weeks, 125 mg for 12 weeks) and were followed-up for a further 4 weeks. The microvasculature was assessed in several ways including structural nailfold capillaroscopy and microscopy capillary permeability. Citing too much variability between capillary permeability imaged at the nailfold in previous studies, this study utilized fluorescence videodensitometry at the ankle (2 × 3 mm image, ×100 magnification, immersion oil applied to the skin surface). Post NaF administration, images were taken every 20 s and digitized from analogue tape with calculation of arbitrary light intensity (automatic gain had been disabled). A curve of relative % fluorescence intensity was plotted over the first 7 min after the bolus arrived and the area under the curve calculated for baseline and weeks 8, 16 and 20. There was a non-significant decrease in dye arrival time and an increase in the area under the curve between baseline and 8 weeks but differences were no longer present at 16 and 20 weeks. No statistically significant change in capillary density at the nailfold was observed over the time period [15].

Permeability Measures in Relation to Other Diseases

The measurement of microvascular permeability, is not limited to studies of SSc and RP but indeed has relevance in other microvascular diseases. Sometimes referred to as videofluorangiography in other fields, this has been used to study several microvascular diseases including diabetes, fibromyalgia, vasculitis, heart failure and renal transplantation [10, 16–19]. It is probable that vasculopathy-related mechanisms overlap between these studies. In diabetes, increased permeability has been reported in comparison to age- and sex-matched healthy controls and relationships have been identified between permeability and vascular endothelial growth factor serum levels (a potential biomarker for SSc [20, 21].

Healthy control studies also enable increased understanding of the physiological effects of drugs on permeability that are potentially relevant to SSc. A study by Herrig et al., proposed administration of drugs via microneedles at the nailfold monitored by fluorescence videomicroscopy. Using this novel technique in 12 healthy controls demonstrated the effects of histamine and the antihistamine cetirizine [22]. Histamine increases vascular permeability via an interaction between H1 receptors and endothelial cells, and potentially plays a key role in skin inflammation and fibrosis [23]. The increased permeability induced by histamine was reduced by cetirizine, improving understanding of mechanistic processes [23]. This was later followed by a dose dependence study using a similar protocol [24]. Costanzo et al. studied interleukin-2 (IL-2), a cytokine involved in immune responses (linked to inflammation and potentially fibrosis and known to be increased in SSc). In a study of 12 healthy controls increased permeability was identified following subepidermal injection of IL-2 when imaged at the tibial plateau [25]. The authors proposed that the increased oedema after administration was related to this increase in permeability.

Capillary Permeability Measured at the Ankle

Following on from the Bollinger et al. studies at the nailfold, others proceeded to monitor permeability over larger areas at the ankle in order to determine whether differences in permeability were systemic as opposed to local to the nailfold. Using methods initially developed in healthy controls and then used in patients with diabetes [26–28], Hettema et al., identified significantly decreased permeability at the ankle in 38 patients with SSc (conversely to previous nailfold measures) as compared to 20 age matched healthy controls. The relationship between permeability and capillary density was suggested as a possible explanation [29].

Sublingual Capillary Imaging and the Relation of the Glycocalyx to Increased Permeability

Sublingual imaging can be carried out with a camera similar to that used for nailfold capillaroscopy. The erythrocytes are easily observed enabling morphological assessment. Morphological sublingual changes appear to correlate with those at the nailfold and functional changes in sublingual microcirculation appear to precede structural alteration [30–33]. One advantage of sublingual over nailfold imaging is the opportunity to measure the glycocalyx, lining the inner capillary wall. The glycocalyx has multiple roles including passively inhibiting capillary fluid leakage and consequential oedema as well as inhibiting coagulation, both relevant to SSc. It is suggested that chronic ischemia-reperfusion induces glycocalyx damage via reactive oxygen species (observed across several microvascular diseases including SSc, diabetes and cardiovascular disease) [34]. In addition, the glycocalyx mediates shear stress, supports nitric oxide production and is the location of 'vascular protective enzymes and a wide range of anticoagulant factors' [32]; this means that its degradation probably feeds directly into SSc-related vasculopathy. Compromised glycocalyx (thinned layer depth) has been demonstrated in patients with SSc as compared to control cohorts in several studies sublingually [30] and it is hypothesized that this directly contributes to both vascular leakage and oedema. Whilst it is not easy to visualize the glycocalyx in the nailfold, these changes are almost certainly systemic and as such account for some of the alterations in permeability discussed above.

Relevance of Permeability to Oedema and the Wider Disease Process

Capillary permeability potentially relates more widely to oedema, which has strong relevance in connective tissue diseases. The presence of puffy fingers is a red flag for the VEDOSS [35], and is an independent predictor for SSc [36]. Puffy fingers also can occur in mixed connective tissue disease and as a possible side effect of calcium channel blockers used in the treatment of Raynaud's phenomenon [37, 38].

In the early stages of SSc and prior to fibrotic alterations, puffy fingers, when present may represent one aspect of systemic oedema. Grassi et al., hypothesized that diffuse endothelial damage may initiate the progression from Raynaud's phenomenon to SSc; citing the work of Bollinger in identifying increased capillary permeability in early disease, prior to morphological changes [12]. It is hypothesised that the chronic cycle of Raynaud's related ischaemic episodes leads to hypoxia and endothelial alteration contributing to upregulation of hypoxia inducible factor, transforming growth factor β and vascular endothelial growth factor [39]. Combined with glycocalyx damage, this leads to interstitial oedema due to increased vascular leak and this contributes to the puffy fingers, in turn leading to fibrosis. At the nailfold capillary level, these functional changes likely occur early, prior to the architectural capillary changes observed as the 'scleroderma pattern'. Giant capillaries and capillary drop out (and later compensatory neovascularisation) are routinely observed within the nailfold at different stages of the SSc disease process: mechanical stretching of the vessel walls in giant capillaries probably contributes to increased permeability, as does the natural process of loosening of tight junctions in angiogenic capillaries [40, 41]. Frech et al. identified abnormalities and damage in the endothelium with consequent interstitial oedema via analysis of forearm biopsies in patients with SSc, but not in patients with primary Raynaud's phenomenon or controls (as expected); building evidence of systemic vascular leak in SSc [42]. Sfikakis et al. suggested that deposition of iron in the tissue surrounding the capillaries, due to haemorrhages, also directly contributes to fibrosis [43].

Indocyanine Green to Visualize Capillary Plasma

Contemporaneously with NaF being first used to measure permeability, indocyanine green [ICG], (also used for retinal angiography) was used to label plasma and plasma mapping in capillaries. ICG binds to plasma/serum proteins, therefore enabling visualization of plasma location under fluorescence. As with NaF this requires a light source, here near infrared light (excitation 780 nm, emission 820 nm). NaF and ICG highlight different aspects of the microvasculature, NaF highlights the permeability of the vessels and diffuses quickly through the capillary wall. ICG highlights the plasma, crossing the microvascular wall or filling the pericapillary area of the interstitial space. ICG binding to the proteins enables the visualization of the capillary wall (otherwise invisible during conventional and NaF fluorescence nailfold capillaroscopy).

Moneta et al. [44] utilized ICG to measure the diameter of capillaries as compared to the erythrocyte column measurement made in conventional capillaroscopy. They found that the erythrocytes were 68% of the diameter as measured by ICG, suggestive of several microns of plasma between the red blood cells and the capillary wall; this work confirmed results from a similar earlier study by Mahler et al. [45]. A further study of the delivery of ICG in a study of 12 healthy controls and 38 patients with SSc or connective tissue disease identified microaneurysms (bulges in the capillary walls) in the patient group [46]. Authors identified the aneurysms as erythrocytes moving outside of the main capillary 'loop' structures due to heterogenous structural expansion. Alongside the expected scleroderma pattern related morphological changes observed in the patient group as compared to the controls, there was a significant difference in the number of aneurysms in patients as compared to controls. Many of these aneurysmal lesions (dilations) could not be identified by conventional capillaroscopy, implying that they only contained plasma rather than erythrocytes.

Brülisauer and Bollinger combined both ICG and NaF in a study of 12 healthy controls and 12 patients with SSc, to identify both permeability and capillary dimensions. A wider plasma layer at the capillary apex and in both limbs was measured for the patients as compared to the controls and an increased halo size was observed in patients at the apex as compared to controls [47].

More recently, the use of ICG for enhanced visualization is seeing a revival via the related technique of fluorescence optical imaging which uses intravenously injected ICG to assess capillary permeability over the whole hand. Imaging can be indicative of areas of vasculopathy and inflammation (more widespread fluorescence representing increased inflammatory-related vascular permeability) [48]. The technique is discussed further in chapter "Using Nailfold Capillaroscopy in Combination with Other Non-invasive Imaging Techniques".

Expert Opinion

In conclusion, measurement of capillary permeability has been shown to be a useful tool in understanding mechanisms for pathogenesis of Raynaud's phenomenon and SSc and to understand response to drugs. Technological advances, including image analysis automation with machine and deep learning potentially make this technique more accessible than when it was first developed and offer a potential route to increasing understanding of microvascular (dys)function even if invasive.

Capillary Perfusion Assessments

Introduction and History

The impact of capillaroscopy has increased dramatically since the 1980s with technological advancements in video microscopy and computer assisted image analysis methods [49]. It has moved the study of the human cutaneous microcirculation beyond the then standard methods of perfusion assessment including plethysmography volumetric / flow changes (see chapter "Using Nailfold Capillaroscopy in Combination with Other Non-invasive Imaging Techniques") as well as radionuclide measurement of Xenon 133 clearance in tissue [50]. Dynamic capillaroscopy measurements have been used to assess microcirculatory blood flow in human skin including at the nailfold. This has enabled the quantification of blood flow dynamics in the nutritional skin capillaries at rest and in response to physiological challenges (such as following the release of arterial occlusion, during application of venous occlusion of the finger, and local cooling tests) [51–53]. Synchronous comparative assessments have shown broad comparability, for example of capillary blood flow with laser Doppler flowmetry (LDF) [54].

Blood Flow Estimation Techniques—Red Blood Cell (RBC) Velocity

Assessment of capillary 'blood flow' in skin, i.e. perfusion, usually concerns the estimation of red blood cell velocity (RBC) [54–58]. However, RBC velocity measurement by conventional optical capillaroscopy is challenging. It is vital to get good quality image sequences for flow related assessments. These images are usually collected at higher magnifications (i.e. giving a capillaroscopy image of 1–2 mm across its width). The digit under study might need gently clamping to reduce movement artefact and improve image quality. Monochrome or colour imaging systems can be utilized. Tresadern et al. have noted that optical 'flow' algorithms may be applied, although without a ground truth (i.e. known blood flow) it is hard to evaluate their accuracy [59]. These authors proposed an image model that generates realistic capillaroscopy videos with known flow. They used this to quantify the effect of flow rate, cell density and contrast (among other measures on estimated flow). Their model aims to help researchers to design capillaroscopy systems that are under real world conditions [59].

The advent of digital computing has helped revolutionize image analysis from the early days of using 'analog' video tape storage media. Simple visual inspection can be used, for example to check for flow-stop conditions although this is a subjective assessment [58]. Specific methods for determining continuous measurements of capillary blood flow velocity have included the Spatial Shift Alignment (SSA) technique [54]. With SSA a capillaroscopic image is digitized by means of a frame grabber. Within the lumen of a suitable capillary limb a region of interest known as a slot is placed. At a frame frequency of 25 per second, this slot is copied in a free part of the frame grabber store along a horizontal axis. A static space-time image is obtained with light diagonal bands representing the passage of plasma gaps through the capillary limb. By determining the gradient of the diagonal bands, a measure of the capillary RBC velocity can be obtained. Other researchers have also estimated the RBC velocity using frame-to-frame determination of the position of capillary plasma gaps for their systemic sclerosis research [60]. Correlation methods have also been employed to determine flow including the Capiflow technique which can quantify the diameter, density and perfusion, i.e., the RBC velocity in the nutritional skin capillary [58]. There is also the CapiScope system (KK Technology Ltd., Devon, UK). This utilizes the grey level pattern along each line and is compared to the pattern from the previous frame(s). A comparison is then performed by calculating the correlation coefficient for every possible shift of the previous grey level profile relative to the new profile. The shift which produces the highest correlation indicates the distance travelled between the two grey level profile measurements, and hence the velocity. RBC velocities from 0 to 2 mm/s can be measured using this video correlation approach which can cover the expected range of resting flow rate in capillaries. As well as their correlation approach KK Technology also have the Capillary CAM1 device (KK Technology Ltd., Devon, UK) which uses a near infrared laser anemometer system to give a velocity recording at a single loop apex (Fig. 3). This allows velocities of 0.05 mm/s to 14.6 mm/s to be measured on targeted capillaries, for example for studying high RBC velocities in tissue inflammation and hyperaemia. There is also the Optical Flow Estimation (OFE) technique of RBC velocity estimation. This uses an image registration function based on a Mutual Information algorithm for stabilizing capillary images to deal with slight finger movements during video acquisition. After image alignment, a skeleton extraction algorithm implemented using thinning enables the tracking of perfusion in the arteriolar and venular limbs, as well as the curved segment of a capillary. OFE

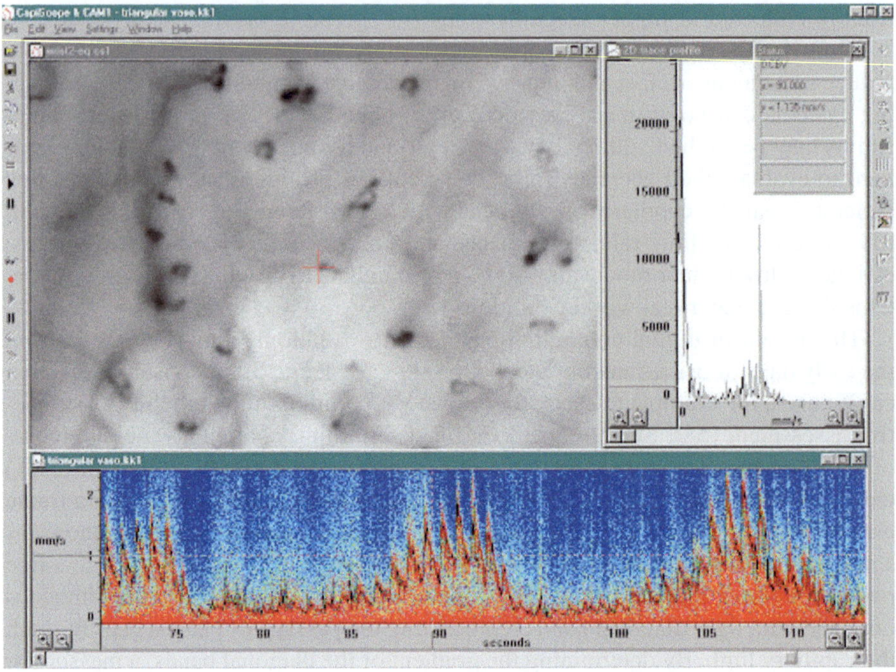

Fig. 3 Skin capillaries imaged with the KK Technology Capillary CAM1 anemometer system (KK Technology Ltd., Devon, UK) giving a velocity recording at a single loop apex. Note the pulsatile component which is superimposed on low frequency vasomotor activity. (Reproduced with kind permission from KK Research Technology Ltd.)

is not only independent to the direction of flow, but it is also able to calculate the intensity displacement of all pixels, looking to provide complete velocity information for the whole vessel limb [61]. High-speed videocapillaroscopy has also been developed and evaluated, with interesting insights into the reverse blood flow effect in capillaries during upper arm occlusion challenge [62]. Technology is advancing all the time, for example, Ye et al. have implemented a deep neural network to automatically classify and distinguish capillaries from images and used this network in conjunction with a spatiotemporal diagram analysis for flow velocity calculation [63].

Capillaroscopy perfusion assessment remains challenging especially at the low basal flow rates. The clinical researcher should therefore also consider other microvascular techniques that can assess RBC velocities/flow and there is a place for these such as with LDF, laser speckle contrast analysis (LASCA) imaging and Tissue Viability Imaging (TIVI) [64, 65]. Laser-based methods of measuring skin perfusion are also discussed in chapter "Using Nailfold Capillaroscopy in Combination with Other Non-invasive Imaging Techniques".

Applications in SSc and Other Clinical Conditions

SSc is usually assessed using static morphological assessments from capillaroscopy imaging for classification and for the study of vascular remodeling [66], but blood flow could also be evaluated in assessing the disease as reduced RBC velocity is a hallmark of SSc. In a key study of 127 SSc patients by Mugii et al., this measure of flow was decreased in patients with SSc compared to healthy controls and patients with other conditions, with mean blood velocity similar for patients with dcSSc and lcSSc subsets [60]. Those SSc patients with normal or non-specific nailfold video-capillaroscopic patterns or an 'early' scleroderma pattern exhibited a significantly lower RBC velocity compared to healthy controls, but patients with the 'active' or 'late' patterns showed a more decreased RBC velocity. There is a role for capillaroscopy and laser techniques together as microvascular damage and a decrease in peripheral blood perfusion are typical features of the disease with serious clinical implications for early diagnosis and for monitoring disease progression [65]. Automated techniques are being developed that assess combined morphology and perfusion for SSc classification. Berks et al., have developed a novel capillaroscopy system that generates high-quality nail-fold images and provides fully automated measurements of capillary structure (i.e. capillary density, mean width, maximum width, shape score, derangement) and mean RBC velocity. The differences between patients with SSc and controls (primary Raynaud's patients and healthy controls) have been quantified and statistically significant differences found [67]. Combining all five structural measurements was found to give better classification than the best single measurement (area under Receiver Operator Characteristic curve = 0.919 ± 0.026), whilst adding flow further improved the classification (to 0.930 ± 0.024). Their reported technique using combined capillary features holds promise for developing clinical trial outcome measures for assessing treatments aimed at improving finger blood flow or microvascular modelling. Taking these works forward, from a clinical perspective, increased uptake of nailfold capillaroscopy by general rheumatologists could be achieved via low-cost hand-held devices with cloud-based automated analysis (see chapters "Nailfold Capillaroscopy—Image Acquisition" and "Quantitative Analysis"). From a research perspective, automated analysis could facilitate large-scale prospective studies using capillaroscopic parameters as possible biomarkers of systemic sclerosis-spectrum disorders [68].

Although findings of nailfold capillary changes and reduced RBC velocity in SSc patients are well established, studies in adult-onset dermatomyositis are scarce. Mugii et al. studied 50 patients with dermatomyositis using nail-fold video capillaroscopy with the RBC velocity evaluated using frame-to-frame determination of the position of capillary plasma gaps. Thirty-seven (74%) of the patients showed the scleroderma pattern and the severity of structural changes in the nail-fold capillaries reflected disease activity. Mean RBC velocity however was not significantly reduced in the dermatomyositis patients compared to healthy controls and was not changed by treatment [69]. The measurement of RBC velocity may be useful in evaluating

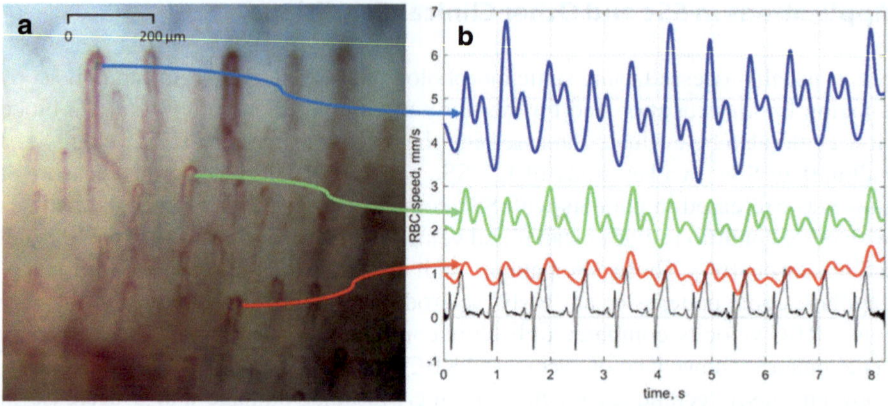

Fig. 4 (**a**) Dynamic capillaroscopy to study the red blood cell (RBC) speed modulation in three exemplary capillaries, clear photoplethysmographic (PPG), (**b**) pulsatile waveforms can be seen in different regions for proximal and distal rows. This image analysis can be used to mechanistically study the origins of the PPG waveform. (From Volkov et al [75] (image taken from Open Access article licensed under a Creative Commons Attribution 4.0 International License))

therapeutic effects on microcirculation, for example assessing iloprost in the treatment of patients with Raynaud's and systemic sclerosis [70].

Other capillaroscopic flow-related assessments that could in future be explored in rheumatological disease include: studying vasomotion and the vascular reactivity of the skin microcirculation [71, 72]; assessing endothelial function [73]; studying capillary pressure alongside morphology, density and blood flow velocity assessments, with direct cannulation using glass micropipettes [74]; and mechanistic determination of the photoplethysmographic (PPG) pulsatile waveform measured at the skin surface (Fig. 4) [75].

Expert Opinion

Capillary perfusion measurements (i.e., RBC velocity estimation) using capillaroscopy can be challenging to perform but with careful technique it can add value in the study of skin microcirculatory blood flow in systemic sclerosis. It also allows assessment of vascular reactivity and offers a potential route to increasing understanding of microvascular (dys)function. Technological advances in the image analysis can improve technique reliability, for example by reducing the impact of movement artefact on velocity (flow) measurements and advancing automation. Intelligent image processing has great potential for moving RBC velocity estimation beyond research and towards routine clinical use, including integrating with other functional measures as well as structural features.

Tissue Oxygenation Assessment at the Capillary Level

Single Point Spectroscopy and Multi Spectral Imaging

As discussed above, in relation to permeability and blood flow, tissue hypoxia potentially plays a key role in the transition to fibrosis in SSc. Thus, measuring oxygenation is of great interest in terms of potentially aiding early diagnosis and as an outcome in clinical trials, as well as in increasing understanding of pathophysiology.

The basis of most non-invasive oxygenation measurement or imaging in the cutaneous vasculature, are spectroscopic techniques that measure the light absorption properties of hemoglobin. When broadband light (white/infrared) is shone onto skin blood vessels, the haemoglobin within absorbs light in different ways according to whether it is deoxygenated or bonded to oxygen (See Fig. 4 in chapter "Using Nailfold Capillaroscopy in Combination with Other Non-invasive Imaging Techniques"). At certain key wavelengths the absorption is either (a) unaffected by oxygen bonding (an isosbestic or spectra crossing point point) or (b) very different for deoxy- and oxygenated haemoglobin. The difference between curves offers the opportunity to determine the level of oxygenation saturation, with isosbestic points enabling a relative calibration of the measurements [76].

Technological advances have facilitated measurement of oxygenation beyond single point measures with spectrometers (discussed in chapter "Using Nailfold Capillaroscopy in Combination with Other Non-invasive Imaging Techniques"). Multispectral imaging uses multiwavelength or broadband light sources to illuminate the skin and cameras with filters at specific wavelengths to capture images at these specific wavelengths and build up a set of images. Alternatively multiple light wavelengths can be used in succession over different frames. Recombining the filtered frames or the frames gathered under different illumination in a specific way then enables oxygenation images to be generated. The technique is used almost exclusively in ophthalmological multimodal imaging technologies to assess the eye's microvascular oxygenation.

The oximetry aspect of pulse oximetry is a basic form of spectral measurement carried out at the finger. A calibrated portable device containing two light emitting diodes (LEDs) at different wavelengths, usually red and near infrared (e.g. 660 and 940 nm) take advantage of the difference in absorption of oxy- and deoxyhemoglobin and devices are calibrated using the difference in the optical response curves to provide a measure of oxygen saturation (SpO2).

In a study to determine correlation between pulse oximeter readings and nailfold capillary patterns ('early', 'active', 'late'), measures of SpO2 were taken from two fingers from 55 patients with SSc [77]. In 47 fingers from 20 patients no signal could be obtained and significant intra-person variation between fingers was identified. There was no correlation to nailfold capillaroscopy pattern but there was a relationship to lung function measurements (Forced Vital Capacity).

Multispectral Imaging of Nailfold Capillaries

To date little has been pursued in terms of developing an oxygenation sensitive system for nailfold capillaroscopy. Multispectral imaging has been used in one study; Taylor-Williams et al. [78] designed and tested a low-cost system using LED illumination of the capillaries. Combining wavelengths of 505, 572 and 590 nm, the authors were able to image healthy control capillaries at the nailfold. The same authors have gone on to utilize a multispectral imaging camera with white light to demonstrate the feasibility of imaging the oxygenation in patients with SSc as compared to a control group (Fig. 5) [79].

One limitation to imaging in the visible spectrum (400–700 nm) is that imaging can be impeded by absorption of melanin which also absorbs in the same wavelength range. Thus, it is difficult to image capillary structure and to measure the oxygenation in capillaries of people with skin in the Fitzpatrick type VI category [80]. These studies show the potential of measuring oxygenation in nailfold

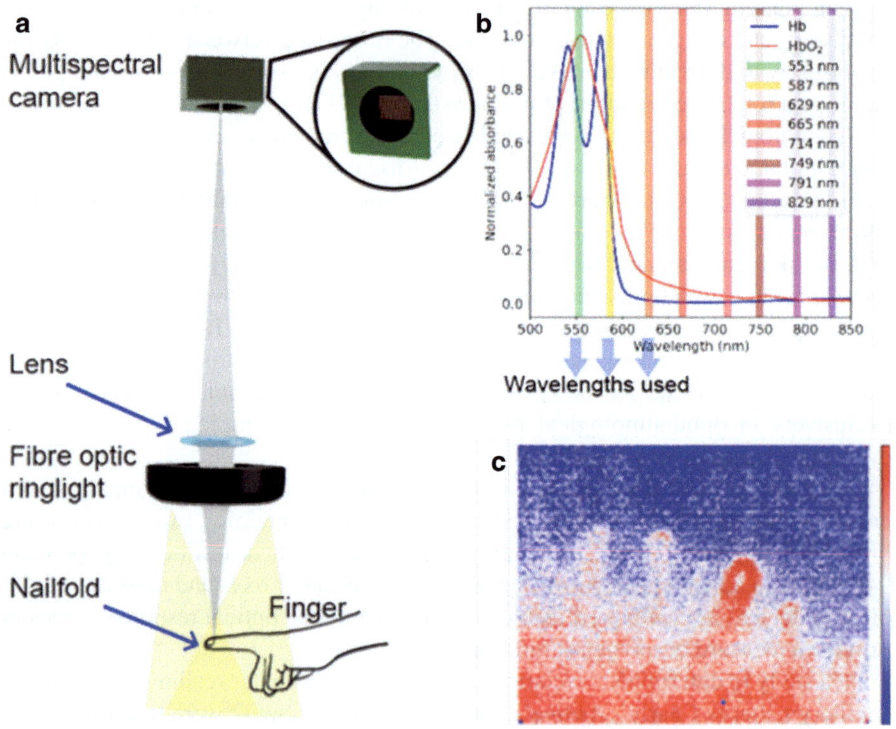

Fig. 5 Multispectral imaging of nailfold capillaries; (**a**) schematic of equipment set-up, (**b**) spectrum of absorption for oxyhaemoglobin (HbO2) and deoxyhaemoglobin (Hb), also showing the available wavelengths within the multispectral camera and those selected for the final image analysis, (**c**) example of false colour image of nailfold capillaries representing relative oxygenation (scale blue to red with red being higher oxygenation). (Courtesy of Michaela Taylor-Williams and Sarah Bohndiek)

capillaries via multispectral imaging, but more work is required to fully prove the principle and overcome melanin absorption.

One possible route to enable imaging skin vasculature through melanin is to image in the near infra-red rather than visible spectrum. This technique collects data from the near infrared wavelengths (e.g. 670 nm, 730 nm, 890 nm and 940 nm), and is potentially less dependent on skin tone [81]. Using near infrared imaging, Gargani et al. found reduced oxygenation in the fingers (but not nailfold capillaries specifically) of 40 patients with SSc as compared to 21 controls both at baseline and after 3 min of brachial occlusion [82].

Photoacoustic Imaging of Nailfold Capillaries

Another imaging technique that has been used to measure oxygenation in the nailfold capillaries is multispectral photoacoustic imaging (a multispectral adaption of ultrasound and optical imaging combined to enable three dimensional imaging, discussed further in chapter "Using Nailfold Capillaroscopy in Combination with Other Non-invasive Imaging Techniques"). Eisenbrey et al. measured oxygenation using a photoacoustic technique; however, whilst this study imaged at the nailfold measurements were made on images taken into the skin cross sectionally (B-mode, perpendicular to the surface of the skin) rather than en-face mode (parallel to the surface of the skin) as would be done with nailfold capillaroscopy [83]. In a study of 7 patients with SSc and 15 controls authors measured oxygenation at baseline and following cold challenge (water at 15 °C, fingers submerged for 1 min; imaging at 5, 15 and 30 min). Patients had a significant decrease in nailfold oxygenation following cold challenge as compared to controls. Receiver Operator Characteristic analysis resulted in a differentiation accuracy of 0.72. In a similar study Daoudi et al., also imaging in B-mode, identified decreased oxygenation at the nailfold of 5 patients with SSc as compared to 9 controls; oxygen saturation correlated with nailfold capillary density [84]. High resolution systems to image at the nailfold and visualise capillaries are now available [85] but to date multispectral devices have not been used to measure oxygenation in the capillaries directly in the rheumatic diseases.

Expert Opinion

The increased combination of multispectral techniques in multimodal imaging systems (evaluating morphology plus function of the microcirculation) will undoubtedly drive capillary imaging forwards. The cost and complexity of systems such as photoacoustic make them unlikely to be the main route of nailfold capillary oxygenation imaging but add to our understanding of pathophysiology and microvascular function in the realm of research. Low-cost, portable LED-based systems, using hand-held cameras, combined with software to automate oxygenation measurements are likely to be the route to systems used in the mainstream.

Overall Summary

Functional measures derived from capillaroscopy offer exciting avenues of new research. We have seen above that a range of characteristics of the microcirculation can be studied beyond conventional structural assessments, including capillary permeability, perfusion i.e. blood flow, and oxygenation in SSc and beyond, contrasted to people without this disease. Capillaroscopy at the nailfold as well as at other skin sites offers important insights. There is still work to do but the added focus on these functional measures should help in the quantification of disease and in understanding the pathological changes that occur by looking at the microvascular level, particularly in early disease before structural changes. Besides exciting challenges there are also opportunities to grasp, e.g., to perform skin imaging across the visible wavelengths and to develop automated AI analytics including multi-dimensional capillary features (e.g. combined permeability, perfusion and oxygenation), moving such technologies through the development pathway from proof-of-concept to formal device evaluation in patients with rheumatological diseases.

References

1. van den Hoogen F, Khanna D, Fransen J, Johnson SR, Baron M, Tyndall A, et al. 2013 classification criteria for systemic sclerosis: an American college of rheumatology/European league against rheumatism collaborative initiative. Ann Rheum Dis. 2013;72:1747–55.
2. Smith V, Herrick AL, Ingegnoli F, Damjanov N, De Angelis R, Denton CP, et al. EULAR study group on microcirculation in rheumatic diseases and the scleroderma clinical trials consortium group on Capillaroscopy. Standardisation of nailfold capillaroscopy for the assessment of patients with Raynaud's phenomenon and systemic sclerosis. Autoimmun Rev. 2020;19:102458.
3. Bharathi PG, Berks M, Dinsdale G, Murray A, Manning J, Wilkinson S, et al. A deep learning system for quantitative assessment of microvascular abnormalities in nailfold capillary images. Rheumatology. 2023;62:2325–9.
4. Berks M, Dinsdale G, Marjanovic E, Murray A, Taylor C, Herrick AL. Comparison between low cost USB nailfold capillaroscopy and videocapillaroscopy: a pilot study. Rheumatology. 2021;60:3862–7.
5. Gracia Tello B, Ramos Ibañez E, Fanlo Mateo P, Sáez Cómet L, Martínez Robles E, Ríos Blanco JJ, et al. The challenge of comprehensive nailfold videocapillaroscopy practice: a further contribution. Clin Exp Rheumatol. 2022;40:1926–32.
6. Bellando-Randone S, Del Galdo F, Lepri G, Minier T, Huscher D, Furst DE, et al. Very early diagnosis of systemic sclerosis collaborators. Progression of patients with Raynaud's phenomenon to systemic sclerosis: a five-year analysis of the European scleroderma trial and research group multicentre, longitudinal registry study for very early diagnosis of systemic sclerosis (VEDOSS). Lancet Rheumatol. 2021;3:e834–43.
7. Trombetta AC, Pizzorni C, Ruaro B, Paolino S, Sulli A, Smith V, Cutolo M. Effects of long-term treatment with bosentan and iloprost on nailfold absolute capillary number, fingertip blood perfusion, and clinical status in systemic sclerosis. J Rheumatol. 2016;43:2033–41.
8. Haverkort DA, Kersten BE, van Rhenen A, van der Velden WJFM, Vonk MC. Case report: a successful second autologous hematopoietic stem cell transplantation in refractory systemic sclerosis, with positive effect on skin involvement, pulmonary function and microcirculation. Front Immunol. 2022;13:925776.

9. Bollinger A, Jäger K, Siegenthaler W. Microangiopathy of progressive systemic sclerosis. Evaluation by dynamic fluorescence videomicroscopy. Arch Intern Med. 1986;146:1541–5.
10. Shirshin EA, Gurfinkel YI, Matskeplishvili ST, Sasonko ML, Omelyanenko NP, Yakimov BP, et al. In vivo optical imaging of the viable epidermis around the nailfold capillaries for the assessment of heart failure severity in humans. J Biophotonics. 2018;11:e201800066.
11. Kohner EM, Dollery CT. Fluorescein angiography of the fundus in diabetic retinopathy. Br Med Bull. 1970;26:166–70.
12. Bollinger A, Jäger K, Roten A, Timeus C, Mahler F. Diffusion, pericapillary distribution and clearance of Na-fluorescein in the human nailfold. Pflugers Arch. 1979;382:137–43.
13. Grassi W, Core P, Cervini C. Increased capillary permeability in systemic sclerosis: help or hindrance? Ann Rheum Dis. 1996 Sep;55(9):603–6.
14. Grassi W, Core P, Carlino G, Cervini C. Acute effects of single dose nifedipine on cold-induced changes of microvascular dynamics in systemic sclerosis. Br J Rheumatol. 1994;33:1154–61.
15. Hettema ME, Zhang D, Stienstra Y, Smit AJ, Bootsma H, Kallenberg CG. No effects of bosentan on microvasculature in patients with limited cutaneous systemic sclerosis. Clin Rheumatol. 2009;28:825–33.
16. Bollinger A, Frey J, Jäger K, Furrer J, Seglias J, Siegenthaler W. Patterns of diffusion through skin capillaries in patients with long-term diabetes. N Engl J Med. 1982;307:1305–10.
17. Grassi W, Core P, Carlino G, Salaffi F, Cervini C. Capillary permeability in fibromyalgia. J Rheumatol. 1994;21:1328–31.
18. Hachulla E, Perez-Cousin M, Flipo RM, Houvenagel E, Cardon T, Catteau MH, et al. Increased capillary permeability in systemic rheumatoid vasculitis: detection by dynamic fluorescence nailfold videomicroscopy. J Rheumatol. 1994;21:1197–202.
19. Bongard O, Weimer D, Lemoine R, Bolle JF, Leski M, Bounameaux H. Cyclosporine toxicity in renal transplant recipients detected by nailfold capillaroscopy with Na-fluorescein. Kidney Int. 2000;58:2559–63.
20. Zinellu A, Mangoni AA. Vascular endothelial growth factor as a potential biomarker in systemic sclerosis: a systematic review and meta-analysis. Front Immunol. 2024;15:1442913.
21. Brausewetter F, Jehle PM, Jung MF, Boehm BO, Brueckel J, Hombach V, Osterhues HH. Microvascular permeability is increased in both types of diabetes and correlates differentially with serum levels of insulin-like growth factor I (IGF-I) and vascular endothelial growth factor (VEGF). Horm Metab Res. 2001;33:713–20.
22. Herrig I, Hoffmann U, Fischer M, Franzeck UK, Bollinger A. Microinjection technique for pharmacological evaluation of microvascular permeability in human skin. Eur J Clin Pharmacol. 1996;4:365–9.
23. Lin L, Yamagata K, Nakayamada S, Sawamukai N, Yamaoka K, Sakata K, et al. Histamine inhibits differentiation of skin fibroblasts into myofibroblasts. Biochem Biophys Res Commun. 2015;463:434–9.
24. Läuchli S, Franzeck UK, Leu AJ, Hoffmann U. Dose-dependent increase of transcapillary diffusion of sodium fluorescein after histamine microinjections. Vasa. 1999;28:79–83.
25. Costanzo U, Franzeck U, Fischer M, Bollinger A, Hoffmann U. Interleukin-2 increases transcapillary diffusion of sodium fluorescein in human skin. J Cardiovasc Pharmacol. 1997;29:81–6.
26. Baer-Suryadinata C, Bollinger A. Transcapillary diffusion of Na-fluorescein measured by a 'large window technique' in skin areas of the forefoot. Int J Microcirc Clin Exp. 1985;4:217–28.
27. Jager J, Oomen PH, Sluiter WJ, Reitsma WD, Smit AJ. Improved reproducibility of the 'large-window' method of assessing transcapillary and interstitial fluorescein diffusion in the skin in healthy subjects and in subjects with insulin-dependent diabetes mellitus. Int J Microcirc Clin Exp. 1997;17:150–8.
28. Oomen PH, Kant GD, Dullaart RP, Tervaert JW, Reitsma WD, Smit AJ. No effects of acute hyperglycaemia and hyperinsulinaemia on skin microcirculation and endothelial markers in type II diabetes mellitus. Scand J Clin Lab Invest. 2004;64:119–27.
29. Hettema ME, Zhang D, Stienstra Y, Oomen PN, Smit AJ, Kallenberg CG, Bootsma H. Decreased capillary permeability and capillary density in patients with systemic

sclerosis using large-window sodium fluorescein videodensitometry of the ankle. Rheumatology. 2008;47:1409–12.
30. Miranda S, Armengol G, Le Besnerais M, Lévesque H, Benhamou Y. New insights into systemic sclerosis related microcirculatory dysfunction by assessment of sublingual microcirculation and vascular glycocalyx layer. Results from a preliminary study. Microvasc Res. 2015;99:72–7.
31. Radic M, Thomas J, McMillan S, Frech T. Does sublingual microscopy correlate with nailfold videocapillaroscopy in systemic sclerosis? Clin Rheumatol. 2021;40:2263–6.
32. Bellando-Randone S, Matucci-Cerinic M. The measurement of the endothelial glycocalyx as a new biomarker of endothelial derangement in systemic sclerosis: a challenge for the future. J Rheumatol. 2017;44:1572–4.
33. Machin DR, Gates PE, Vink H, Frech TM, Donato AJ. Automated measurement of microvascular function reveals dysfunction in systemic sclerosis: a cross-sectional study. J Rheumatol. 2017;44:1603–11.
34. Abassi Z, Armaly Z, Heyman SN. Glycocalyx degradation in ischemia-reperfusion injury. Am J Pathol. 2020;190:752–67.
35. Minier T, Guiducci S, Bellando-Randone S, Bruni C, Lepri G, Czirják L, et al. EUSTAR co-workers; EUSTAR co-workers. Preliminary analysis of the very early diagnosis of systemic sclerosis (VEDOSS) EUSTAR multicentre study: evidence for puffy fingers as a pivotal sign for suspicion of systemic sclerosis. Ann Rheum Dis. 2014;73:2087–93.
36. Tanaka Y, Kuwana M, Fujii T, Kameda H, Muro Y, Fujio K, et al. 2019 diagnostic criteria for mixed connective tissue disease (MCTD): from the Japan research committee of the ministry of health, labor, and welfare for systemic autoimmune diseases. Mod Rheumatol. 2021;31:29–33.
37. Ennis H, Hughes M, Anderson ME, Wilkinson J, Herrick AL. Calcium channel blockers for primary Raynaud's phenomenon. Cochrane Database Syst Rev. 2016;2:CD002069.
38. Luggen M, Belhorn L, Evans T, Fitzgerald O, Spencer-Green G. The evolution of Raynaud's phenomenon: a longterm prospective study. J Rheumatol. 1995;22:2226–32.
39. Mingyuan X, Qianqian P, Shengquan X, Chenyi Y, Rui L, Yichen S, Jinghong X. Hypoxia-inducible factor-1α activates transforming growth factor-β1/Smad signaling and increases collagen deposition in dermal fibroblasts. Oncotarget. 2017;14(9):3188–97.
40. Bruni C, Frech T, Manetti M, Rossi FW, Furst DE, De Paulis A, et al. Vascular leaking, a pivotal and early pathogenetic event in systemic sclerosis: should the door be closed? Front Immunol. 2018;9:2045.
41. Lambova SN, Müller-Ladner U. Capillaroscopic pattern in systemic sclerosis—an association with dynamics of processes of angio- and vasculogenesis. Microvasc Res. 2010;80:534–9.
42. Frech TM, Revelo MP, Drakos SG, Murtaugh MA, Markewitz BA, Sawitzke AD, Li DY. Vascular leak is a central feature in the pathogenesis of systemic sclerosis. J Rheumatol. 2012;39:1385–91.
43. Sfikakis PP, Vlachogiannis NI, Ntouros PA, Mavrogeni S, Maris TG, Karantanas AH, Souliotis VL. Microvasculopathy-related hemorrhagic tissue deposition of iron may contribute to fibrosis in systemic sclerosis: hypothesis-generating insights from the literature and preliminary findings. Life. 2022;16(12):430.
44. Moneta G, Brülisauer M, Jäger K, Bollinger A. Infrared fluorescence videomicroscopy of skin capillaries with indocyanine green. Int J Microcirc Clin Exp. 1987;6(1):25–34.
45. Mahler F, Nagel G, Saner H, Kneubühl F. In vivo comparison of the nailfold capillary diameter as determined by using the erythrocyte column and FITC-labelled albumin. Int J Microcirc Clin Exp. 1983;2(2):147–55.
46. Bollinger A, Saesseli B, Hoffmann U, Franzeck UK. Intravital detection of skin capillary aneurysms by videomicroscopy with indocyanine green in patients with progressive systemic sclerosis and related disorders. Circulation. 1991;83:546–51.
47. Brülisauer M, Bollinger A. Measurement of different human microvascular dimensions by combination of videomicroscopy with Na-fluorescein (NaF) and indocyanine green (ICG) in normals and patients with systemic sclerosis. Int J Microcirc Clin Exp. 1991;10:21–31.

48. Pfeil A, Drummer KF, Böttcher J, Jung C, Oelzner P, Renz DM, et al. The application of fluorescence optical imaging in systemic sclerosis. Biomed Res Int. 2015;2015:658710.
49. Bollinger A, Fagrell B. Clinical Capillaroscopy: a guide to its use in clinical research and practice. Toronto: Hogrefe & Huber; 1989.
50. Fagrell B. Dynamics of skin microcirculation in humans. J Cardiovasc Pharmacol. 1985;7(Suppl 3):S53–8.
51. Gasser P. Video-nailfold-microscopy and local cold test: morphological and hemodynamic correlates in 124 healthy subjects. Vasa. 1991;20:244–51.
52. Klyscz T, Hahn M, Beck W, Blazek V, Rassner G, Jünger M. Development of a computer-assisted thermoelectric Peltier cold test procedure with integrated photoplethysmography unit for noninvasive evaluation of acral skin circulation. Biomed Tech. 1997;42:234–9.
53. Pache M, Schwarz HA, Kaiser HJ, Wüest P, Klöti M, Dubler B, Flammer J. Elevated plasma endothelin-1 levels and vascular dysregulation in patients with rheumatoid arthritis. Med Sci Monit. 2002;8:CR616–9.
54. Tooke JE, Ostergren J, Fagrell B. Synchronous assessment of human skin microcirculation by laser Doppler flowmetry and dynamic capillaroscopy. Int J Microcirc Clin Exp. 1983;2:277–84.
55. Ostergren J, Fagrell B. Videophotometric capillaroscopy for evaluating drug effects on skin microcirculation—a double-blind study with nifedipine. Clin Physiol. 1984;4:169–76.
56. Rosén L, Ostergren J, Fagrell B, Stranden E. Skin microvascular circulation in the sympathetic dystrophies evaluated by videophotometric capillaroscopy and laser Doppler fluxmetry. Eur J Clin Investig. 1988;18:305–8.
57. Lentner A, Berger F, Wienert V. Spatial shift alignment (SSA)—a new method for determining blood flow velocity in video capillary microscopy. Biomed Tech. 1994;39:170–5.
58. D'Emilia I, Biava G, Delfino M, Galiano P, Modica M, Camera A, Del Porto R. Usefulness of computerized dynamic capillaroscopy in the monitoring of treatment of progressive systemic sclerosis with synthetic prostacyclin. Recenti Prog Med. 1996;87:106–9.
59. Tresadern PA, Berks M, Murray AK, Dinsdale G, Taylor CJ, Herrick AL. Simulating nailfold capillaroscopy sequences to evaluate algorithms for blood flow estimation. In: 2013 35th Annual International Conference of the IEEE Engineering in Medicine and Biology Society (EMBC). New York: IEEE; 2013. p. 2636–9.
60. Mugii N, Hasegawa M, Hamaguchi Y, Tanaka C, Kaji K, Komura K, et al. Reduced red blood cell velocity in nail-fold capillaries as a sensitive and specific indicator of microcirculation injury in systemic sclerosis. Rheumatology. 2009;48:696–703.
61. Wu CC, Zhang G, Huang TC, Lin KP. Red blood cell velocity measurements of complete capillary in finger nail-fold using optical flow estimation. Microvasc Res. 2009;78:319–24.
62. Dremin V, Kozlov I, Volkov M, Margaryants N, Potemkin A, Zherebtsov E, et al. Dynamic evaluation of blood flow microcirculation by combined use of the laser Doppler flowmetry and high-speed videocapillaroscopy methods. J Biophotonics. 2019;12:e201800317.
63. Ye F, Yin S, Li M, Li Y, Zhong J. In-vivo full-field measurement of microcirculatory blood flow velocity based on intelligent object identification. J Biomed Opt. 2020;25:1–11.
64. Allen J, Howell K. Microvascular imaging: techniques and opportunities for clinical physiological measurements. Physiol Meas. 2014;35:R91–R141.
65. Ruaro B, Nallino MG, Casabella A, Salton F, Confalonieri P, De Tanti A, Bruni C. Monitoring the microcirculation in the diagnosis and follow-up of systemic sclerosis patients: focus on pulmonary and peripheral vascular manifestations. Microcirculation. 2020;27:e12647.
66. Murray AK, Moore TL, Manning JB, Taylor C, Griffiths CE, Herrick AL. Noninvasive imaging techniques in the assessment of scleroderma spectrum disorders. Arthritis Rheum. 2009;61:1103–11.
67. Berks M, Dinsdale G, Murray A, Moore T, Manning J, Taylor C, Herrick AL. Automated structure and flow measurement—a promising tool in nailfold capillaroscopy. Microvasc Res. 2018;118:173–7.
68. Herrick AL, Berks M, Taylor CJ. Quantitative nailfold capillaroscopy-update and possible next steps. Rheumatology. 2021;60:2054–65.

69. Mugii N, Hasegawa M, Matsushita T, Hamaguchi Y, Horie S, Yahata T, et al. Association between nail-fold capillary findings and disease activity in dermatomyositis. Rheumatology. 2011;50:1091–8.
70. Rademaker M, Cooke ED, Almond NE, Beacham JA, Smith RE, Mant TG, Kirby JD. Comparison of intravenous infusions of iloprost and oral nifedipine in treatment of Raynaud's phenomenon in patients with systemic sclerosis: a double blind randomised study. BMJ. 1989;298:561–4.
71. Fagrell B. Microcirculatory methods for the clinical assessment of hypertension, hypotension, and ischemia. Ann Biomed Eng. 1986;14:163–73.
72. Gasser P, Bühler FR. Nailfold microcirculation in normotensive and essential hypertensive subjects, as assessed by video-microscopy. Hypertens. 1992;10:83–6.
73. Bouskela E. Kraemer de Aguiar LG, Nivoit P, Bahia LR, Villela NR, Bottino DA vascular dysfunction in metabolic disorders: evaluation of some therapeutic interventions. Bull Acad Natl Med. 2007;191:475–93.
74. Shore AC. Capillaroscopy and the measurement of capillary pressure. Br J Clin Pharmacol. 2000;50:501–13.
75. Volkov MV, Margaryants NB, Potemkin AV, et al. Video capillaroscopy clarifies mechanism of the photoplethysmographic waveform appearance. Sci Rep. 2017;7:13298.
76. Feather JW, Hajizadeh-Saffar M, Leslie G, Dawson JB. A portable scanning reflectance spectrophotometer using visible wavelengths for the rapid measurement of skin pigments. Phys Med Biol. 1989;34:807–20.
77. Akdogan A, Kilic L, Dogan I, Karadag O, Bilgen SA, Kiraz S, Ertenli I. Effect of capillaroscopic patterns on the pulse oximetry measurements in systemic sclerosis patients. Microvasc Res. 2015;98:183–6.
78. Taylor-Williams M, Mead S, Sawyer TW, Hacker L, Williams C, Berks M, Murray A, Bohndiek SE. Multispectral imaging of nailfold capillaries using light-emitting diode illumination. J Biomed Opt. 2022;27:126002.
79. Taylor-Williams M, Khalil I, Dinsdale G, Manning J, Berks M, Murray A, Bohndiek SE. Multispectral imaging in nailfold capillaroscopy for the detection of systemic sclerosis. Proc SPIE. 2024:PC128270M.
80. Fitzpatrick TB. The validity and practicability of sun-reactive skin types I through VI. Arch Dermatol. 1988;124:869–71.
81. Hartwig V, Marinelli M, Gargani L, et al. Two-dimensional near infrared spectroscopic imaging of the hand to assess microvascular abnormalities in systemic sclerosis: a pilot study. J Near Infrared Spectrosc. 2015;23:59–66.
82. Gargani L, Bruni C, Barskova T, Hartwig V, Marinelli M, Trivella MG, et al. Near-infrared spectroscopic imaging of the whole hand: a new tool to assess tissue perfusion and peripheral microcirculation in scleroderma. Semin Arthritis Rheum. 2019;48:867–73.
83. Eisenbrey JR, Stanczak M, Forsberg F, Mendoza-Ballesteros FA, Lyshchik A. Photoacoustic oxygenation quantification in patients with Raynaud's: first-in-human results. Ultrasound Med Biol. 2018;44:2081–8.
84. Daoudi K, Kersten BE, van den Ende CHM, van den Hoogen FHJ, Vonk MC, de Korte CL. Photoacoustic and high-frequency ultrasound imaging of systemic sclerosis patients. Arthritis Res Ther. 2021;23:22.
85. Nitkunanantharajah S, Haedicke K, Moore TB, Manning JB, Dinsdale G, Berks M, et al. Three-dimensional optoacoustic imaging of nailfold capillaries in systemic sclerosis and its potential for disease differentiation using deep learning. Sci Rep. 2020;10:16444.

Nailfold Capillaroscopy as a Biomarker for Monitoring Disease and Treatment Response

Ariane L. Herrick and Andrea Murray

Key Points

- By providing a non-invasive window into the microcirculation, nailfold capillaroscopy has the potential to provide a biomarker for monitoring disease progression and treatment response in patients with systemic sclerosis or dermatomyositis (and related conditions).
- Capillaroscopic abnormality has to be measurable if it is to be developed as a biomarker: substantial progress is being made here, for example in automated measurement.
- Nailfold capillaroscopy is already being used in some centres to monitor treatment response in patients with dermatomyositis.

A. L. Herrick
Centre for Musculoskeletal Research, Division of Musculoskeletal and Dermatological Sciences, The University of Manchester, Manchester Academic Health Science Centre, Manchester, UK

Northern Care Alliance NHS Foundation Trust, Salford, UK

National Institute for Health and Care Research (NIHR) Manchester Biomedical Research Centre, Manchester, UK

Department of Rheumatology, Aberdeen Royal Infirmary, NHS Grampian, Aberdeen, UK

Centre for Arthritis and Musculoskeletal Health, University of Aberdeen, Aberdeen, UK

A. Murray (✉)
Centre for Musculoskeletal Research, Division of Musculoskeletal and Dermatological Sciences, The University of Manchester, Manchester Academic Health Science Centre, Manchester, UK

Northern Care Alliance NHS Foundation Trust, Salford, UK

National Institute for Health and Care Research (NIHR) Manchester Biomedical Research Centre, Manchester, UK
e-mail: andrea.murray@manchester.ac.uk

A. L. Herrick et al. (eds.), *Nailfold Capillaroscopy in Rheumatological Diseases*,
https://doi.org/10.1007/978-3-032-03970-5_11

- Several studies in patients with systemic sclerosis have examined nailfold capillary changes in response to drug treatment, for example haematopoietic stem cell transplantation and vasoactive therapies.
- Technical challenges include difficulties in measuring capillary density (the parameter most often used to gauge abnormality) and in visualising capillaries in darker skin tones.
- Assessing reliability of capillaroscopic measures is complex: studies of test-retest reliability (image acquisition) and of intra- and interobserver reliability of image interpretation demonstrate that good reliability (a prerequisite for a biomarker) is achievable.
- Recent and future technological advances hold promise for allowing development of nailfold capillaroscopy as a biomarker.

Introduction

One of the key challenges to clinicians is to gauge whether a disease is progressing and/or responding to treatment. This is important in both clinical practice and research. Biomarkers can often help in providing a way forwards. A biomarker has been defined as "A defined characteristic that is measured as an indicator of normal biological processes, pathogenic processes or responses to an exposure or intervention" [1]. Different subtypes of biomarker have been defined, as described in a U.S. Food and Drug Administration (FDA) and National Institutes of Health (NIH) resource: 'Biomarkers, EndpointS and other Tools (BEST)' [1, 2]. In this chapter we shall focus on monitoring biomarkers and response biomarkers.

To give context to the subsequent sections, a *monitoring* biomarker can used to assess disease progression or (more generally) a change in disease severity, either worsening or 'improvement'. This may include assessment of treatment response. A *response* biomarker is used to assess biological response after exposure to (for example) a drug, including pharmacodynamic response or as a surrogate endpoint in clinical trials. However, it must be emphasised that a biomarker is not a clinical outcome assessment: it does not measure how an individual feels, functions or survives. However, a response biomarker could be a surrogate endpoint which might predict clinical benefit based on scientific evidence.

This chapter will describe how advances in nailfold capillaroscopy hold promise for biomarker development. We shall first discuss the rationale for exploring nailfold capillaroscopy as a biomarker. Then we shall discuss the technical challenges, bearing in mind the stringent requirements for biomarker validation. This will be followed by discussion of the use of nailfold capillaroscopy as a biomarker in current clinical practice, primarily in childhood dermatomyositis. The evidence supporting the use of nailfold capillaroscopy as a biomarker in the research (including clinical trial) setting will then be described. Finally, areas of future research, including next steps to validation as a response biomarker, will be discussed.

Rationale for Nailfold Capillaroscopy as a Biomarker

Nailfold capillaroscopy gives unique, direct visualisation of the microcirculation, allowing assessment of microcirculatory structure and (as discussed in chapter "Research Methods; Functional Measures of Nailfold Capillaroscopy Including Permeability, Perfusion and Oxygenation") different aspects of microcirculatory function including capillary blood flow and permeability. It is non-invasive, allowing repeat assessments over time. Therefore, development of nailfold capillaroscopy as a biomarker 'makes sense' because different capillaroscopic parameters, including capillary density, fit the definition of "A defined characteristic that is measured as an indicator of normal biological processes, pathogenic processes or responses to an exposure or intervention." This is especially true in the context of diseases such as systemic sclerosis (SSc) and dermatomyositis when microvascular abnormalities are well recognised and most likely drive the disease process. Indeed, nailfold capillaroscopy has long been proposed as a biomarker for SSc [3] and as discussed below is already used to inform clinical decision making in patients with juvenile dermatomyositis. However, a key and defining feature of a biomarker is that is has to be measurable. And here lies the major challenge: can we measure capillary abnormality? Figure 1 shows the capillaries of patients with SSc. There is no doubt that these are abnormal. But that is not sufficient. We need to be able to measure the degree of abnormality and make precise measurements of any changes over time. In other words, we need to quantify the abnormality/abnormalities reliably, and demonstrate that the measured parameters are sensitive to change. Up until very recently, this has not been possible, and so although it is well recognised that (at least in dermatomyositis) capillary abnormalities can regress, it has proved

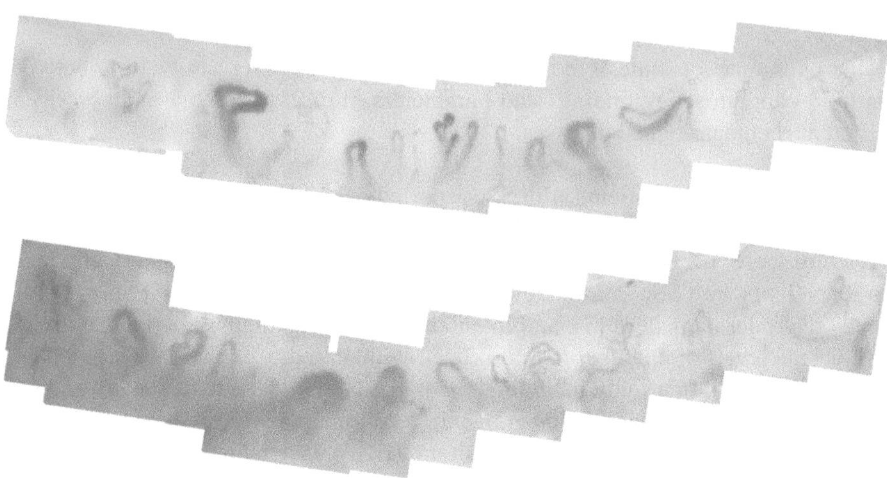

Fig. 1 Panoramic mosaic images showing very abnormal nailfold capillaries in SSc: enlarged capillaries, areas of avascularity, and distortion of the capillary architecture. The challenge is to quantify these abnormalities

difficult to quantify change. However, advances in methodology, including assessment of capillary structure automatically using a machine learning approach as discussed in chapter "Quantitative Analysis" and as discussed below under 'Future technologies', allow us to be optimistic that a way forward can be found.

In this chapter, we shall focus on nailfold capillaroscopy as a biomarker to monitor and assess response to treatment in patients with SSc and with dermatomyositis, because these are the two diseases in which there has been most interest and in which nailfold capillaroscopy is likely to have most potential. However, it should be noted that nailfold capillaroscopy has been suggested as a biomarker in other diseases, including 'non-rheumatological' diseases as diverse as diabetic nephropathy [4] and paediatric inflammatory bowel disease [5].

Two further points will be considered in this chapter in making the case for nailfold capillaroscopy as a biomarker in different rheumatological diseases. First, different investigators have looked for associations between the severity of nailfold capillaroscopic change and other potential biomarkers, primarily circulating biomarkers of vasculopathy. Some of these studies will be briefly described, because they contribute to the rationale of nailfold capillaroscopy as a biomarker. Second, several studies have examined associations between nailfold capillaroscopy change and (degree of) pulmonary arterial hypertension (PAH), which is one of the vascular manifestations of connective tissue disease, in particular of SSc. Nailfold capillaroscopy in PAH will be discussed briefly here, because the literature adds further weight to nailfold capillaroscopy as a biomarker of (connective tissue disease-related) systemic vascular disease.

Associations Between Nailfold Capillaroscopy Findings and Other Markers of Rheumatological Diseases

Table 1 summarises some of the studies which have looked for associations between nailfold capillaroscopy findings and parameters of disease activity and severity in different rheumatological diseases.

SSc In a study of 18 patients with SSc reported over 20 years ago [6], serum levels of E-selectin, a marker of endothelial cell activation, correlated with capillaroscopic 'deletion score' i.e. the greater the loss of capillaries, the higher the E-selectin level. In 99 patients with SSc, plasma levels of endothelin-1 were highest in those with a 'late' scleroderma pattern [7], and in another study including 60 patients with SSc [8] plasma levels of endothelin-1 correlated with an index of capillary size ('capillary dimension'). In a study including 103 patients (divided into discovery and replication cohorts) [9], endothelial progenitor cell counts were reduced and serum levels of vascular endothelial growth factor (VEGF) were increased in patients with 'late' scleroderma pattern (compared to those with 'early'/'active' patterns). Cutolo and Smith in 2013 [3] reviewed the literature examining links between nailfold capillaroscopy pattern and angiogenic and angiostatic factors. Di Martino et al. [10] subsequently reported that numbers of circulating endothelial cells (which are

Table 1 Some of the studies investigating associations between nailfold capillaroscopy findings and other markers predominantly of vasculopathy in different rheumatological diseases. Only associations within disease groups are described here (i.e. results from healthy controls are not tabulated)

Reference	Disease(s)	Number of subjects	NFC technique	Nailfold parameters evaluated	Links/biomarkers examined	Key findings/ conclusions
Systemic sclerosis						
Valim et al. 2004 [6]	SSc	18	Wide-field capillaroscopy. Magnification 16X. 8 fingers	'Ectasia' and 'deletion' scores	Serum E-selectin	E-selectin levels correlated with the deletion score i.e. higher levels were found in those patients with the greatest loss of capillaries.
Sulli et al. 2009 [7]	SSc	99	Video-capillaroscopy. Magnification 200X. 8 fingers	'Early', 'active', 'late' patterns. Semiquantitative ratings of: Enlarged/giant capillaries Haemorrhages Loss of capillaries Ramified capillaries Disorganisation	Plasma endothelin-1	Endothelin-1 levels were highest in patients with a 'late' scleroderma pattern. Negative correlation between number of capillaries and endothelin-1 levels.

(continued)

Table 1 (continued)

Reference	Disease(s)	Number of subjects	NFC technique	Nailfold parameters evaluated	Links/biomarkers examined	Key findings/ conclusions
Kim et al. 2010 [8]	SSc	60	Light microscope. Magnification 100X and 400X. 8 fingers	Quantitative scoring of capillary density and dimensions including 'capillary dimension' (the sum of pixel numbers of a defined area at the capillary apex)	Plasma endothelin-1	Positive correlation between level of endothelin-1 and 'capillary dimension' .
Avouac et al. 2013 [9]	SSc	103: 60 (discovery cohort) + 43 (replication cohort)	Videocapillaroscopy. Magnification 200X. 8 fingers	'Early', 'active' and 'late' scleroderma patterns	Circulating endothelial progenitor cells. Circulating endothelial cells. Serum levels of eight endothelial markers	Reduced counts of endothelial progenitor cells, and increased levels of VEGF in patients with 'late' scleroderma pattern.
Di Martino et al. 2021 [10]	SSc	50	Not stated	'Unspecific alteration', 'early', 'active' and 'late' scleroderma patterns	Peripheral blood circulating endothelial cells	Numbers of circulating endothelial cells were highest in patients with a 'late' capillaroscopic pattern.
Idiopathic inflammatory myopathy (IIM)						
Papadopoulou et al. 2021 [11]	Juvenile dermatomyositis	90	Otoscope. Magnification 10x. 8 fingers	Normal capillaries (n=38) vs abnormal (n=52)	Included markers of endothelial injury (including circulating endothelial cells) and inflammation markers	Patients with abnormal capillaries had higher numbers of circulating endothelial cells and higher galactin-9 levels than those with normal capillaries.

Tang et al. 2025 [12]	IIM	55	Videocapillaroscopy. 8 fingers	Semi-quantitative scoring system	A panel of interferon-stimulated genes, cytokines and chemokines	Positive correlations between NFC scores and expression of certain interferon-stimulated genes and certain cytokine levels.
SLE						
Kuryliszyn-Moskal et al. 2009 [13]	SLE	80	Stereomicroscope. Magnification 200X. 8 fingers	Changes graded as: 0 (no changes), 1 (mild changes), 2 (moderate changes), 3 (severe changes)	Serum endothelial cell activation markers and disease activity (by SLEDAI)	Significant correlation between SLEDAI and severity of capillary abnormality. Patients with moderate/severe capillaroscopic abnormalities had higher serum VEGF levels than those with no/mild changes
Berkcamp et al. 2024 [14]	Childhood onset SLE	47 (32 of whom had NFC data available). Patients examined twice (median time between visits 14.5 months)	Videocapillaroscopy. Magnification 200X. 8 fingers	Capillaroscopy pattern: Normal Microangiopathy Scleroderma pattern	15 serum markers of endothelial function	A weak positive correlation between levels of angiopoietin-2 and a scleroderma pattern at the second time-point (6 patients had a scleroderma pattern).

IIM Idiopathic imflammatory myopathy, *NFC* nailfold capillaroscopy, *SLE* systemic lupus erythematosus, *SLEDAI* Systemic Lupus Erythematosus Disease Activity Index, *VEGF* vascular endothelial growth factor increased with endothelial damage) were highest in patients with a 'late' scleroderma pattern in a study of 50 patients (of whom 23 had a 'late' pattern') [10].

Idiopathic Inflammatory Myopathies (IIM) In 90 patients with juvenile dermatomyositis [11], the 52 patients with abnormal nailfold capillaries (as assessed using an otoscope i.e. with low magnification) had higher levels of circulating endothelial cells than the 38 with normal capillaries. A recent study of 55 patients with IIM [12] reported correlations between semi-quantitative capillaroscopy score and certain interferon-stimulated genes and cytokines: the authors suggested that capillaroscopy might be a marker for interferon pathway activation in patients with IIM.

Systemic Lupus Erythematosus (SLE) In 80 patients with SLE [13], patients with moderate/severe changes on nailfold capillaroscopy had higher VEGF levels than those with no or only mild changes, and a correlation was reported between SLE disease activity and the severity of nailfold capillary change. In a study of childhood-onset SLE [14], correlations were examined between nailfold capillaroscopy pattern ('normal', 'microangiopathy', 'scleroderma pattern') and 15 different serum markers of endothelial function. No correlations were found other that a weak correlation between levels of angiopoietin-2 and a scleroderma pattern (present in 6 of 32 patients). No quantitative capillaroscopy analyses were undertaken.

In conclusion, several studies have examined levels of circulating (bio)markers, including markers of endothelial cell activation, and related these to presence or absence, or different grades of capillary abnormality. However, these groupings/gradings are often subjective, and are highly unlikely to be sensitive to change over time. What are required are parameters which measure the degree of capillary abnormality as a continuous variable and which are likely to be sensitive to change. This will allow more detailed examination of associations between severity of nailfold capillaroscopy change and other markers of vasculopathy. More definite evidence that the degree of capillaroscopic change is linked to circulating markers of vasculopathy will strengthen the case for capillaroscopy as a biomarker, always bearing in mind that associations may depend on which disease is being studied and also on stage/duration of disease.

Associations Between Nailfold Capillaroscopy Findings and Pulmonary Arterial Hypertension

It is outside the remit of this chapter to review the literature on nailfold capillaroscopy in patients with PAH. However, it is worth highlighting here that amongst patients with SSc, nailfold capillary density has been shown to be reduced in those with PAH compared to those without PAH [15]. Although this finding has not been replicated in all studies [16], several studies suggest that those patients with SSc who also have PAH have the more marked capillary changes [17, 18]. This raises the question as to whether abnormalities on nailfold capillaroscopy might be a biomarker of a more 'general' (or systemic) vasculopathy, at least in patients with SSc, and provides further weight to the concept of nailfold capillaroscopy as a biomarker of vasculopathy.

Relevant to this argument is the finding that severity of SSc-related telangiectases (in terms of size and number) has been found to be associated with severity of nailfold capillary change [19]. Telangiectases, similarly to PAH, are a manifestation of SSc-related vasculopathy.

Technical Challenges

There are several technical challenges when considering nailfold capillaroscopy as a biomarker. These can be considered in terms of image acquisition and of interpretation. The key point for the clinician to note is that capillaries can only be assessed and measured if they are well visualised, and so it is important to ensure the highest possible quality of images. Acquisition difficulties mainly revolve around user experience/training, choice and use of equipment (hardware and software interface), image collection protocols, and actual collection of images from the patient (which can be difficult if patients have finger contractures, or if there is skin fibrosis or oedema). Thumbs are generally omitted. Interpretation of images heavily relies on acquisition, since good quality images of the desired number across the nailfold and in the preselected number of fingers are essential. However, even when provided with clear images of nailfold capillaries, deciding how best to assess or measure these has long been debated with many options available. Ensuring good inter- and intra-observer reliability of image interpretation can be challenging. Here, we consider the challenges of image acquisition and interpretation (including interpretation in different skin tones), and their impact on capillaroscopy as a biomarker. Finally we discuss reliability (in relation to both image acquisition and interpretation): good reliability is a prerequisite for any potential biomarker.

The Challenges of Image Acquisition

Choice of Nailfold Capillaroscopy System

Obtaining a 'Good' Image In terms of acquiring images one of the key first choices is in equipment, often a trade-off between expense and lack of sophisticated features (discussed further in chapter "Nailfold Capillaroscopy—Image Acquisition"); however, even low-cost systems can offer similar imaging quality, magnification and outcomes to more expensive ones [20–24]. Another consideration is low vs high magnification systems, low magnification (which can be lower cost) enables a wider field of view, but less detail can be resolved. And low magnification systems may not offer the opportunity to record the image digitally. Higher magnification systems enable higher resolution, often leading to capillary abnormality being graded more severely than with lower magnification, and subtle early changes may be observed more easily. However, high magnification systems are limited in their field of view and as such several frames are required to cover the full nailfold. Handheld systems are now available at low cost but still enabling good quality, high magnification imaging. It is worth noting that when we talk about magnification, we refer here to the optical magnification of the system which relates to the lenses used; however, it is usually possible to then add digital magnification in terms of viewing these images on a larger screen.

Most systems include illumination with a ring of LEDs (around the camera), which can illuminate skin. These can cause specular reflections, or bright spots from the oil on the image (placing a small amount of oil on the skin is key to ensure good visualisation through skin surface), but the more expensive systems have polarizers which can remove these, enhancing image quality. Imaging is generally carried out with white light but can also be with green light, which can enhance the contrast of the capillaries in black and white images. Several capillaroscopy systems come with software enabling easy measurement of capillary width. Different users will prefer different systems. Some techniques are contact, submerging the tip of the camera in the oil; this offers stability but may also blanche the skin if too much pressure is applied and may cause discomfort. Practise is key in improving quality of images, understanding best positioning and becoming accomplished at focusing well. Lower magnification systems such as dermatoscopes (approximately x10 magnification), which can be used with digital cameras or mobile phones for image capture, enable visualisation of the whole nailbed and tend to be easier to focus than higher magnification systems. Handheld microscopes (approximately 200x magnification) allow visualisation of approximately 1.5 mm of the nailbed per image, enabling a view of the capillaries at higher resolution and facilitating measurement but their depth of focus is smaller, meaning that it can be more difficult to initially find the correct focus. In addition, imaging capillaries at the edge of the finger, where the finger curves downwards often can be difficult, the curvature meaning that a whole frame (from left edge to right) cannot remain in focus. These points are included under 'technical challenges' because it is important that any investigator seeking to use nailfold capillaroscopy as a biomarker has a full understanding of how to acquire high quality images and chooses (and becomes expert in using) a system which allows acquisition of sufficiently high-quality images to allow tracking of change over time.

Even with adequate training and the correct equipment, some factors preclude acquisition of images that can be interpreted. Thickened skin and oedema can obscure capillaries and visualisation can be difficult even in some healthy controls due to skin that does not transmit light well or poor contrast in capillaries. Another issue is visualisation of capillaries in darker skin tones, which can be difficult as we describe below.

Number of Fingers

The number of fingers to be imaged varies according to the intended purpose of imaging. One can argue that for diagnosis observation of even only one finger with characteristic changes may be sufficient. However, for a biomarker and/or for full assessment of severity (scleroderma pattern or quantitative density and width) an assessment across all fingers is required due to the heterogeneity of structural changes both across one nailfold and also across all 8 digits (excluding thumbs). Dinsdale et al. assessed the sensitivity to diagnostic criteria in a study of 173 participants when different numbers and combinations of fingers were examined (discussed further in chapter "Nailfold Capillaroscopy—Image Acquisition"), sensitivity increased from 31.7% to 46.6% for one finger to 59.8% for bilateral ring fingers and 74.6% for all 8 fingers [25].

The Challenges of Image Interpretation

Image Quality or Evaluability

As discussed above, whether an image is of good enough quality to be assessed is a key issue and is addressed in several studies. The study reported by Dinsdale et al. [26], in which 10 observers interpreted subsets of 1650 images, included 'ungradable' as part of the image categorisation. Observers assessed the percentage of evaluable measures (density, width, presence of giants) from images. They found that density could be measured in 73% of images but that overall grade ('normal', 'early', 'active', 'late') could only be assessed in 46.2% of images. The authors acknowledged the challenge of obtaining evaluable images. A study comparing dermoscopy and nailfold videocapillaroscopy included a 'classifiable' category ('poor visualization/cannot be categorized'). Higher resolution images from videocapillaroscopy had a higher level of classifiability; 84% versus 70% for dermoscopy [22]. Many studies only include images that are 'evaluable' as a first step in examining, for example, reliability [27, 28]. If capillaroscopy is to be used as a biomarker, then it is important that investigators take into account that in any one study, there will be a proportion of capillaroscopic images/ parameters that cannot be evaluated, even if all steps are taken to ensure image quality. Investigators should also make it clear in their reporting how this issue was 'handled'.

Assessment of Density

Another technical challenge within quantitative analysis is determining the distal row and calculating capillary density [29]. From both a diagnostic perspective and for tracking disease (either via the 'early', 'active' and 'late' patterns or capillary counting), density is the parameter which has the strongest support. For this reason, several strategies to determine which capillaries should be included for counting have been tested (Fig. 2—showing different annotations for density) [27, 30, 31]. Hofstee et al. [30] proposed a 90° method, whereby 'a capillary loop was considered to be a distal loop if the apex of the capillary made an angle of ≥90° with the apex of its adjacent capillaries'. Comparison of the 90° technique with the density calculated as per 'observer choice' in the distal row gave slightly lower values for the 90° technique (90° 7.06 caps/mm vs 'observer choice' 7.78) but improved interobserver reliability (Interclass correlation coefficient (ICC) 90° 0.87 vs 'observer choice' 0.71). Wildt et al. [31] compared three capillaroscopy systems to

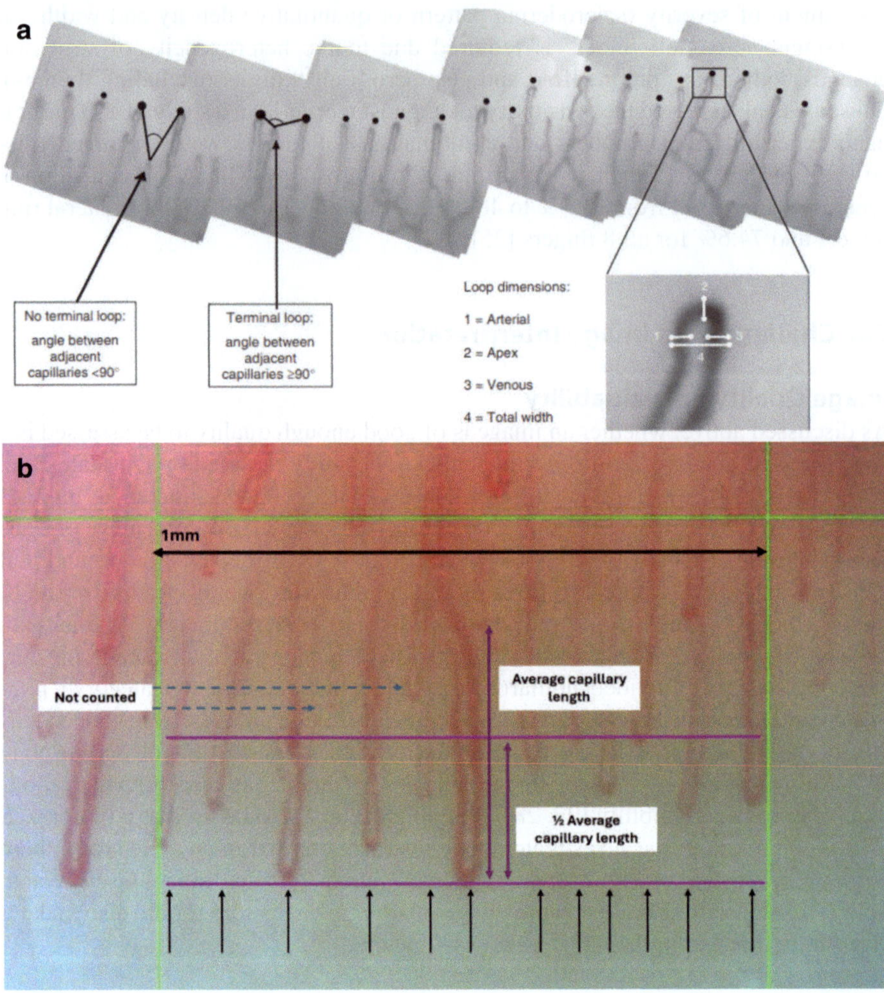

Fig. 2 Measuring capillary density. Different proposals for determining the density of distal row capillaries including (**a**) 90° rule between capillary apices. Reproduced by permission of Oxford University Press on behalf of the British Society for Rheumatology [30]. (**b**) using the half height of distal capillaries to binarize distal apices [27]. (Courtesy of Vanessa Smith and Ramona Govender)

measure density in images taken sequentially on the non-dominant ring finger (40 patients with SSc and 21 healthy controls). The first system was a stereomicroscope with zoom, x20, visualised by eye alone, the second system was the stereomicroscope with digital software to enable digital magnification, the final system was videocapillaroscopy at x300 magnification which generated panoramic mosaics across the whole nailfold. The 90° rule was used to assess the distal row. The differences in density were reported in subgroups, e.g. 4.3, 5.4 and 6.1 loops/mm for systems 1–3 in limited cutaneous SSc. Density differences were larger between the systems for the patients with SSc than for controls; there was no significant difference between the techniques in healthy control density. In patients, the difference between techniques (1) and (2) was believed to be due to the different magnifications (e.g. viewed through the microscope vs displayed on a screen). The difference between (2) and (3) was believed to be due to the averaging of frames over time with the videocapillaroscopy system: because capillary walls are transparent and only red blood cells are observed during imaging, averaging frames with time can enable unfilled or partially filled capillaries to be observed more easily, leading to a higher density measurement. Smith et al. [27] propose drawing a horizontal line across the image at the vertical midpoint of the capillaries and selecting only those capillaries that have apices above that threshold (Fig. 2b).

Age may influence capillary density. Several studies have measured both width and density in different age groups in control populations. Some studies suggest that apical width and density tend not to change with age, but venous and arterial limb increase with age (6–15 years) [32, 33]. Other studies indicate potential increases in density with age [34]. Studies in paediatric patients are discussed in chapter "Nailfold Capillaroscopy in Children".

In summary, determining density is an important factor for capillaroscopy as a biomarker. The choice of imaging technique (magnification/resolution and software used) can influence this as can interpretation of the images. Automation of analysis should facilitate density measurements in the future, with machine learning algorithms deciding which capillaries belong to the distal row, and counting capillaries (discussed further below in 'Future Technologies').

The Challenge Posed by Darker Skin Tones

Melanin in the skin resides in the epidermal layer above the capillaries and presents in vertical lines, parallel with the capillary limbs (Fig. 3), obfuscating visualisation and measurement. In a study of 800 healthy controls (aged 12–77 years), who were categorised as white (n = 468) or non-white (n = 332), skin pigmentation was acknowledged to be one of several factors that can influence visualisation of capillaries [35]. Periungual colour and colour of the skin behind the capillaries, referred to as 'background' were strongly correlated with visibility. There was a statistically significant difference in visibility between the groups (with capillaries in the white group being more easily observed). Skin tone was associated with capillary density; the white group having a mean of 9.33 capillaries/mm versus 8.77 in the non-white group. A study in healthy controls carried out in India, in Fitzpatrick skin types III-VI (Table 2) [36], highlighted the potential issues around capillaroscopy in darker skin tones and identified that capillary density decreased with increasing skin type and that in type VI skin, sometimes capillaries cannot be observed at all [37].

In a study from the Netherlands, 145 healthy children underwent capillaroscopy to examine the influence of age and ethnicity related data on capillary density. Density was assessed and averaged over 8 fingers (2 frames per finger), following acclimatization. No effect was found for age; however, for skin pigmentation (scored 1–3) density significantly decreased from paler (1) to darker skin tones (3) [33]. Decreased visualisation in darker skin was also shown in a study of

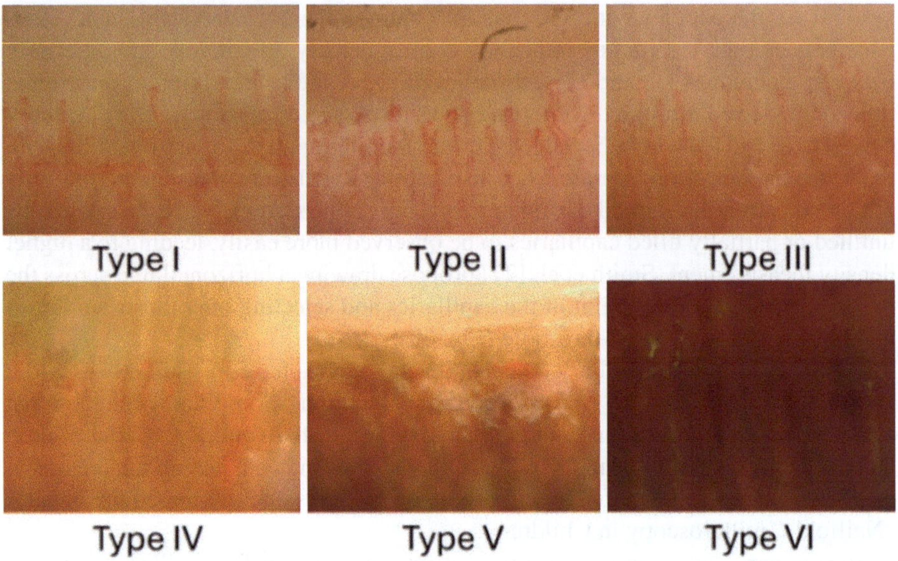

Fig. 3 Examples of nailfold images taken in different Fitzpatrick skin types

Table 2 Fitzpatrick skin types [36]

Skin type	Description
Type I	Very fair skin, often with red or blonde hair and blue eyes. This type always burns and never tans.
Type II	Fair skin, often with red or blonde hair and blue, hazel, or green eyes. This type usually burns and tans with difficulty.
Type III	Fair skin, often with brown or blonde hair and blue, brown, or hazel eyes. This type can sometimes burn and gradually tans.
Type IV	Light brown skin. This type rarely burns and tans easily.
Type V	Brown skin. This type never burns and tans very easily.
Type VI	Dark brown to black skin. This type never burns and tans very easily.

capillaroscopy in patients with diabetes as compared to a control group, noting a significant decrease between Fitzpatrick skin tones IV and V [38].

These studies highlight an important point about the about the applicability of nailfold capillaroscopy across different skin tones. Pending further research and development, with the aim of trying to ensure equal access to nailfold capillaroscopy for all patients, data from the studies described provide a good baseline to understand what is likely to be visualised and what is 'normal' in terms of density across skin tones, enabling clinicians to adjust expectations accordingly.

Other studies report data including from cohorts from a range of ethnicities, including Asian and black patients or healthy controls, with no mention of difficulty in viewing capillaries [34, 39–42]. Bhakuni et al. [39] reported a study of 42 patients with SSc and 42 controls carried out in India; the images which are included in their report are indicative of good visualisation and their capillary densities (healthy control, 8.7 capillaries/mm; SSc 5.3 capillaries/mm) fit well within the ranges reported in larger cohorts with lower skin types. Terreri et al. [34] reported a study of 329 children (binarising skin tone as white [n = 217] or non-white); with mean (SD) capillary density of 7.1 (0.8) loops/mm. They stated that capillary visualisation was good (n = 227), regular (79) or poor (23) but reported no relationship to skin colour or ethnicity. There was no significant difference in capillary density between the white and non-white groups. Torres-Ruiz et al. [42] specified that there were no differences in capillaroscopic parameters (categorized as 'early', 'active', and 'late' patterns) between ethnicities. In a case series describing 14 black patients with dermatomyositis who underwent capillaroscopy, 6/14 patients were reported to have abnormalities, without any mention of any difficulties in visualization [41]. That these studies did not report issues in visualization due to skin tone may be because images with poorly visualised capillaries were excluded or because in some cohorts this was not a problem. As mentioned above, if capillaries can be clearly visualised then they can be assessed with confidence.

In conclusion, visualisation of capillaries potentially becomes more difficult in skin types V and VI. Visualisation of certain abnormalities (e.g. large or giant loops) may be easier in darker skin tones than identifying areas of avascularity or making accurate density measurements. Since there is currently no solution to this problem, caution should be applied when imaging in darker skin tones to avoid underestimating density and overestimating avascular areas. Possible solutions are discussed in the Future Technologies section below.

Reliability

An important issue that straddles both acquiring and analysing/interpreting images is reliability. Good reliability is essential to be reassured that the same outcome can be obtained by different observers or at different time points; knowing that changes that are observed with time or following intervention are real and not due to poor reliability. There are several aspects of reliability which need to be considered in relation to capillaroscopy: in acquisition, this includes the field of view captured per finger (magnification [high-, low-resolution systems], number of frames) and the number of fingers imaged. In interpretation this relates to the data extracted from the images (semi-quantitative scale ['early', 'active', 'late'], quantitative, e.g. density and width) and how these are combined (capillary-, finger- or patient-level).

Reliability of Image Acquisition

In terms of image acquisition, the same (or a different) observer being able to return to capture the same area of the nailfold is key. Good test-retest reliability is essential if capillaroscopy is to be used as a biomarker when, for example in a clinical trial, the same or a different observer may be acquiring the nailfold images at the patient's next visit.

Maximising the chance of good reliability in image acquisition can be achieved by taking several frames across the whole nailfold (to produce a panoramic mosaic image, at high magnification/resolution that captures as much of the nailfold as possible); however, this is time consuming across all 8 fingers. Many studies specify at least 2 frames in the centre of the nailfold.

A small number of studies have assessed reliability of image acquisition (more studies have examined reliability of image interpretation). A study of 58 patients with SSc [43] aimed to assess test-retest reliability (same observer) of image acquisition as well as inter- and intra-observer reliability of image interpretation (Fig. 4). Two panoramic mosaic images were obtained from the non-dominant ring finger, with finger removed from under the microscope between images (image set 1 and 2). Capillary apices for set 1 were marked across the whole image by two observers

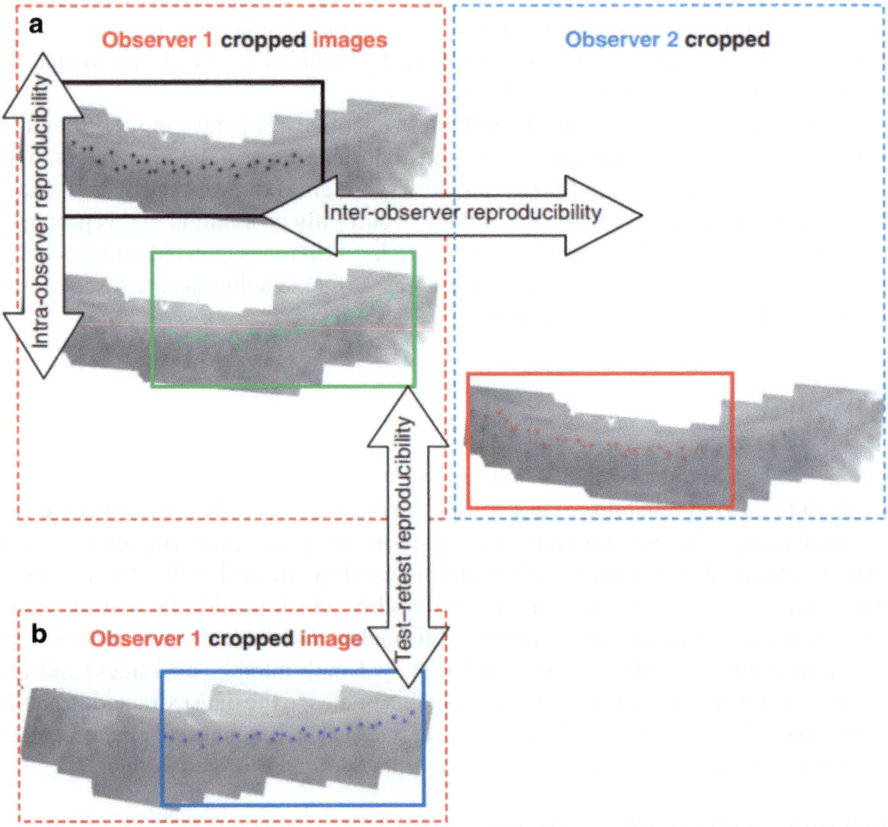

Fig. 4 Example of how images are used to assess reliability; (**a**) The same image (image **a**) assessed twice by Observer 1 for intra-observer reproducibility; image (**a**) assessed by Observers 1 and 2 for inter-observer reproducibility; image (**a**) and image (**b**) assessed by Observer 1 for test-retest reliability. This process was carried out for both the full image and on a cropped version, with the area selected at each time by the observer. (Reproduced by permission of Oxford University Press on behalf of the British Society for Rheumatology from Murray et al. [43])

(to test inter-observer reliability of image interpretation). Observer one marked the set 1 images twice (to test intra-observer reliability of image interpretation). Observer 1 also marked the set 2 images (test-retest reliability of image acquisition). In addition, observers were asked to mark-up apices in a fixed length, cropped area, chosen by them to contain a unique capillary that could be tracked by them with time (to mimic imaging in a portion but not the whole nailfold). Structural measures including width and density were assessed. For capillary density the inter-observer agreement ICCs were 0.85 for cropped images and 0.98 for the whole images, intra-observer ICCs were 0.89 for cropped images and 0.98 for whole images and the test-retest ICCs were 0.80 for cropped images and 0.93 for whole images. The study demonstrated the great improvement in reliability with images that spanned the nailfold as compared to cropped images and this was due to the fact that when cropped often a different area had been selected (Fig. 4) [43].

In another study including patients with SSc, primary RP and healthy controls, 41 participants had all 10 fingers imaged 1 week apart (i.e. test-retest of image acquisition with no expected changes due to disease within the short timeframe [44]). High magnification mosaic images were assessed by a blinded observer generating grading of scleroderma pattern (normal, 'early', 'active', 'late') and quantitative outcomes of density, apex width, number of giant vessels. Intra-observer intra-visit (same image assessed twice) gave ICCs 0.68–0.97 and intra-observer inter-visit (baseline vs. 1 week), gave 0.56–0.90 (image grading being highest and presence of giant vessels being lowest). The study's conclusion was that capillaroscopy was reproducible and suitable as an outcome for clinical trials.

Reliability of Image Interpretation

In terms of inter- and intra-observer agreement in grading or measuring capillary features, different studies have assessed this in various ways (qualitative and semi-quantitative) and across different cohorts [35, 45–50]. Some of these will be described here.

Boulon et al. [51] assessed inter and intra-observer agreement of capillaroscopy assessment for the categorisation and diagnosis of patients with SSc. Eleven expert observers all assessed images from 8 fingers from 50 patients with SSc and 50 patients with Raynaud's but no underlying connective tissue disease. Images were binarized to SSc pattern or not SSc pattern (presence of giant capillaries, avascular areas and disorganization). Seven of the eleven experts repeated this process 2 weeks later. Excellent inter-observer agreement was identified (κ 0.86) for the first assessment and a similar outcome was also found for intra-observer agreement. The study suggests differentiation between presence or absence of the scleroderma pattern is highly reliable. A contemporaneous study, that reported two observers assessing images for categories relevant to the Maricq and Cutolo patterns (8 fingers in 100 patients with SSc), identified initially poor inter-observer agreement (κ 0.47–0.49) [52]. Agreement improved after a second meeting (κ 0.64–0.69), when observers assessed a subset of images from the 8 fingers (ring finger, left hand) and also assessed at the patient level (assessing all 8 fingers). Various iterations of assessment occurred after several meetings and the authors concluded that assessments of certain features (giant capillaries, microhaemorrhages and density) tend to be more reliable than that of others (disorganisation or bushy capillaries) which may be more subjective. Assessments of the Maricq and Cutolo patterns had similar levels of agreement. The study suggested that training and consensus meetings greatly improve reliability.

Smith et al. [27] formulated a fast-track algorithm, at a consensus meeting, designed to improve diagnosis of a SSc pattern for those who may not be experts. The algorithm was shown to provide excellent reliability (κ 0.92–1).

Hofstee et al. [30] assessed inter- and intra-observer reliability of assessing nailfold capillary images from patients with SSc, primary RP and healthy controls (50 images in total, non-dominant ring finger). Images were assessed by 6 blinded observers from 3 sites (inter-observer reliability) and each observer assessed images twice (intra-observer variability). Images were scored under quantitative (various measures of width, density) and qualitative outcomes (e.g. avascularity, giant, tortuous). Inter- and intra-observer reliability was excellent for quantitative data (inter-observer ICCs 0.67–0.94, intra-observer ICCs 0.92–0.98). Agreement for qualitative data was lower (inter-observer weighted κ 0.21–0.84, intra-observer 0.68–0.92). The authors suggested combining the individual features (here, total width and presence of giant capillaries) with the most reliability when considering future studies. The higher reliability of quantitative compared to qualitative measures reported in this study [30] is relevant to capillaroscopy as a biomarker because this lends further weight to the argument that quantitative (continuous variable) parameters are more likely to be useful as biomarkers than qualitative assessments,

In a multicentre study involving ten expert observers, each observer assessed batches of images (from 1650 mosaic images from cohorts of patients with SSc, primary RP and healthy controls, who had 10 fingers imaged, including thumbs). Observers graded images (normal, 'early', 'active', 'late', 'non-specific', ungradable), marked the apex location (to generate density), measured the apex width and assessed shape, using bespoke software [26]. Images were assessed by diagnostic subgroup: SSc, primary RP or healthy control. Intra-observer reliability was better than inter-observer reliability (ICCs 0.71–0.93 vs 0.41–0.78). The highest ICC related to the image grade and the lowest to presence of giant capillaries; density ICCs were 0.65–0.92.

Comparing Reliability of Image Interpretation Between Different Capillaroscopy Systems

Several studies have compared different systems to assess how magnification influences inter- and intra-observer variability [21, 22, 53, 54]. Sekiyama et al. [53] compared inter- and intra-observer reliability of interpreting images obtained with stereo microscopy (x10–25 magnification) to that obtained with videomicroscopy (x200). Images from 20 participants were examined (8 fingers), and measurements were repeated at a period <4 weeks separation (to assess intra-observer reliability). Images were assessed as normal, non-specific or SSc; for the stereomicroscope both inter- and intra-observer agreement were perfect ($\kappa = 1$), for videocapillaroscopy the intra-observer agreement was perfect and inter-observer agreement was 0.917. Mazzotti et al. [21] compared dermoscopy and stereomicroscopy and found moderate to good agreement in assessing the SSc pattern, higher in stereomicroscopy with its higher magnification (κ 0.71, vs 0.6 for dermoscopy). Another study compared dermoscopy to videocapillaroscopy (0–3 scale of severity, from normal (0) to grossly abnormal (3) or an unclassifiable category); 40 images were assessed by 48 observers [22]. The study identified similar intra-observer 'classifiability rates' (from a linear mixed model) in image interpretation between techniques (dermoscopy 0.75 vs videocapillaroscopy 0.61) and inter-observer (0.39 vs 0.31). Of note, the investigators noted that more of the videocapillaroscopy images could be graded than dermoscopy images and that videocapillaroscopy images tended to be graded as a more severe pattern (potentially due to higher magnification providing more detail); flagging the importance of selecting the optimal system used to capture images if using as a biomarker.

Conclusions—Reliability

In conclusion, assessing reliability of nailfold capillaroscopy image acquisition and interpretation is complex because many different factors have to be taken into account. Test-retest (of image acquisition) appears to be relatively reliable with the same system over time as long as the whole (or majority) of the nailfold is captured [43, 44]. Regarding reliability of image interpretation, intra-observer reliability tends to be higher than inter-observer reliability, which is to be expected. Qualitative data shows variability in agreement, with more simple and easy to define concepts such as presence or absence of SSc pattern or giant capillaries being more reliable than categorising avascular areas, shape change or patterns of severity. Training and consensus discussion improve agreement. Measuring quantitative density and width tend to rely on software (manual assessment is labour intensive for width measurement) but offer more objective measures than some of the other parameters discussed.

Monitoring of Disease in the Clinical Setting

As discussed in chapter "Clinical Indications", nailfold capillaroscopy is used in the clinical setting not only for diagnosis, but also to inform management of patients with dermatomyositis, many of whom have marked nailfold capillary changes. It has long been recognised [55] that in dermatomyositis, the degree of nailfold capillary abnormality correlates with disease activity, and that appearances can 'improve' with effective treatment. This is particularly relevant when it is unclear whether there might be some ongoing subclinical disease activity because if so, then this would be an indication not to reduce treatment. Clinical monitoring of disease activity in dermatomyositis is fully discussed in chapter "Nailfold Capillaroscopy in Idiopathic Inflammatory Myopathies", and is perhaps particularly important in children, when the risks and benefits of continuing treatment have to be especially finely balanced. It is possible that in childhood dermatomyositis, seeing that the nailfold capillaries remain abnormal may encourage children and their parents to continue with their treatment i.e. nailfold capillaroscopy might aid compliance. This is a subject of ongoing research.

At present, many adult and paediatric rheumatologists do not use nailfold capillaroscopy in their clinical practice [56, 57] and so although monitoring of disease activity in dermatomyositis and in other IIMs associated with nailfold capillary changes (chapter "Nailfold Capillaroscopy in Idiopathic Inflammatory Myopathies") makes good sense, this application is currently most likely to be confined to specialist centres. Although a UK survey suggested that most paediatric rheumatologists looked at nailfold capillaries, this was in children with Raynaud's phenomenon and most used an opthalmoscope [57], which may not allow sufficiently good visualisation of capillaries to detect changes over time. It will be interesting to see whether the use of nailfold capillaroscopy to monitor IIM changes over the next 10 years as uptake of nailfold capillaroscopy increases, facilitated by advances in image acquisition and interpretation.

At present, there is no defined role for nailfold capillaroscopy in monitoring patients with established SSc in the clinical setting. Nailfold capillary changes do not occur over short time frames in patients with SSc in the same way as in those with dermatomyositis [58], although they can change over longer time intervals [59] (Fig. 5). This is because the microangiopathy of SSc is non-inflammatory, in contrast with nailfold capillary changes in IIMs which are thought to be driven by perivascular inflammation [60], and which are therefore likely to be (at least partly) reversible with treatment with immunosuppressant and/or corticosteroid therapy. However, whether nailfold capillary abnormalities in patients with SSc can be 'normalised' with drugs with potential to remodel the vasculature is a key question and a subject of intense interest which is discussed below.

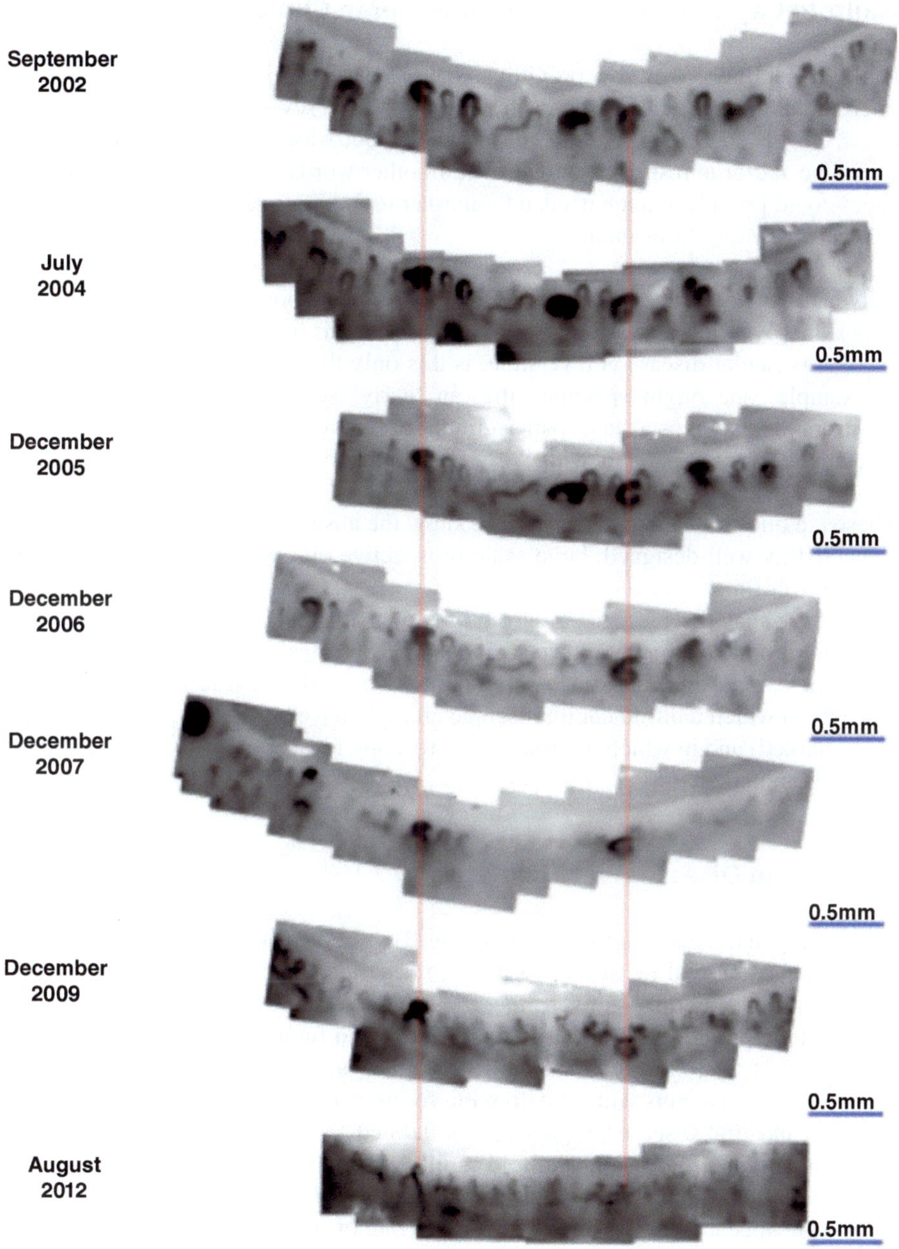

Fig. 5 High-magnification nailfold mosaic sequence covering a near 10-year period. (Reproduced by permission of Oxford University Press on behalf of the British Society for Rheumatology from Dinsdale et al. [59])

Nailfold Capillaroscopy as a Biomarker in Clinical Research

Nailfold capillaroscopy, by providing a non-invasive window into the aberrant microcirculation which is a characteristic feature of several rheumatological diseases, affords enormous potential to study how microvascular disease might change over time and/or in response to treatment. In other words, nailfold capillary appearances could provide a much needed biomarker to facilitate research including clinical trials. Key questions include:

'In what way does microvascular disease progress, and how quickly?'
'Does microvascular disease regress, and if so can this happen spontaneously?
'If microvascular disease is reversible, is this only the case if 'caught' early?' For example, one might speculate that an 'early' scleroderma pattern might be reversible, whereas a 'late' pattern might be irreversible. This question is especially relevant in patients with 'Very Early Diagnosis of SSc' (VEDOSS' [61].

These are questions to which we do not know the answers, but all of them could be answered by well-designed, large scale prospective observational studies studying change over time.

Here we shall discuss what is currently known about nailfold capillaroscopy as a potential biomarker for monitoring disease and response to treatment. As already mentioned, we shall focus on SSc and dermatomyositis because these are the two diseases in which nailfold capillaroscopic changes have been most studied (and are most marked) and in which nailfold capillaroscopy is most likely to provide a long-awaited biomarker.

Monitoring Disease Over Time

Monitoring disease over time is challenging. Two studies of SSc and one of juvenile dermatomyositis will be discussed here, to describe some of the previous experience in monitoring disease over time, the challenges faced, and how these studies contribute to providing a platform on which to build future research programmes.

Avouac et al. [62] examined nailfold capillaroscopic change over time (over 3 years) in 140 patients with SSc, looking for associations between capillaroscopic changes and SSc disease progression as defined by development of new digital ulcers and organ progression. Nailfold capillaroscopy was performed annually, with most patients (89%) having 4 nailfold examinations. 'Progression' in nailfold capillaroscopic appearances was reported in 72 (51%) of patients during the 3 year time interval. The main conclusion of the study was that reduction in the number of capillaries was associated with disease progression, specifically with overall disease progression, occurrence of new digital ulcers, lung vascular progression, skin fibrosis progression, and worsening of the Medsger severity score [63]. Also, development (or increase in the numbers of) giant capillaries was associated with reduced risk of development of new digital ulcers. This study therefore supports the concept of nailfold capillaroscopic appearances as a biomarker of disease.

It is worth considering how the investigators assessed changes in nailfold capillaries over time [62]. In each patient, 8 digits (thumbs were excluded) were examined using videocapillaroscopy (magnification 200x). In each digit, two 1 mm 'consecutive fields' were examined, meaning that 16 images were examined in each patient. Four quantitative parameters were examined across all 16 images: the number of capillaries (capillary density/mm, with severe loss of capillaries defined as <4 capillaries/mm), the number of giant capillaries, the number of microhaemorrhages and the number of 'neoangiogenic' capillaries. Progression in nailfold capillaroscopic appearances was defined as either incident (first time) occurrence of any of these 4 abnormalities ('severe capillary loss' being the abnormality relating to capillary density) or progression in any of these 4 parameters. For each of the 4 abnormalities, the authors reported the numbers of patients who developed new 'lesions', who developed worsening of lesions, or in whom lesions regressed. This was a complicated task, involving assessment of abnormalities in 16 images per patient and (as in all studies looking for change over time) there would be a concern that the two images per finger might not always have been from exactly the same section of the nailfold on each occasion. But there was a clear signal that patients progressing during the 3 year period to severe loss of capillaries (< 4/mm) were those most likely to experience clinical progression. The protection which development of giant capillaries afforded against digital ulcer development was interpreted by the authors as being suggestive of a 'benign' disease course in this subset. From a practical perspective, counting numbers of giant capillaries, which are easy to define, is a relatively simple task. Counting the total number of capillaries (i.e measuring capillary density) is more complex (as discussed above under 'technical challenges'). Counting haemorrhages and counting/defining 'neoangiogenesis' are probably even more complex. It would be interesting to know whether measuring capillary density and analysing this as a continuous variable would have strengthened the results.

Sulli et al. [64] also examined associations between progression of nailfold capillaroscopic change and organ involvement. This was an extension of a previous study [65] and although only 34 patients were included, a strength of the study was the long duration of follow-up (12 years, standard deviation 2 years). Nailfold capillaroscopy was performed annually. All 34 patients recruited had an 'early' scleroderma pattern on nailfold capillaroscopy. Of these 34 patients, 8 (24%) remained with an 'early' pattern, 9 (26%) progressed to an active pattern, 13 (38%) progressed to a 'late' pattern and 4 (12%) 'improved' to non-specific abnormalities. A key finding was that the 13 patients progressing to a 'late' pattern took a median of 59 months to do so, but transitioned through an 'active' pattern by a median of 11 months. This was a much shorter time than in the 9 patients who had an active pattern at last follow-up, who took a median of 55 months to reach this. The authors concluded that early transition to an active pattern put the patient at high risk of going on to develop a 'late' pattern, which was associated with increased prevalence of internal organ involvement. The authors also documented 'microvascular evolution score' at the different timepoints. This study therefore provided further support that nailfold capillaroscopy may be a useful tool to monitor disease progression in that changes occur over time and are related to severity of internal organ involvement. The challenge is how to measure that change over time reliably and accurately.

Both these studies [62, 64] were single centre. Single centre studies have the advantage of maximising the likelihood of consistency in image acquisition and interpretation, and Avouac included assessments of inter-rater reliability of image acquisition (3 investigators acquired images) and intra-rater reliability of image evaluation (one investigator analysed all images) [62]. It is likely that to validate nailfold capillaroscopy as a biomarker, large scale multicentre studies will be required. An analysis from the European Scleroderma Trials and Research group (EUSTAR) database demonstrates the appetite for this approach. Velauthapillai et al. [66] sought to address whether there was an association between change in capillaroscopy pattern and development of interstitial lung disease (ILD), studying 275 patients from the EUSTAR database with a median follow-up duration of 2 years and a median number of nailfold capillaroscopy examinations of 2 during this follow-up. The authors concluded that increasing severity of nailfold capillaroscopy pattern ('early', 'active' and 'late') was associated with an increased annual risk of developing ILD. This was an ambitious study, and had a number of limitations, including being a post hoc analysis, no central reading of images, and only qualitative rating of images. As the authors pointed out, including measurement of capillary density would have added value to the study, but had this been included it would have been important to ensure standardisation of image acquisition and interpretation [67]. Nonetheless, this study is important because it demonstrates the feasibility of international collaboration in longitudinal studies of nailfold capillaroscopy. Future studies using large datasets could benefit from automated analysis of images as discussed in chapter "Quantitative Analysis".

These three studies have all examined nailfold capillaroscopy as a potential biomarker for monitoring SSc. As mentioned above, its use as a biomarker in dermatomyositis is already recognised clinically, based upon the many studies, reviewed in chapter "Nailfold Capillaroscopy in Idiopathic Inflammatory Myopathies", describing associations between nailfold capillaroscopic abnormalities and disease activity and severity. Many of these reports relate to childhood dermatomyositis. One recent study will be mentioned here. Kjojah et al. [68] in a single centre retrospective study of 68 patients with juvenile dermatomyositis followed over at least 5 years and with at least 4 capillaroscopy assessments, reported that the number of capillary end row loops/mm (measured over 3 mm on each finger) was a marker of disease progression. For example, end row loop count showed more change in 'monocyclic short' than in patients with chronic disease, increasing from 4.8 ± 1.5 /mm at baseline to 6.7 + 1.5/mm at 12 months. The authors concluded that a goal of new treatments should be to restore end row loop counts to values comparable to those of healthy controls (in whom end row loop count was 7.9 ± 0.9/mm), consistent with the belief that nailfold capillaroscopy could be a biomarker in future research studies including clinical trials.

The studies described above demonstrate how different groups of investigators, in different ways, have all made the case for nailfold capillaroscopy to be used as a research tool to monitor disease progression. The challenge now is to build upon this work as described below.

Studying Treatment Response

A key question is whether nailfold capillaroscopy can be used as a biomarker/surrogate endpoint in studies assessing treatment response, including clinical trials. This would make sense, because if a drug can lead to 'improvement' in microvascular structural change then this would provide evidence of effectiveness in modifying the underlying disease process. As discussed in chapter "Nailfold Capillaroscopy in Idiopathic Inflammatory Myopathies", in patients with dermatomyositis nailfold capillary abnormalities tend to regress alongside disease activity and so there is a strong rationale for exploring capillaroscopic parameters (for example capillary density) as surrogate endpoints. However, there is very little in the dermatomyositis literature examining nailfold capillaroscopic change in response to specific drug treatments or in clinical trials. In patients with SSc, any changes in nailfold capillary appearances in response to treatment are likely to occur over longer timeframes, given the non-inflammatory nature of the micro-angiopathy in most patients. Nonetheless several studies, including the SENSCIS trial [69] have examined nailfold capillary change in response to drug treatment in patients with SSc. Some of these are summarised in Table 3.

An important question is whether, in patients with early diffuse cutaneous SSc in whom there is thought to be immune activation and inflammation, immunosuppressive therapy might favourably influence microvascular change. A second question is whether drugs with vascular remodelling potential might either stabilise or reverse nailfold capillary structural change. This second question might be especially pertinent in patients with early limited cutaneous disease, including patients with VEDOSS (very early diagnosis of SSc) in whom microvascular change might be more likely to be reversible than in patients with more established disease. These two questions will be discussed in turn because both have been addressed in a small number of studies which demonstrate the potential of nailfold capillaroscopy as a biomarker and also some of the challenges and potential pitfalls. The increasing interest in nailfold capillaroscopy as a biomarker is demonstrated by nailfold capillary density being chosen as the primary outcome measure in a randomised placebo-controlled trial of intravenous methylprednisolone in very early SSc [70]. No change in capillary density was observed at 12 weeks in either treatment group [71].

Nailfold Capillary Changes in Response to Autologous Haematopoietic Stem Cell Transplantation in Patients with SSc

If immunosuppression favourably influences the abnormal nailfold capillaries in patients with SSc, then this is likely to be seen with haematopoietic stem cell transplantation (HSCT), an intense immununosuppressive procedure which tends to be

Table 3 Some of the studies (in chronological order) examining nailfold capillaroscopic change in response to drug treatment in patients with SSc

Reference	Treatment (including duration of treatment)	Study design	Number of subjects	Nailfold capillaroscopy method	Main nailfold parameters evaluated	Key findings/ conclusions
Moore et al. 2007 [77]	Bosentan. 6 months	Open-label	18	Videocapillaroscopy. Magnification 300x. Non-dominant ring finger	Capillary density, total capillary width, arterial diameter, venous diameter, apical diameter	No changes in any of these quantitative parameters after 6 months' treatment
Aschwanden et al. 2008 [72]	Autologous HSCT. Patient with SSc re-examined after 5 months	Observational	2 (one had mixed connective tissue disease)	'A relatively large field of view'. Serial images included for one finger.	Visual assessment of pattern.	Substantial improvement in appearances (to almost normal in the patient with SSc)
Miniati et al. 2009 [74]	HSCT (6 patients) or cyclophosphamide (10 patients). Cyclophosphamide given for 1 year.	Observational	16 (all had a 'late' scleroderma pattern on nailfold capillaroscopy)	Videocapillaroscopy. Magnification 200x or 100x. 10 fingers Capillaroscopy pre-treatment, then 3 months, then 6 monthly post-treatment	Pattern + semiquantiative grading	Pattern changed from 'late' to 'active' in the 6 patients treated with HSCT within 3 months. In the 6 patients treated with HSCT, the number of enlarged/ giant capillaries increased, and capillary loss reduced (i.e. number of capillaries increased).

Shah et al. 2011 [78]	IV iloprost (5 days' treatment)	Observational	10	Videocapillaroscopy. Magnification 300x. Non-dominant ring finger	Capillary density, total capillary width, apical width. Assessments pre-treatment, then 3 days, 5 days and 12 months post-treatment	Trend for capillary density to increase immediately post-treatment and for apical width to decrease at 12 months.
Cutolo et al. 2013 [79]	IV iloprost with or without addition of bosentan. 3 year follow-up	Observational	30 (15 of whom received bosentan)	Videocapillaroscopy. Magnification 200x. 8 fingers	Scleroderma pattern. Semi-quantitative scoring including of number of capillaries, giant capillaries, microhaemorrhages, ramifications, disorganisation	Capillary loss reduced (i.e. number of capillaries increased) in patients receiving bosentan.
Trombetta et al. 2016 [80]	IV iloprost with or without addition of bosentan (prescribed for PAH or for digital ulcers). 4 year follow-up.	Observational	30 (15 of whom received bosentan)	Videocapillaroscopy. Magnification 200x. 8 fingers (Four 1mm fields per finger)	Capillary density (number of capillaries/mm)	Capillary density increased significantly after 4 years in patients receiving bosentan.

(continued)

Table 3 (continued)

Reference	Treatment (including duration of treatment)	Study design	Number of subjects	Nailfold capillaroscopy method	Main nailfold parameters evaluated	Key findings/ conclusions
Santana-Goncalves et al. 2022 [73]	Autologous HSCT	Retrospective study	27	Stereomicroscope. Magnification10X to 40X 8 fingers. Capillaroscopy performed before HSCT, and after 6 and 12 months.	Included capillary density/mm and number of giant capillaries	Capillary density increased at 12 months, and number of giant capillaries reduced.
Kersten et al. 2025 [71]	IV methylprednisolone vs placebo. 12 weeks	RCT (in patients with very early SSc)	30	Videocapillaroscopy. Magnification 200x. 8 fingers (two images per finger)	Capillary density was the primary endpoint.	No changes in capillary density or number of megacapillaries/mm in either treatment group.

IV Intravenous; *HSCT* Haematopoietic stem cell transplantation, *PAH* Pulmonary arterial hypertension, *RCT* Randomised controlled trial, *SSc* Systemic sclerosis reserved for highly selected patients usually with early diffuse cutaneous SSc. There have been several reports of regression of nailfold capillaroscopic abnormality following HSCT (Table 3). The report by Aschwanden et al. [72] showed striking improvement in appearances following HSCT in a patient with early diffuse cutaneous SSc as well as in a patient with mixed connective tissue disease. Changes were convincing because a large section of the nailfold was visualised, and so there was no doubt from visual inspection of the images that microvascular remodelling had occurred, and similarly in the example illustrated in the report by Santana-Goncalves et al. [73] when a widefield view of the same finger was shown before and after treatment, demonstrating improvement after HSCT. This is the advantage of the widefield view (of which Maricq was a proponent as discussed in chapter "History of Nailfold Capillaroscopy"): the whole nailfold can be seen at a glance, and the clinician can be confident of seeing all the capillaries. Conversely in the report by Miniati et al. [74] when example images are of single high magnification frames, there would be concern that the same area of the nailfold might not always have been captured. Miniati et al. reported that in 6 patients treated with HSCT, a 'late' scleroderma pattern converted to 'early' within 3 months of treatment. Nailfold capillaroscopic pattern is a secondary outcome measure in the multicentre UPSIDE study in patients with early diffuse cutaneous SSc [75]: the results of this study are awaited with interest because this study, in which 120 patients with early diffuse cutaneous SSc will be randomised to receive either HSCT or cyclophosphamide followed by mycophenolate mofetil, will provide the opportunity to examine nailfold capillaries sequentially over time in a much larger number of patients than in previous studies.

The message from the studies up until now examining nailfold capillary changes in response to HSCT is that the microvasculature can be remodelled in SSc, at least in patients with early diffuse cutaneous SSc. Some of the serial images shown as exemplars [72, 73] are very convincing. This is potentially very exciting. The challenge now is to quantify this change in future studies, because precise quantification of abnormality might allow detection (and measurement) of improvement in response to less intense immunosuppressant regimes as has been suggested to occur, for example, in response to mycophenolate mofetil [76].

Nailfold Capillary Changes in Response to Drugs Which Have Vascular Remodelling Potential in Patients with SSc

Several drugs used in the treatment of SSc-related digital vasculopathy and PAH have vascular modelling potential. A small number of studies have looked for nailfold capillary change in response to the endothelin-1 receptor antagonist bosentan, and to intravenous iloprost (Table 3) [77–80], as reviewed by Lemmers et al. [81]. As examples, in a study of 18 patients with SSc treated with bosentan for 6 months [77], there was no change in any of the quantitative parameters assessed in a single nailfold. However, this was an uncontrolled study, all patients had well-established disease, and the duration of treatment was short. In two studies from Genoa [79, 80], bosentan in combination with iloprost, but not iloprost alone, led to reduced capillary loss/increased capillary density after 3–4 years. Patient numbers were small (15 patients treated with bosentan in each study) but the promising signal suggests the need for further research. In the study by Trombetta et al. [80], capillary density was calculated from four 1 mm images from each of 8 fingers (32 images), thus capturing much of the nailfold in each finger and so especially likely to be a 'true' result. If nailfold capillaroscopy can provide evidence for microvascular remodelling, always bearing in mind that this may be disease-stage dependent, then this paves the way to use nailfold capillaroscopy as a biomarker not only in treatment studies of vasoactive therapy but also in studies of early prevention, for example in patients with VEDOSS.

In summary, several studies have provided evidence to suggest that nailfold capillaries can change in response to treatment not only in dermatomyositis but also in SSc. Better, more effective treatments for both of these rare diseases are badly needed. Nailfold capillaroscopy has potential as a biomarker in studies not only of immunosuppression (in dermatomyositis and early diffuse cutaneous SSc) but also of vasoactive therapies. However, care must be paid to study design, ensuring (as discussed earlier in this chapter) that (a) image acquisition allows comparison between the same sections of the nailfold at each visit (ideally capturing most of the nailfold) and (b) image interpretation includes quantitative measures on a continuous scale, because these are most likely to be precise and sensitive to change (c) factors influencing interpretation of capillary density e.g. skin tone are taken into account.

Future Directions and Technologies

To validate capillaroscopy as a biomarker/surrogate endpoint will require a number of different steps, including demonstrating that parameters of interest (for example capillary density) are sensitive to change and are able to detect treatment effect. Capillaroscopy also needs to be feasible in the clinical trial setting.

This section will focus on development of technologies which are likely to facilitate acquisition and interpretation of capillaroscopy data/measurements which are objective, reliable and sensitive to change, as well as feasible.

In terms of future technologies to improve nailfold capillaroscopy as a biomarker, there are several likely advances which we shall divide into advances in image acquisition, and advances in image interpretation.

Acquisition

The advent of low-cost devices is likely move capillaroscopy beyond specialist/tertiary referral centres to general rheumatology clinics, particularly alongside bespoke capture software. This will make longitudinal measurements more feasible in multicentre clinical trials. It is even possible that in the future patient self-imaging, with devices that connect to mobile phones, may be possible outside of the laboratory or hospital (with training).

As discussed in chapter "Research Methods: Functional Measures of Nailfold Capillaroscopy Including Permeability, Perfusion and Oxygenation", assessment of capillary function, including permeability, perfusion and oxygenation, potentially adds sensitivity to detecting subtle changes in capillaries. These functional measures are likely to change over much shorter periods of time (minutes-hours) than structural measures. They thus increase the possibilities for capillaroscopy as a biomarker to measure change in response to treatment. Technological developments such as cameras capable of faster frame rates, over a widefield area will enable whole nailfold imaging at high resolution, facilitating practical, functional measures of capillary flow and oxygenation. Work is also ongoing to develop methods of acquiring images that improve evaluability, including in improving imaging in darker skin tones. This may involve moving to other wavelengths (colours) of light, including near infrared light which can penetrate through the melanin in the skin; however. it remains to be seen as to whether these wavelengths provide enough contrast between the capillaries and their surrounding tissue and whether this will be a useful tool. Imaging with infrared light has been shown to be useful to visualise larger vessels in the skin (e.g. for intravenous access) [82] but requires further validation in relation to capillaries at the nailfold.

Interpretation

The main future technology to aid interpretation, is already in development; the use of 'Artificial intelligence' (AI). Advances in this field are very likely to improve the chances of development of reliable, sensitive to change nailfold capillaroscopic surrogate endpoints. Although AI is discussed in chapter "Quantitative Analysis", we shall also describe some recent advances here, as these give pointers to future developments.

The increasing role of computer vison and machine learning potentially offers an excellent opportunity to improve on objective measures, given that capillaries tend to be well defined within images; however, even here there are complexities both in the data used to train algorithms and then how best to interpret and categorise these, particularly in 'borderline' cases where even expert clinicians may struggle to categorise capillary patterns.

Computer vision, machine learning, deep learning (under the umbrella term of artificial intelligence or AI) have all been used in several studies of nailfold capillaroscopy and are of importance for capillaroscopy as a biomarker as they remove observer variability. The distinct patterns and generally good contrast between capillaries and surrounding tissue lend themselves well to edge finding and pattern recognition algorithms. Thus, automatic measurement of capillary number (density), width and shape become an objective measure, removing much of the inter and intra-observer variability. Objective measurement and categorisation become within reach. Caution must be taken, however, as algorithms are only as good as their training data, which need to be based on a large number of images, representing good examples over a range of health and disease. Quality assurance of results is essential to ensure that automated interpretation fits with expectation (e.g. assessment of capillaries being identified and widths and densities being measured).

The AUTOCAPI system [83] is an automated system to assess capillary density (capillary number) within a defined area of the nailfold image. Software was developed using 150 images for testing and 80 for training from patients with SSc, and primary RP and healthy controls. Manual versus automated measurements were compared in a boxed region, 1 mm wide. ICCs for manual versus automated capillary number for four observers varied between 0.88–0.94 for SSc images, 0.62–0.85 for primary RP and 0.56–0.91 for controls. Subsequent to this, the CAPI-score algorithm for automated measurement of density and capillary shape was developed using nearly 22,000 images from patients with primary RP and SSc (with input from nine observers) [28, 84, 85]. The algorithm, utilising the EULAR 'Smith fast track algorithm', (discussed above) as a starting point [27] enables differentiation between normal, non-specific, and SSc 'early', 'active' and 'late' patterns. Differentiation of non SSc vs SSc had an accuracy of 0.88 and normal vs non-specific 0.73. A follow-on study [86] used images categorised into SSc patterns by consensus to train a machine learning algorithm. The model achieved accuracy of 0.91 in differentiating non-SSc and SSc patterns.

A EUSTAR collaboration using deep learning analysed over 17, 000 images from 234 patients with SSc and 55 with VEDOSS. The study based its algorithm on the Smith fast track algorithm, and assessed width, density and microhaemorrhages [87]. Automation performed well, the area under the Receiver Operating Curve (ROC, sensitivity plotted against 1-specificity) was 85.8–93.5% differentiating 'early', 'active' or' late' patterns. Comparing a subset of images for automated versus expert manual assessment, agreement was high (72–91%).

In parallel, another study used deep learning software that was trained with 111 images from a high-resolution system [88]. Testing of the algorithm was on high-resolution images from 132 participants and low-cost microscope images from 66 participants. Participants were split approximately 50:50 SSc: primary RP or healthy control. Quantitative measures of density, width and shape were extracted from images. Differentiating the SSc data from that of primary RP/controls, the area under the ROC curve was 91% for high-resolution images, 89% for the low cost system images. The sensitivity and specificity for expert observers was 82% and 73% respectively. The deep learning automation was shown to be as good as expert assessment and low-cost microscopes were demonstrated to provide high enough quality images, with software processing these to a high specificity and sensitivity.

Ozturk et al. [89] assessed the difference between both supervised (trained and tested with manual input of image assessment for training) machine learning and then unsupervised deep learning on images from a cohort of patients with SSc. The study followed on from previous reliability work [51, 52]. Deep learning exceeded the accuracy of machine learning with an accuracy >0.87 to differentiate between SSc and no SSc (healthy controls and primary RP).

Unsupervised machine learning has also been used to compare images from 76 patients with dermatomyositis, 26 with anti-synthetase syndrome and 33 with SSc [90]. Patients were categorised into 2 clusters using hierarchical clustering analysis, identifying significant differences in the incidence of ILD. The study provides further evidence towards nailfold capillary changes being associated with systemic disease.

These studies together demonstrate the capability of AI to differentiate between different capillaroscopic patterns. It therefore seems a reasonable assumption that AI methods may also hold promise for quantifying capillaroscopic change over time (i.e. provide a monitoring/response biomarker). If future research proves this to be the case, then this would be a major advance for several reasons First, automated measurement saves time (manual measurement is very time-consuming) and so image interpretation becomes feasible in the clinical trial setting. Second, automated measurement is objective. Third, it allows for standardisation across multiple centres. And the fact that AI methods can be applied in low-cost systems is an important development because this makes image collection feasible in multicentre trials. This is especially relevant because studies in patients with SSc and dermatomyositis, the diseases for which nailfold capillaroscopy is most likely to be useful as a biomarker, are often multicentre due to the rarity of both diseases.

In validating capillaroscopy as a monitoring/response biomarker, an important next step will be to apply automated measures in a variety of different longitudinal studies, examining sensitivity to change and correlating capillaroscopic changes with other measures of disease status.

Expert Opinion Statement on Future Directions

Future technologies will enable capillaroscopy to be more readily available to a wider range of interested parties, including for clinical trials. Improved imaging technology will allow improved evaluability (including in darker skin tones) and incorporation of functional measures (flow, oxygenation). Machine and deep learning will, along with international collaboration (facilitating access to large image banks and expert observers), remove much of the subjectivity in interpretation and provide automated longitudinal measurements for use in clinical trials.

Conclusions and Expert Opinion

Nailfold capillaroscopy has the potential for providing one or more biomarkers for monitoring of SSc and dermatomyositis, and related diseases, in both clinical practice and in clinical research. Future biomarkers could be measures of capillary structure, and also of capillary function such as blood flow although functional measures require considerably more refinement than structural measures before they can be considered ready for validation studies. Biomarkers have to be measurable, and reliable, and there are challenges to be overcome such as optimising capillary density measurement and assessing capillaries in different skin tones. However, progress is being made. Advances in technologies which allow image acquisition at relatively low cost, alongside AI methods which allow automated interpretation of images avoiding human subjectivity, are paving the way for feasible capillaroscopy-based biomarkers. A next step will be to validate these in longitudinal, and multi-centre studies, including in clinical trials.

References

1. Califf RM. Biomarker definitions and their applications. Exp Biol Med. 2018;243(3):213–21.
2. FDA-NIH Biomarker Working Group. BEST (biomarkers, EndpointS, and other tools) resource [internet]. Silver Spring (MD): Food and Drug Administration (US); 2016. Available from: https://www.ncbi.nlm.nih.gov/books/NBK326791/ Co-published by National Institutes of Health (US), Bethesda (MD)
3. Cutolo M, Smith V. State of the art on nailfold capillaroscopy: a reliable diagnostic tool and putative biomarker in rheumatology? Rheumatology. 2013;52:1933–40.
4. Hsu PC, Liao PY, Huang SW, Chang HH, Chiang JY, Lo LC. Nailfold capillary abnormalities as indicators of diabetic nephropathy progression: a cross-sectional study in type 2 diabetes. Ann Med. 2025;57:2458766.
5. Kurowski JA, Patel SR, Wechsler JB, et al. Nailfold capillaroscopy as a biomarker in the evaluation of pediatric inflammatory bowel disease. Crohn's Colitis. 2021;360(3):1–5.
6. Valim V, Assis LS, Simoes MF, Trevisani VF, Pucinelli ML, Andrade LE. Correlation between serum E-selectin levels and panoramic nailfold capillaroscopy in systemic sclerosis. Braz J Med Biol Res. 2004;37:1423–7.
7. Sulli A, Soldano S, Pizzorni C, et al. Raynaud's phenomenon and plasma endothelin: correlations with capillaroscopic patterns in systemic sclerosis. J Rheumatol. 2009;36:1235–9.
8. Kim HS, Park MK, Kim HY, Park SH. Capillary dimension measured by computer-based digitalized image correlated with plasma endothelin-1 levels in patients with systemic sclerosis. Clin Rheumatol. 2010;29:247–54.
9. Avouac J, Vallucci M, Smith V, et al. Correlations between angiogenic factors and capillaroscopic patterns in systemic sclerosis. Arthritis Res Ther. 2013;15:R55.
10. Di Martino ML, Frau A, Losa F, et al. Role of circulating endothelial cells in assessing the severity of systemic sclerosis and predicting its clinical worsening. Sci Rep. 2021;11:2681.
11. Papadopoulou C, Hong Y, Krol P, et al. The vasculopathy of juvenile dermatomyositis: endothelial injury, hypercoagulability, and increased arterial stiffness. Arthritis Rheumatol. 2021;73:1253–66.
12. Tang M, Shi J, Pang Y, et al. Nailfold videocapillaroscopy findings are associated with IIM subtypes and IFN activation. Arthritis Res Therapy. 2025;27:62.
13. Kuryliszyn-Moskal A, Ciolkiewicz M, Klimiuk PA, Sierakowski S. Clinical significance of nailfold capillaroscopy in systemic lupus erythematosus: correlation with endothelial cell activation markers and disease activity. Scand J Rheumatol. 2009;38:38–45.
14. Bergkamp SC, Bergkamp ND, Wahadat MJ, et al. Learning from serum markers reflecting endothelial activation: longitudinal data in childhood-onset systemic lupus erythematosus. Lupus Sci Med. 2024;11:e001190.
15. Hofstee HM, Vonk Noordegraaf A, Voskuyl AE, et al. Nailfold capillary density is associated with the presence and severity of pulmonary arterial hypertension in systemic sclerosis. Ann Rheum Dis. 2009;68:191–5.
16. Lemmers JM, van Caam AP, Kersten B, et al. Nailfold capillaroscopy and candidate-biomarker levels in systemic sclerosis-associated pulmonary hypertension: a cross-sectional study. J Scleroderma Relat Disord. 2023;8:221–30.
17. Smith V, Vanhaecke A, Vandecasteele E, et al. Nailfold videocapillaroscopy in systemic sclerosis–related pulmonary arterial hypertension: a systematic literature review. J Rheumatol. 2020;47:888–95.

18. Arvanitaki A, Giannakoulas G, Triantafyllidou E, et al. Nailfold videocapillaroscopy: a novel possible surrogate marker for the evaluation of peripheral microangiopathy in pulmonary arterial hypertension. Scand J Rheumatol. 2021;50:85–94.
19. Hurabielle C, Avouac J, Lepri G, de Risi T, Kahan A, Allanore Y. Skin telangiectasia and the identification of a subset of systemic sclerosis patients with severe vascular disease. Arthritis Care Res. 2016;68:1021–7.
20. Dogan S, Akdogan A, Atakan N. Nailfold capillaroscopy in systemic sclerosis: is there any difference between videocapillaroscopy and dermatoscopy? Skin Res Technol. 2013;19:446–9.
21. Mazzotti NG, Bredemeier M, Brenol CV, Xavier RM, Cestari TF. Assessment of nailfold capillaroscopy in systemic sclerosis by different optical magnification methods. Clin Exp Dermatol. 2014;39:135–41.
22. Hughes M, Moore T, O'Leary N, et al. A study comparing videocapillaroscopy and dermoscopy in the assessment of nailfold capillaries in patients with systemic sclerosis-spectrum disorders. Rheumatology. 2015;54:1435–42.
23. Dinsdale G, Peytrignet S, Moore T, et al. The assessment of nailfold capillaries: comparison of dermoscopy and nailfold videocapillaroscopy. Rheumatology. 2018;57:1115–6.
24. Berks M, Dinsdale G, Marjanovic E, Murray A, Taylor C, Herrick AL. Comparison between low cost USB nailfold capillaroscopy and videocapillaroscopy: a pilot study. Rheumatology. 2021;60:3862–7.
25. Dinsdale G, Roberts C, Moore T, et al. Nailfold capillaroscopy-how many fingers should be examined to detect abnormality? Rheumatology. 2019;58:284–8.
26. Dinsdale G, Moore T, O'Leary N, Tresadern P, Berks M, Roberts C, et al. Intra-and interobserver reliability of nailfold videocapillaroscopy—a possible outcome measure for systemic sclerosis-related microangiopathy. Microvasc Res. 2017;112:1–6.
27. Smith V, Vanhaecke A, Herrick AL, et al. EULAR study group on microcirculation in rheumatic diseases. Fast track algorithm: how to differentiate a "scleroderma pattern" from a "nonscleroderma pattern". Autoimmun Rev. 2019;18:102394.
28. Gracia Tello BDC, Sáez Comet L, Lledó G, et al. Capi-score: a quantitative algorithm for identifying disease patterns in nailfold videocapillaroscopy. Rheumatology. 2024;63:3315–21.
29. Emrani Z, Karbalaie A, Fatemi A, Etehadtavakol M, Erlandsson BE. Capillary density: an important parameter in nailfold capillaroscopy. Microvasc Res. 2017;109:7–18.
30. Hofstee HM, Serné EH, Roberts C, et al. A multicentre study on the reliability of qualitative and quantitative nail-fold videocapillaroscopy assessment. Rheumatology. 2012;51:749–55.
31. Wildt M, Wuttge DM, Hesselstrand R, Scheja A. Assessment of capillary density in systemic sclerosis with three different capillaroscopic methods. Clin Exp Rheumatol. 2012;30:S50–4.
32. Herrick AL, Moore T, Hollis S, Jayson MI. The influence of age on nailfold capillary dimensions in childhood. J Rheumatol. 2000;27:797–800.
33. Bergkamp SC, Smith V, Kuijpers TW, Cutolo M, van den Berg JM, Schonenberg-Meinema D. Correlations between capillary density and degree of skin pigmentation in healthy children analysed by nailfold video capillaroscopy. Quant Imaging Med Surg. 2023;13:3938–47.
34. Terreri MT, Andrade LE, Puccinelli ML, Hilário MO, Goldenberg J. Nail fold capillaroscopy: normal findings in children and adolescents. Semin Arthritis Rheum. 1999;29:36–42.
35. Andrade LE, Gabriel Júnior A, Assad RL, Ferrari AJ, Atra E. Panoramic nailfold capillaroscopy: a new reading method and normal range. Semin Arthritis Rheum. 1990;20:21–31.
36. Fitzpatrick TB. The validity and practicability of sun-reactive skin types I through VI. Arch Dermatol. 1988;124:869–71.
37. Bairwa D, Kavadichanda CG, Dunga S, Mathew A, Aishwarya G, Gayathri MS, et al. Effect of skin phototype on quantitative nailfold capillaroscopy. J Scleroderma Relat Disord. 2022;7:197–203.
38. Ahmad S, Pai VV, Sharath A, Ghodge R, Shukla P. Qualitative analysis of nailfold capillaries in diabetes and diabetic retinopathy using dermatoscope in patients with coloured skin. Indian J Dermatol Venereol Leprol. 2023;1:1–8.

39. Bhakuni DS, Vasdev V, Garg MK, Narayanan K, Jain R, Mullick G. Nailfold capillaroscopy by digital microscope in an Indian population with systemic sclerosis. Int J Rheum Dis. 2012;15:95–101.
40. Melsens K, Cutolo M, Schonenberg-Meinema D, Foeldvari I, Leone MC, et al. EULAR study group on microcirculation in rheumatic diseases. Standardized nailfold capillaroscopy in children with rheumatic diseases: a worldwide study. Rheumatology. 2023;62:1605–15.
41. Ezeofor AJ, O'Connell KA, Cobos GA, Vleugels RA, LaChance AH, Nambudiri VE. Distinctive cutaneous features of dermatomyositis in black adults: a case series. JAAD Case Rep. 2023;37:106–9.
42. Torres-Ruiz J, Pinal-Fernandez I, Selva-O'Callaghan A, Campbell B, Muñoz-Braceras S, Mejía-Domínguez NR, et al. Nailfold capillaroscopy findings of a multicentric multiethnic cohort of patients with idiopathic inflammatory myopathies. Clin Exp Rheumatol. 2024;42:367–76.
43. Murray AK, Vail A, Moore TL, Manning JB, Taylor CJ, Herrick AL. The influence of measurement location on reliability of quantitative nailfold videocapillaroscopy in patients with SSc. Rheumatology. 2012;51:1323–30.
44. Dinsdale G, Moore T, O'Leary N, Berks M, Roberts C, Manning J, et al. Quantitative outcome measures for systemic sclerosis-related microangiopathy—reliability of image acquisition in nailfold capillaroscopy. Microvasc Res. 2017;113:56–9.
45. Anderson ME, Allen PD, Moore T, Hillier V, Taylor CJ, Herrick AL. Computerized nailfold video capillaroscopy—a new tool for assessment of Raynaud's phenomenon. J Rheumatol. 2005;32:841–8.
46. Smith V, Pizzorni C, De Keyser F, et al. Reliability of the qualitative and semiquantitative nailfold videocapillaroscopy assessment in a systemic sclerosis cohort: a two-centre study. Ann Rheum Dis. 2010;69:1092–6.
47. Hudson M, Masetto A, Steele R, Arthurs E, Baron M, Canadian Scleroderma Research Group. Reliability of widefield capillary microscopy to measure nailfold capillary density in systemic sclerosis. Clin Exp Rheumatol. 2010;28:S36–41.
48. Smith V, Beeckman S, Herrick AL, Decuman S, Deschepper E, De Keyser F, et al. EULAR study group on microcirculation. An EULAR study group pilot study on reliability of simple capillaroscopic definitions to describe capillary morphology in rheumatic diseases. Rheumatology. 2016;55:883–90.
49. Cutolo M, Melsens K, Herrick AL, Foeldvari I, Deschepper E, De Keyser F, et al. EULAR study group on microcirculation in rheumatic diseases. Reliability of simple capillaroscopic definitions in describing capillary morphology in rheumatic diseases. Rheumatology. 2018;57:757–9.
50. Guillén-Del-Castillo A, Simeón-Aznar CP, Callejas-Moraga EL, Tolosa-Vilella C, Alonso-Vila S, Fonollosa-Pla V, Selva-O'Callaghan A. Quantitative videocapillaroscopy correlates with functional respiratory parameters: a clue for vasculopathy as a pathogenic mechanism for lung injury in systemic sclerosis. Arthritis Res Ther. 2018;20:281.
51. Boulon C, Blaise S, Lazareth I, et al. Reproducibility of the scleroderma pattern assessed by wide-field capillaroscopy in subjects suffering from Raynaud's phenomenon. Rheumatology. 2017;56:1780–3.
52. Boulon C, Devos S, Mangin M, et al. Reproducibility of capillaroscopic classifications of systemic sclerosis: results from the SCLEROCAP study. Rheumatology. 2017;56:1713–20.
53. Sekiyama JY, Camargo CZ, Eduardo L, Andrade C, Kayser C. Reliability of widefield nailfold capillaroscopy and video capillaroscopy in the assessment of patients with Raynaud's phenomenon. Arthritis Care Res. 2013;65:1853–61.
54. Ma Z, Mulder DJ, Gniadecki R, Cohen Tervaert JW, Osman M. Methods of assessing nailfold capillaroscopy compared to video capillaroscopy in patients with systemic sclerosis-a critical review of the literature. Diagnostics. 2023;13:2204.
55. Silver RM, Maricq HR. Childhood dermatomyositis: serial microvascular studies. Pediatrics. 1989;83:278.

56. Eden M, Wilkinson S, Murray A, et al. Nailfold capillaroscopy: a survey of current UK practice and 'next steps' to increase uptake among rheumatologists. Rheumatology. 2023;62:335–40.
57. Anderson C, Leone V, Pain C. Comment on: Nailfold capillaroscopy: a survey of current UK practice and 'next steps' to increase uptake among rheumatologists. Rheumatology. 2023;62:e303–4.
58. De Angelis R, Cutolo M, Gutierrez M, Bertolazzi C, Salaffi F, Grassi W. Different microvascular involvement in dermatomyositis and systemic sclerosis. A preliminary study by a tight videocapillaroscopic assessment. Clin Exp Rheumatol. 2012;30(Suppl 71):S67–70.
59. Dinsdale G, van Roon AM, Murray A, Taylor C, Herrick AL. Longitudinal nailfold capillaroscopy tracking of microangiopathic changes in systemic sclerosis. Rheumatology. 2018;57(9):1554.
60. Kubo S, Todoroki Y, Nakayamada S, et al. Significance of nailfold videocapillaroscopy in patients with idiopathic inflammatory myopathies. Rheumatology. 2019;58:120–30.
61. Bellando-Randone S, Del Galdo F, Lepri G, et al. Progression of patients with Raynaud's phenomenon to systemic sclerosis: a five-year analysis of the European scleroderma trial and research group multicentre, longitudinal registry study for very early diagnosis of systemic sclerosis (VEDOSS). Lancet Rheumatol. 2021;3:e834–43.
62. Avouac J, Lepri G, Smith V, et al. Sequential nailfold videocapillaroscopy examinations have responsiveness to detect organ progression in systemic sclerosis. Sem Arthritis Rheum. 2017;47:86–94.
63. Medsger TA Jr, Silman AJ, Steen VD, et al. A disease severity scale for systemic sclerosis: development and testing. J Rheumatol. 1999;26:2159–67.
64. Sulli A, Paolino S, Pizzorni C, et al. Progression of nailfold capillaroscopic patterns and correlation with organ involvement in systemic sclerosis: a 12 year study. Rheumatology. 2020;59:1051–8.
65. Sulli A, Pizzorni C, Smith V, Zampogna G, Ravera F, Cutolo M. Timing of transition between capillaroscopic patterns in systemic sclerosis. Arthritis Rheum. 2012;64:821–5.
66. Velauthapillai A, de Vries-Bouwstra JK, Henes J, et al. Longitudinal association between nailfold capillaroscopy and incident interstitial lung disease: A EUSTAR database analysis. J Scleroderma Relat Disord. 2025; (online ahead of print)
67. Smith V, Herrick AL, Ingegnoli F, et al. EULAR study group on microcirculation in rheumatic diseases and the scleroderma clinical trials consortium group on Capillaroscopy. Standardisation of nailfold capillaroscopy for the assessment of patients with Raynaud's phenomenon and systemic sclerosis. Autoimmun Rev. 2020;19(3):102458.
68. Khojah A, Morgan G, Klein-Gitelman MS, Pchman LM. Juvenile dermatomyositis: association between nail fold capillary end row loop– area under the curve– and disease damage indicators. Pediatr Rheumatol. 2023;21:137.
69. Distler O, Highland KB, Gahlemann M, et al. Nintedanib for systemic sclerosis-associated interstitial lung disease. N Engl J Med. 2019;380:2518–28.
70. Van den Hombergh WMT, Kersten BE, Knaapen-Hans HKA, et al. Hit hard and early: analysing the effects of high-dose methylprednisolone on nailfold capillary changes and biomarkers in very early systemic sclerosis: study protocol for a 12-week randomised controlled trial. Trials. 2018;19:449.
71. Kersten BE, Lemmers JM, Vanhaecke A, et al. Efficacy of methylprednisolone in very early systemic sclerosis: results of the 'hit hard and early' randomized controlled trial. Rheumatology. 2025;64:1261–9.
72. Aschwanden M, Daikeler T, Jaeger KA, et al. Rapid improvement of nailfold capillaroscopy after intense immunosuppression for systemic sclerosis and mixed connective tissue disease. Ann Rheum Dis. 2008;67:1057–9.
73. Santana-Goncalves M, Zanin-Silva D, Henrique-Neto A, et al. Autologous hematopoietic stem cell transplantation modifies specific aspects of systemic sclerosis-related microvasculopathy. Therap Adv Musculoskel Dis. 2022;14:1–13.
74. Miniati I, Guiducci S, Conforti ML, et al. Autologous stem cell transplantation improves microcirculation in systemic sclerosis. Ann Rheum Dis. 2009;68:94–8.

75. Spierings J, van Rhenen A, Welsing PM, et al. A randomised, open-label trial to assess the optimal treatment strategy in early diffuse cutaneous systemic sclerosis: the UPSIDE study protocol. BMJ Open. 2021;11:e044483.
76. Wildt M, Andréasson K, Hamberg V, Hesselstrand R, Wuttge DM. Treatment with mycophenolate mofetil is associated with improved nailfold vasculature in systemic sclerosis. Rheumatology. 2024;63:385–91.
77. Moore TL, Vail A, Herrick AL. Assessment of digital vascular structure and function in response to bosentan in patients with systemic sclerosis-related Raynaud's phenomenon. Rheumatology. 2007;46:363–4.
78. Shah P, Murray AK, Moore TL, Herrick AL. Effects of iloprost on microvascular structure assessed by nailfold videocapillaroscopy: a pilot study. J Rheumatol. 2011;38:2079–80.
79. Cutolo M, Zampogna G, Vremis L, Smith V, Pizzorni C, Sulli A. Longterm effects of endothelin receptor antagonism on microvascular damage evaluated by nailfold capillaroscopic analysis in systemic sclerosis. J Rheumatol. 2013;40:40–5.
80. Trombetta AC, Pizzorni C, Ruaro B, et al. Effects of longterm treatment with bosentan and iloprost on nailfold absolute capillary number, fingertip blood perfusion, and clinical status in systemic sclerosis. J Rheumatol. 2016;43:2033–41.
81. Lemmers JMJ, Velauthapillai A, van Herwaarden N, Vonk MC. Change of the microvascularization in systemic sclerosis, a matter of air. Best Pract Res Clin Rheumatol. 2021;35:101683.
82. Cuper NJ, Klaessens JH, Jaspers JE, et al. The use of near-infrared light for safe and effective visualization of subsurface blood vessels to facilitate blood withdrawal in children. Med Eng Phys. 2013;35:433–40.
83. Cutolo M, Trombetta AC, Melsens K, et al. Automated assessment of absolute nailfold capillary number on videocapillaroscopic images: proof of principle and validation in systemic sclerosis. Microcirculation. 2018;25:e12447.
84. Gracia Tello B, Ramos Ibañez E, Fanlo Mateo P, et al. The challenge of comprehensive nailfold videocapillaroscopy practice: a further contribution. Clin Exp Rheumatol. 2022;40:1926–32.
85. Gracia Tello BC, Ramos Ibañez E, Saez Comet L, Guillén Del Castillo A, Simeón Aznar CP, Selva-O'Callaghan A, et al. External clinical validation of automated software to identify structural abnormalities and microhaemorrhages in nailfold videocapillaroscopy images. Clin Exp Rheumatol. 2023;41:1605–11.
86. Lledó-Ibáñez GM, Sáez Comet L, Freire Dapena M, Mesa Navas M, Martín Cascón M, Guillén Del Castillo A, et al. CAPI-detect: machine learning in capillaroscopy reveals new variables influencing diagnosis. Rheumatology. 2025;7:keaf073.
87. Garaiman A, Nooralahzadeh F, Mihai C, et al. Vision transformer assisting rheumatologists in screening for capillaroscopy changes in systemic sclerosis: an artificial intelligence model. Rheumatology. 2023;62:2492–500.
88. Bharathi PG, Berks M, Dinsdale G, et al. A deep learning system for quantitative assessment of microvascular abnormalities in nailfold capillary images. Rheumatology. 2023;62:2325–9.
89. Ozturk L, Laclau C, Boulon C, et al. Analysis of nailfold capillaroscopy images with artificial intelligence: data from literature and performance of machine learning and deep learning from images acquired in the SCLEROCAP study. Microvasc Res. 2025;157:104753.
90. Xu H, Qian J. The role of nailfold video-capillaroscopy in the assessment of dermatomyositis. Rheumatology. 2025;64:2987–94.

Using Nailfold Capillaroscopy in Combination with Other Non-invasive Imaging Techniques

Andrea Murray and Cristiane Kayser

Abbreviations

RP	Raynaud's phenomenon
SSc	Systemic sclerosis
LDF	Laser Doppler flowmetry
LDI	Laser Doppler imaging
LSCI	Laser speckle contrast imaging
LASCA	Laser speckle contrast analysis
NVC	Nailfold videocapillaroscopy
IR	Infrared
IRT	Infrared thermography
DU	Digital ulcer
PPG	Photoplethysmography
CDUS	Colour Doppler ultrasonography
PDUS	Doppler ultrasound
OCT	Optical coherence tomography

A. Murray (✉)
Centre for Musculoskeletal Research, Division of Musculoskeletal and Dermatological Sciences, The University of Manchester, Manchester Academic Health Science Centre, Manchester, UK

Northern Care Alliance NHS Foundation Trust, Salford, UK

National Institute for Health and Care Research (NIHR) Manchester Biomedical Research Centre, Manchester, UK
e-mail: andrea.murray@manchester.ac.uk

C. Kayser
Rheumatology Division, Escola Paulista de Medicina, Universidade Federal de São Paulo—UNIFESP, São Paulo, Brazil
e-mail: cristiane.kayser@unifesp.br

A. L. Herrick et al. (eds.), *Nailfold Capillaroscopy in Rheumatological Diseases*,
https://doi.org/10.1007/978-3-032-03970-5_12

OCTA	Optical coherence tomography angiography
MRI	Magnetic resonance imaging
MRA	Magnetic resonance angiography

Key Points

- There are many non-invasive imaging techniques that can add value to capillaroscopy
- Laser Doppler techniques and thermography measure skin blood flow and are relatively well validated; they can help to differentiate between healthy controls and patients with SSc and primary RP
- Laser Doppler techniques and thermography sometimes, but not always, show correlations between lower blood flow in the fingers and more severe nailfold capillaroscopy changes
- Studying Doppler ultrasound and/or magnetic resonance imaging in combination with nailfold capillaroscopy allows comparisons between microvascular and larger vessel disease.
- Other more novel techniques such as optical coherence tomography and photoacoustic imaging are now being applied to the study of rheumatological diseases, but these require further validation to translate to clinical benefit.

Introduction

Several non-invasive imaging techniques have been used alone or in combination with nailfold capillaroscopy to investigate the microvasculature of the skin in rheumatic diseases, particularly in patients with Raynaud's phenomenon (RP) and systemic sclerosis (SSc)-spectrum disorders. Most of them have the advantage of assessing other aspects of the peripheral microcirculation beyond the structural abnormalities evaluated by nailfold capillaroscopy, including perfusion, oxygenation and volume of microcirculation.

It is worth noting that techniques assessing microcirculation function are carried out in temperature-controlled laboratories to minimize the effects of environmental conditions on the outcomes. Dynamic challenges can also be used to enhance understanding of physiological differences, including between cohorts, e.g primary RP and SSc, or SSc and controls. These dynamic challenges include heating, cooling and post occlusive hyperaemia.

These techniques and challenges, in addition to nailfold capillaroscopy aid understanding of the relationships between microvascular structure and function or between microvascular structure and macrovascular structure and/or function; furthering knowledge of pathophysiology and disease mechanisms.

Techniques to Assess Perfusion

Laser Based Techniques

Laser Doppler techniques including laser Doppler flowmetry (LDF), laser Doppler imaging (LDI) and, more recently laser speckle contrast imaging (LSCI), and the very similar technique laser speckle contrast analysis (LASCA), are useful tools for the assessment of microvascular perfusion and cutaneous blood flow [1]. The principle of the laser Doppler techniques is based on the Doppler effect, in which changes in wavelength due to movement between red blood cells and the detector are used to determine the speed of blood flow [2]. Depending on the laser wavelength employed, the nutritional capillaries close to the skin surface and the underlying arterioles and venules deeper in the dermis can be assessed [3]. Most systems use red or infrared (IR) wavelengths with a penetration depth of approximately 1mm in the skin [4]. Measurements are described in arbitrary perfusion units. They can be used with dynamic tests of cold challenge, local heating, or occlusion to evaluate the responsiveness of blood flow in patients with primary or secondary RP (Fig. 1). Laser Doppler techniques are mostly used for clinical research, and they are useful for monitoring disease progression and treatment response in clinical trials in patients with primary or secondary RP [4, 5].

LDF, the first method described, provides continuous flow assessment of a single point or vessel. Due to the single-point assessment, a high variability between measurements has been described, given the inherent heterogeneity of the cutaneous microvasculature [6]. Moreover, only a small area can be measured, and most types of the equipment require skin contact, which can change blood flow/blanche skin if too much pressure is applied. LDI has the advantage of being non-invasive and providing tissue perfusion measurement over a wide area of the skin, thus providing more reproducible results [1]. However, LDI does not provide continuous, real-time flow assessment, as LDF, due to laser scanning. Finally, LSCI combines near-continuous flow assessment with a larger field of view by wide-field illumination and snapshot imaging [6] but is very sensitive to unintentional movements and has a limited imaging depth, thus limiting assessment to more superficial microvasculature [4]. LSCI/LASCA is based on the principle that when an object is illuminated by laser light, the backscattered light will form a so-called "speckle pattern" made of dark and bright areas. If there is no movement, this pattern is stationary, but when movement occurs, as in red blood cells within a tissue, the speckle pattern changes in intensity that is related to the blood flow. LSCI has a spatial resolution that is five-fold bigger than that of LASCA, but it has a poorer temporal resolution, and processing takes longer than LASCA [7]. A study comparing LASCA and LDF showed a significant correlation between both methods, but LASCA showed lower intra-operator variability than LDF and was considered less time-consuming and more accepted by the patients [8].

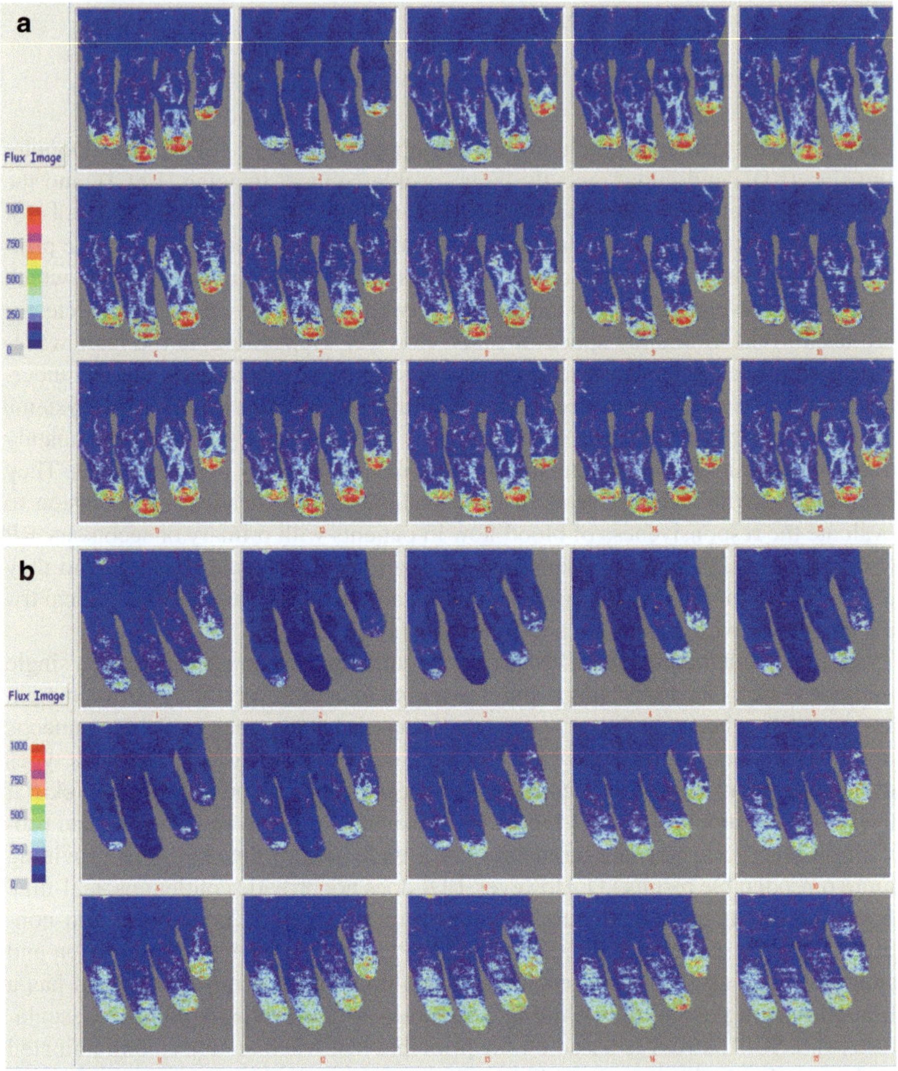

Fig. 1 Sequence of Laser Doppler Imaging (LDI) images (left to right, then top to bottom) of fingertip blood flow. First figure left at upper corner is at baseline, prior to cold challenge. Second image in the top row, immediately after cold stimulus. Image frames were taken 1 min apart for 15 min. (**a**) shows a healthy control and (**b**) a patient with systemic sclerosis (SSc). The top panel ((**a**), healthy control subject) shows increased flow at the distal digits as compared to the dorsum of the hand. Immediately after the cold challenge the overall perfusion decreases in the submerged area but then returns to baseline quickly. The lower panel ((**b**), patient with SSc) shows relatively lower flow at baseline (first frame) as compared to the control, both in the distal digits and dorsum. Return to baseline is slower than for the control post cold challenge and some digits can be seen to be more affected than others (asymmetric rewarming)

The associations between structural abnormalities of the microcirculation observed using nailfold capillaroscopy and the functional abnormalities measured using laser Doppler methods have been explored in some studies, with mixed results. Nonetheless, most of the studies have shown a correlation between the severity of microvascular damage seen by nailfold capillaroscopy and digital flow in patients with SSc that is characterized by morphological and functional vasculopathy even in the early stages of the disease [7].

In a study using LDF to assess perfusion in 34 patients with SSc, a negative correlation was observed between fingertip perfusion and the severity of microangiopathy on nailfold videocapillaroscopy (NVC) [9]. In another study by Rosato et al., in patients with SSc, the late SSc capillaroscopy pattern was associated with absence of skin flow recovery after cold stimulus assessed by LDI [10]. In less severe scleroderma capillaroscopy patterns, the mean perfusion returned to basal values after cold stimulus in patients with early capillaroscopy pattern and recovery was incomplete in patients with the active capillaroscopy pattern on NVC [10].

A study using LASCA, in 61 patients with SSc and 61 healthy subjects, revealed a negative correlation between peripheral perfusion and microangiopathy evolution score values assessed by NVC in patients with SSc [8]. The same authors evaluated the perfusion of 70 patients with SSc and 70 healthy subjects using LASCA [11] in selected skin areas of the hands (the dorsal and volar regions). Patients with SSc showed a significantly lower perfusion than healthy subjects at fingertips, periungual areas, and palm of the hands. The authors correlated LASCA with nailfold capillary damage scores by NVC in patients with SSc. A negative correlation between microangiopathy evolution score on NVC and perfusion values was identified, as well as between loss of capillaries and perfusion.

In contrast, in a cross-sectional study comparing nailfold capillary structure using NVC with LSCI in patients with SSc, primary RP, and healthy controls, no correlation was found between blood flow as measured by LSCI and any of the capillary structure measurements as measured by nailfold capillaroscopy [12]. In another study, a lower digital blood flow before and after cold stimulus by LDI was found in patients with SSc [13]. However, no correlation was found between mean finger blood flow and nailfold capillaroscopy parameters [13]. The authors suggest that LDI and NVC are complementary tools for the evaluation of different microangiopathy aspects in patients with SSc.

A study by Dinsdale et al, from 2020 [14], compared LDI with nailfold capillaroscopy and other methods including oxygenation (spectroscopy) and skin thickness measurements (high frequency ultrasound) in 265 subjects with primary RP, undifferentiated connective tissue disease, SSc and healthy controls. No significant correlation between capillary density (number/mm) and perfusion (distal-dorsum difference, a gradient between the finger and the dorsum of the hand) was found. Nonetheless, skin perfusion showed a significantly positive correlation with finger oxygenation ($r = 0.23$; $p < 0.001$), and capillary density showed a significantly negative correlation with skin thickness ($r = -0.26$; $p < 0.001$) in patients with SSc [14].

In addition, in a small study evaluating the correlation between nailfold capillaroscopy and LDI in patients with juvenile SSc, a positive correlation was found between morphological changes evaluated by the number of capillaries in nailfold capillaroscopy and finger blood flow measured by LDI with a marginal p-value, suggesting a possible association between peripheral microangiopathy and skin blood flow [15].

Few studies have evaluated nailfold capillaroscopy combined with laser Doppler in other rheumatic diseases beyond SSc. In patients with systemic lupus erythematosus, one study using LASCA showed significantly lower perfusion levels in different regions of the hands (fingertip, palm, and periungual) compared to healthy subjects [16]. Furthermore, a positive correlation was observed between perfusion and absolute nailfold capillary number as assessed by NVC, suggesting a correlation between functional and morphological microvascular impairment in patients with systemic lupus erythematosus.

Szabo et al., [17] evaluated capillary morphology by nailfold capillaroscopy and LDI in patients with Sjogren's syndrome and poly/dermatomyositis compared to primary RP and healthy individuals. The authors found a significantly decreased cutaneous perfusion in Sjogren's syndrome and patients with poly/dermatomyositis compared to the control group. As in SSc, patients with poly/dermatomyositis also had significantly decreased cutaneous perfusion compared to patients with primary RP. However, no difference was found between patients with Sjogren's syndrome and those with primary RP. Although nailfold capillaroscopy was performed in all patients, the correlations between nailfold capillaroscopy abnormalities and LDI were not described.

Several studies reported that laser Doppler techniques can help in the differentiation between primary RP and secondary RP present in patients with SSc [12, 18]. However, whether the combination of laser Doppler techniques with nailfold capillaroscopy improves the diagnostic accuracy of the identification of patients with SSc, including distinguishing patients with SSc from those with primary RP and from healthy controls, has not yet been confirmed [19]. The combination of LDI with NVC and thermography showed a better diagnostic accuracy, correctly differentiating patients with SSc, from those with primary RP and controls in 94% of cases, as opposed to 89% using NVC alone [12]. However, of all the techniques, NVC provided the best classification, and the combination of all three techniques improved classification and specificity but did not increase sensitivity. Thus far, when only a single microcirculatory tool is used, NVC seems to be the best discriminator between SSc patients, patients with primary RP, and healthy subjects.

Laser Doppler techniques have also been used to measure response to treatment for digital vasculopathy and RP [20] and to predict the occurrence of digital ulcers (DU) in patients with SSc. One study evaluated the prognostic value of skin perfusion as measured by LDI in predicting new DU occurrence in 58 patients with SSc. As shown in previous studies, the skin perfusion of hands was lower in patients with SSc compared to healthy controls, and skin perfusion decreased according to the severity of nailfold capillaroscopy abnormalities. Lower skin perfusion of hands was associated with the development of new DU, suggesting that LDI could be used in the identification of patients at high risk of developing DUs [21].

Thermography

Thermography utilizes a thermal (or IR) camera to passively image the body's heat (sometimes referred to as IR thermography or IRT) [22]. Heat emitted from the skin is an indirect measure of perfusion. Since IR radiation can penetrate into skin over a few millimeters, inversely, the detected IR radiation likely comes from deeper layers than skin alone, including superficial muscle perfusion. As a passive technique, it is relatively simple to use, eye safe and images in real time over a large area. The disadvantages are that as well as being an indirect measure it can have a blunted (slower) response to rapid changes in perfusion. Worth noting is the recent advent of low-cost (£100s rather than £10,000s), portable thermal cameras that either attach to mobile phones or come as phone-sized standalone devices. Handheld devices offer the possibility of ambulatory monitoring, outside of the laboratory. These devices are yet to be proven in terms of their robustness, being environmentally susceptible (due to the lack of insulation within the small footprint). As with laser Doppler techniques, most previous thermography research studies have been carried out in temperature-controlled rooms after acclimatization, and as such it remains to be seen how useful low-cost cameras will be outside of these criteria but they show great promise [23–27].

A recent review of thermography research studies in rheumatic diseases identified studies in RP, SSc, osteoarthritis, rheumatoid arthritis and juvenile localized scleroderma [28]. Traditionally, when studying patients with RP, thermography has been used alongside a cold challenge, a technique used in several UK clinics as part of the diagnosis process. Participants' (nitrile gloved) hands are placed into cold water for a short period of time (approx. 5–15 °C, 1–5 min, protocols vary) and then allowed to rewarm/recover at room temperature over a longer period (e.g. 15 min at 23 °C). Imaging is carried out both prior to and following the rewarming (Fig. 2). One challenge in comparing studies has been the differences in both the challenge itself and the outcome measures taken from the data [29]. At baseline the outcomes are usually finger temperature or the difference between the finger and hand dorsum skin temperature (since the hand dorsum temperature remains relatively normal, not being affected by the RP; sometimes called distal dorsal difference or finger gradient (Fig. 3)). Post cooling, outcomes include assessment of rewarming, such as maximum temperature reached, percentage recovery, gradient of initial rewarming or area under the rewarming curve [30].

Several studies compare nailfold capillaroscopy to thermography. Miziołek et al. [31] compared thermography (including average finger temperature at the nailfold) to semi quantitative capillary patterns and nailfold capillary density (as per the Capillaroscopic Skin Ulcers Risk Index [CSURI] [32]) in 19 patients with limited cutaneous SSc. There was moderate correlation between the temperature at the

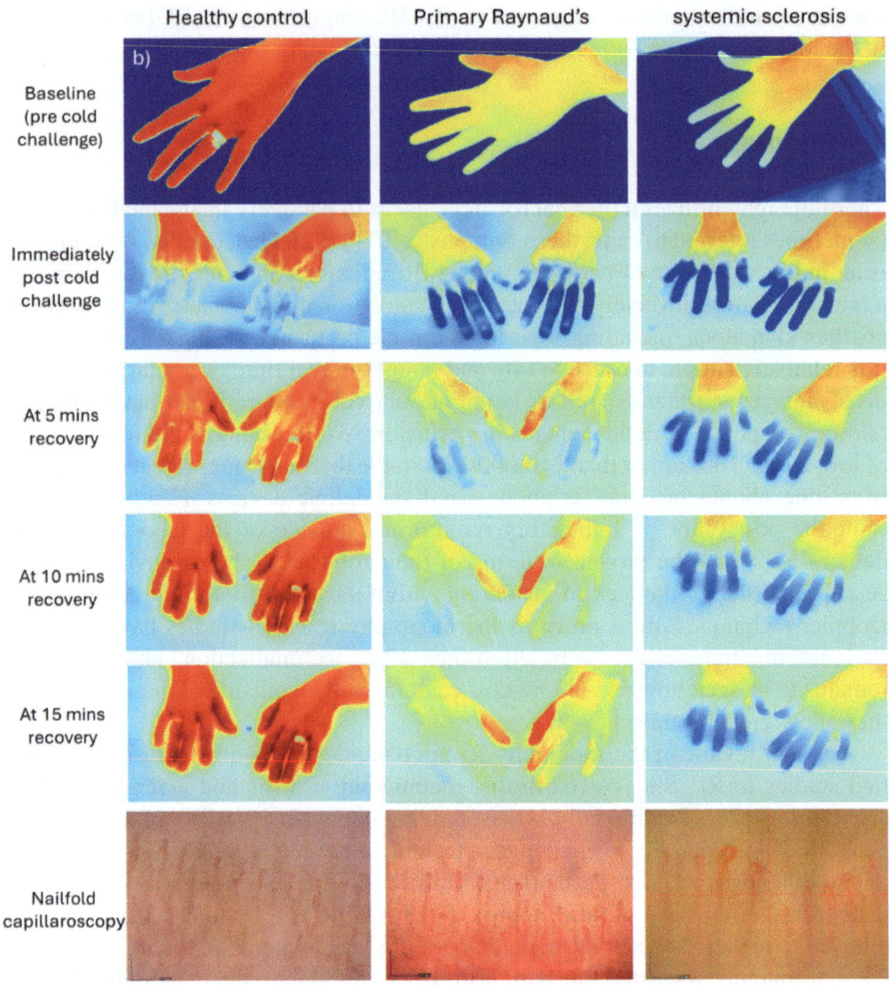

Fig. 2 False coloured thermal images and comparative nailfold capillaroscopy for a healthy control, patient with primary Raynaud's phenomenon a patient with systemic sclerosis. All thermal images are shown on the same temperature scale with red relatively warmer and blue relatively cooler temperatures. Scale bar on capillaroscopy images is 0.2 mm. (Courtesy of Graham Dinsdale and Joanne Manning)

finger nailfold and the number of capillaries per mm (R = 0.5). Finger nailfold skin temperature decreased from early, through active, to late pattern ($p < 0.001$).

Comparing thermal imaging to quantitative nailfold capillaroscopy in a study of 16 patents with SSc, 14 with primary RP and 16 healthy controls, Murray et al. [12] identified a negative correlation between capillary width and baseline finger skin temperature (i.e. as width increases, finger temperature decreases).

Secondary RP as assessed by thermography, has been shown to be associated with the development of DUs in SSc [33], although no nailfold capillaroscopy

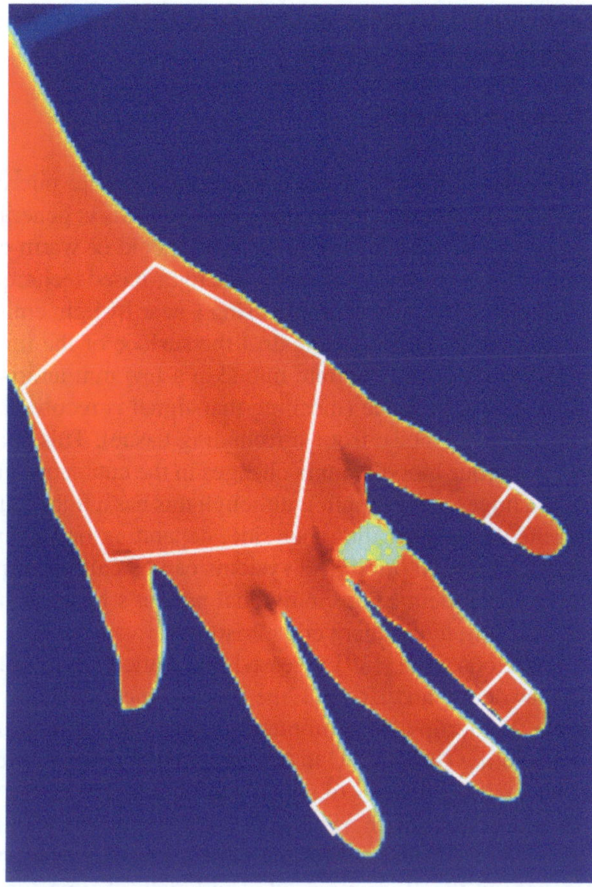

Fig. 3 False coloured thermal image showing the regions of interest for calculating a distal dorsal difference or finger gradient. Regions of interest in the digits are placed to avoid inclusion of the nail. In a healthy control distal temperature is higher than that at the dorsum, thus a distal dorsal difference is positive (distal -dorsal temperature). In a patient with Raynaud's phenomenon this tends to reverse. (Courtesy of Graham Dinsdale and Joanne Manning)

was included for comparison. Nolan et al. [34] compared thermography and nailfold capillaroscopy in 25 patients with SSc-related digital pitting to 25 patients without pitting. Whilst capillaroscopy was more abnormal in those with pitting, the thermal gradient along the finger was not significantly different between the cohorts.

A retrospective study of RP in patients with fibromyalgia [35] assessed 48 patients with primary RP and 18 with fibromyalgia and RP who had undergone clinical thermography with cold challenge (20 °C ±0.1 °C for 1 min with 10 min follow-up). In patients with fibromyalgia baseline finger temperatures were higher than those with primary RP and there was no significant finger temperature gradient. Post cooling, digit and dorsal temperatures were also higher for patients with fibromyalgia versus those with primary RP. Authors identified no significant decreased perfusion induced by cold challenge in patients with fibromyalgia, despite reported skin colour changes during Raynaud's episodes. The authors suggested that a different mechanism may be responsible for RP in fibromyalgia than in primary RP.

Techniques to Assess Microvascular and Macrovascular Volume and Structure

Plethysmography

Plethysmography is a technique used to measure microvascular volume and function [36]. In relation to rheumatic diseases this is generally for measuring perfusion dynamics and is often combined with a cold or warm challenge or occlusion (brachial or finger). Modern systems use light-based techniques known as photoplethysmography (PPG) (for example using a near IR light emitting diode and detector that sit adjacent to each other against the surface of the finger) [37, 38]. Near IR light (800-100 nm) can penetrate into skin a few mm and is preferentially absorbed by haemoglobin in tissue (meaning that signal is recorded from the vessels with little interference or noise from surrounding tissue). This enables PPG to record arterial and/or venous blood volume changes in the cutaneous vasculature (one basic example is a finger pulse monitor, although this has a light source on one side of the finger and the detector on the other side, depending on transmission of light though the finger). Research or clinical systems can be calibrated prior to use making the systems independent of the individual patient's blood volume, skin colour, thickness and enabling interpatient comparisons.

Van Roon et al. [39] assessed 381 patients with RP, performing both nailfold capillaroscopy and IR PPG. the latter to measure microvascular volume at the fingertip. Fingertips were monitored with PPG post heating (33 °C), during whole hand cooling (from 33 °C to 6 °C or until the temperature was not tolerated, in increments of 3 °C). 15 secs of signal was obtained to assess the perfusion of fingers and the recovery of the fingers was then monitored for 10 min at room temperature. The presence of RP was confirmed with a loss of perfusion during cooling or lack of recovery in the 10 min period. The length of time for which ischaemia was measured was significantly increased in patients (particularly during recovery) who had both early and active capillaroscopy patterns as compared to those that had 'normal' capillary pattern (there were no late patterns). Thus, a more severe ischaemia was measured in patients' fingers when they had SSc more advanced capillaroscopy patterns. The capillaroscopy and PPG data, enabled categorization of patients to no underlying disease, early or definite SSc or another classifiable disease (e.g. mixed connective tissue disease, lupus or Sjogren's). A similar protocol was later used to determine the likelihood of a patient having SSc; if all fingers recovered in 10 min, or if the thumb was not involved, then the chance that the patient had SSc was low [40].

Rosato et al. [38], in a large study of 105 patients with SSc, 96 with primary RP and 85 controls compared nailfold capillaroscopy (categorized as early, active, late) and fingertip PPG. Post acclimatisation (20 min, 24 °C), the PPG wave signal was assessed for amplitude and homogeneous digital artery pulsatile pattern across the fingers; homogeneity being accepted as <15% variation. In 96 % of controls and patients with primary RP the signal was found to be homogenous (similar pulsatile flow across all fingers). In the SSc group only 26 % were found to have a homogeneous pattern; 9 % with the early, 6 % with active and 81 % with late nailfold capillary pattern. In the late pattern this was characterized by an absence or large reduction of sphygmic wave signal. The amplitude of the wave pattern lowest in those with primary RP, and highest in the control group. In the SSc group the amplitude was highest in the early group decreasing through active to late (indicating decreased flow). In the control group PPG was homogenous and had high amplitude, in the primary RP group the amplitude was decreased, indicating lower flow. For those with SSc there were differences in the pattern between fingers, potentially due to structural defects in larger vessels but flow was higher than for primary RP, except for those with later capillaroscopy pattern.

The same authors [41], later recruited 100 patients with SSc, 92 patients with primary RP and 80 controls and compared LDI of the dorsal aspect of the hand (at room temperature) to PPG at the fingertips. Lower signal amplitude represented lower flow. Perfusion, as measured by LDI was lowest in the primary RP group and significantly lower than the SSc group ($p<0.0001$). Perfusion in the SSc group was significantly lower than for controls ($p < 0.0001$). This trend held for the PPG amplitude; there was strong correlation between the PPG amplitude and the mean perfusion. A subsequent study compared several techniques including nailfold capillaroscopy, PPG, colour Doppler ultrasonography (CDUS, discussed in the section below) and LDI to assess hand microvasculature in 36 patients with SSc and 20 matched healthy controls. CDUS data showed normal palmar arteries' patterns in controls and patients with early capillaroscopy patterns (although in patients with 'early' disease, SSc blood flow signal was decreased and resistive indices increased). Significant degradation (e.g. narrowing, reduced flow) was identified in patients with SSc with active and late nailfold capillary patterns. A PPG 'dyshomogenous' pattern (indicative of differences in PPG patterns in two or more fingers and therefore non-uniform vascular volume or perfusion over the hand) was found to occur significantly more often in the patient group; particularly in groups categorized with early and active nailfold capillaroscopy; these occurred in >90% of patients. This was mirrored by the LDI data too (indicating decreased flow as in previous studies) [42].

Whilst finger PPG is the most relevant form of plethysmography for the rheumatic diseases, particularly those involving RP, other versions have been used. Not just limited to the peripheries, plethysmography can assess other aspects of physiology relevant to the rheumatic diseases. Barth et al. combined nailfold capillaroscopy (active or late pattern and density) and body plethysmography to look for associations with pulmonary function (total lung capacity) in 58 patients with juvenile dermatomyositis. Twenty one patients had normal capillary density (>6/mm) and there was an association between total lung capacity and nailfold capillary density ($\beta = 0.295$, $P = 0.018$) [43]. This suggested that the peripheral microvasculature is likely related to disease progression in other organs and offers a window on the disease process.

Optical Coherence Tomography

Optical coherence tomography (OCT) is a non-invasive laser-based technique which employs a low-intensity IR laser beam that can produce high-contrast images of skin up to 2-3 mm deep with a resolution of 1–10 μm [6]. OCT is a well-established diagnostic tool in ophthalmology. Due to its high resolution, it is also a valuable tool to explore the most superficial layers of the skin, such as the dermal-epidermal junction and sweat ducts [44]. Previous studies have used conventional OCT, for example, to detect and quantify skin fibrosis in patients with SSc, showing a good correlation between the severity of skin involvement on OCT and the histology obtained from skin biopsies [45]. However, it does not provide information about functional microcirculation or perfusion [6]. Dynamic OCT is a new non-invasive technique that utilizes speckle variance derived from amplitude information to detect cutaneous blood flow *in vivo*. The dynamic OCT technique is sensitive to the movement of blood cells, thereby obtaining integrated information on vascular network morphology and volume as well as flow data to a skin depth usually reaching the mid dermis [46]. Dynamic OCT has shown significant correlation with LCSI flux measurement and was able to reliably image and identify morphologic changes in the vascular network consistent with the induced physiological changes of blood flow in healthy subjects [46].

Dynamic OCT has been shown to be able to visualize the capillary morphology and flow status in the nailfold capillaries, in a case series of 4 participants, including 2 with SSc and one with dermatomyositis [47]. Dynamic OCT was compared to NVC in one case-controlled study with 40 patients with SSc, and 10 age- and sex-matched healthy controls [48]. Patients and controls were stratified into five NVC patterns: normal, nonspecific, and early, active, or late scleroderma patterns. Quantitative analysis of dynamic-OCT images showed excellent reliability and a significant difference in microvascular flow density across controls, SSc patients with normal/nonspecific NVC patterns, and SSc patients with the scleroderma pattern on NVC. Moreover, microvascular flow density evaluated by dynamic OCT showed a significant correlation with the well-known microvascular abnormalities observed on NVC. Despite these promising results, the technique is restricted to a few research centers, and larger studies and standardization are needed to evaluate if this quantitative measure could be used in clinical trials and practice [48].

Optical Coherence Tomography Angiography (OCTA)

Optical coherence tomography angiography (OCTA) has also been used to evaluate the ocular microcirculation and its possible correlation with the peripheral microvascular damage in patients with autoimmune diseases, particularly SSc. One of these studies investigated the correlations between finger microvascular morphology and function and the status of ocular microcirculation by NVC, LASCA, and OCTA in patients with SSc and healthy controls. The authors found significant correlations between the mean capillary number in NVC and the mean perfusion of fingers, as well as with the retinal and choroidal perfusion evaluated by OCTA, indicating that peripheral microvascular damage is correlated with impaired ocular microcirculation in SSc. In addition, significantly reduced retinal and choroidal perfusion was detected in SSc patients compared to controls [49].

Doppler Ultrasound

Variations of Doppler ultrasound (including power Doppler ultrasound [PDUS] and colour Doppler ultrasound [CDUS]) can be used to assess the larger vessels in the limbs. Ultrasound uses ultrasound waves (at MHz frequency) directed into the skin and reflected from internal boundaries to assess structure, including that of blood vessels. The trade-off between depth of imaging and resolution leads to larger vessels such as arteries being imaged in hands and forearms. As with laser Doppler, the Doppler signal in the vessels provides a measure of flow or perfusion. PDUS provides a measure of the signal strength and CDUS provides the direction of flow displayed on a false colour scale. There have been several studies assessing the function of the macrovasculature in the rheumatic diseases and comparing this to nailfold capillaroscopy, aiming to compare micro- and macrovasculopathies, with a particular focus on the vasculopathy underlying or preceding development of DUs. Structural outcome measures are typically intima media thickness and internal diameter which are indicative of occlusion and large vessel disease. Functional measures include measures of systolic and diastolic velocities and vascular resistance, referred to as both resistive or resistivity indices (difference between the peak systolic and end diastolic flow velocities divided by the peak systolic velocity). Study outcomes vary, with some identifying relationships between micro- and macrovascular aspects of disease and other not finding associations.

High-resolution Doppler ultrasound was compared to nailfold capillaroscopy in 33 patients with SSc and 34 controls. Patients with SSc were grouped according to capillaroscopy pattern (early, active, late). Proximal resistive index and the peak systolic velocity were calculated (interdigital artery). The distal resistive index was calculated at the nailfold arteriole. Patients with SSc had slower proximal systolic velocity and higher distal resistive index than the controls (but no difference was found for the proximal resistance). There was no correlation between the US findings and the capillaroscopy grading [50].

Schioppo et al. prospectively studied 106 patients with SSc using both PDUS (2-4 fingers) and nailfold capillaroscopy (8 fingers) to assess presence of ulnar artery occlusion and measure resistivity index in the radial and ulnar palmar arteries. In addition, PDUS measurements were made of finger pulp and nailbed perfusion. These data were compared to conventional nailfold capillaroscopy (capillary number) and history of DU. Seven patients had arterial occlusions. At the finger pulp and nailbed, increased perfusion mapped to higher number of capillaries. Resistive index did not correlate with microvascular measures; however, those with a history of DUs had increased vascular resistance as compared to those with no DUs. Trends in both finger pulp and nailbed perfusion suggested that patients with a history of DUs had lower perfusion [51].

CDUS has been compared to capillaroscopy in a prospective study of 79 patients with SSc to determine a score for predicting DUs (alongside fluorescence optical imaging, a technique discussed in more detail below). DUs were assessed for 12 months after the baseline imaging visit; 29 % of patients developed ulcers. Data were assessed as possible outcomes and receiver operator curves were generated with outcomes included to provide specificity and sensitivity data. Late nailfold capillaroscopy pattern had an odds ratio of 1.476 (0.5–4.0) for development of DUs but was not statistically significant; however, reduced density had an OR 9.0 (1.1–73.6), $p = 0.03$ and was highly sensitive (94.7%) but not specific (33.3%). The occurrence of more than 35% of arteries being narrowed/occluded as observed by CDUS had an OR of 4.3 (1.5–12.4), $p = 0.01$ and specificity and sensitivity of 68.2% and 66. 7% respectively. Capillaroscopy showed low specificity and CDUS moderate sensitivity as predictors of DU. A combination of the imaging techniques (CDSU, capillaroscopy and fluorescence optical imaging) with clinical features including skin involvement, clinical history and presence of DU, gave a predictive sensitivity of 100% and specificity of 74% for new DUs during follow-up; indicative that objective measures of micro and macrovasculopathy may be valuable measures of vascular changes occurring in advance of ulceration [52].

D'Alessandro et al. imaged the radial and ulnar arteries of 43 patients with SSc at the wrist, with CDUS. Twelve patients had ulnar artery occlusions; 42% of these occlusions occurred in late capillaroscopy pattern and 83.3% of these patients had DU. Imaging was also carried out in 23 patients with primary RP and 22 healthy controls. Resistive index in both the radial and ulnar arteries was higher in both SSc and primary RP than controls and peak velocities were lower in the patients with SSc as compared to both those with primary RP and the control group [53]. Another paper prospectively assessing DU occurrence, compared both CDUS and nailfold capillaroscopy. The authors identified nearly 40% of 36 patients had occlusions of palmar digital arteries at baseline. Nineteen patients developed DUs in the 5 year follow-up period. All patients who developed DUs had a history of DUs. Resistive index was higher in those with DUs than those without. Increased resistive index and late capillary pattern were found to be predictive of DUs [54].

A study comparing patients with SSc and those with fibromyalgia (as controls) compared nailfold capillaroscopy and CDUS at the forearm (intima media thickness, internal diameter and resistive indices of the radial and ulnar arteries). Only one of the 23 patients with fibromyalgia had arterial occlusions in contrast to ten of the 50 patients with SSc. Patients with SSc had a significantly higher intima media thickness to internal diameter ratio as compared to the fibromyalgia cohort (0.33 ± 0.17 vs 0.19 ± 0.05, $p = 0.001$). Capillaroscopy was assessed as a composite score of density, disorganization and ramification averaged across both hands. Capillaroscopy was graded as normal for all of the fibromyalgia cohort. The authors found no relationship between nailfold capillaroscopy and CDUS in patients with SSc [55].

These studies suggest that microvascular changes are common and, often macrovascular changes are present in patients with SSc (the latter particularly in those with advanced disease and comorbidities such as DU); however, the micro- and macrovascular changes may have different mechanisms of pathogenesis.

Fluorescence Optical Imaging

Another interesting technique is the use of fluorophore probes for microvascular imaging [6]. Several non-specific fluorescent dyes are currently approved for use in humans, particularly in the determination of cardiac output, liver function diagnostics, and ophthalmic angiography [56]. One of these dyes is the fluorophore indocyanine-green, a fluorescent marker for skin imaging. Although originally used to predominantly contrast superficial skin structures, it can also be used to delineate skin perfusion and vasculature [6].

The fluorescence optical imaging method measures the fluorescence of the fluorophore indocyanine green using light-emitting diodes and a charge-coupled detector (CCD, a high-resolution camera). It was first used in rheumatology to detect *in vitro* and *in vivo* tissue altered by inflammation. Patients studies included those with rheumatoid arthritis [57]. The principle of florescence optical imaging technology is based on translating indocyanine green-time-series images into quantitative measures such as tissue perfusion based on dynamic pattern of indocyanine green, which is mainly dependent on regional tissue perfusion [58].

The first studies evaluating fluorescence optical imaging in patients with SSc and RP were published by Pfeil et al. in 2014 and 2015, in which the potential to detect therapeutic response to treatment with intravenous iloprost or alprostadil was evaluated [59, 60]. In the first study, fluorescence optical imaging of the hands was evaluated in 11 patients with SSc and 11 healthy controls using intravenous indocyanine green. In SSc patients, fluorescence optical imaging was also performed before and after seven days of iloprost. The healthy controls revealed no enhancement of indocyanine green, while SSc patients showed an enhancement of indocyanine green in both hands. A significantly reduced enhancement of fluorescence optical imaging (−39.1%) was observed after treatment with iloprost [59]. In the second study from the same group, a significant reduction in the indocyanine green enhancement after seven days of either iloprost or alprostadil therapy was observed (suggestive of decreased inflammation), which ranged from 40.9% to 24.7%. The study suggests that the fluorescence optical imaging technique was able to visualize soft-tissue inflammation with both high sensitivity and specificity, suggesting that this technique might be promising in the diagnosis and therapy assessment of patients with SSc-associated RP [60].

An association between nailfold capillaroscopy findings and fluorescence optical imaging was found in one previous study. In this study by Friedrich et al, fluorescence optical imaging was able to identify areas of abnormal or decreased microcirculatory flow in the hands and fingers of patients with SSc, which appear as areas of reduced enhancement. Interestingly, a missing or insufficient signal of fluorescence in fingertips during the entire examination, indicating pathologic enhancement distribution, was more frequent in patients with current DUs and/or pitting scars than in those without. Moreover, a missing initial indocyanine green accumulation in the fingertip was significantly associated with the presence of at least one DU and/or pitting scar in the corresponding finger. Thus, fluorescence optical imaging can be considered a promising tool that could be helpful in the assessment and the exact localization of areas with low perfusion in patients with SSc. In addition, fluorescence optical imaging findings were significantly associated with a late capillaroscopic pattern, and a diffuse SSc subtype, suggesting an association with more severe disease [61]. In a prospective study from the same group, a higher risk of DU development in patients with SSc was observed with abnormal fluorescence distribution using fluorescence optical imaging [62]. However, one limitation of fluorescence optical imaging is that the total fluorescence signal varies depending on factors such as the current cardiovascular state of the subject, the speed of the injection, or the effective concentration of the fluorescent dye in the blood. Thus, the signal is represented as a proportion of the strongest signal in the examined area and depicts microvascular disturbances, not exclusively the absolute blood volume in the hands [61].

Magnetic Resonance Imaging (MRI)/Angiography

Beyond microvascular involvement, a high prevalence of abnormalities of digital arteries of the hands has been described using angiography of digital arteries and extremities in patients with SSc [63, 64]. Magnetic resonance angiography (MRA) has the advantage over arteriography in that it is non-invasive and allows the accurate imaging of the small vessels of the wrist and hands. Substantial damage of major arterial and venous vessels, as well as the microcirculation of the hands, was found in patients with SSc using MRA [65]. The Digital Artery Volume Index (DAVIX), using a quantitative, non-invasive imaging score based on time-of-flight MRI angiography, is a new method mainly used to visualize blood flow within vessels without the need to administer a specific contrast agent. Time-of-flight images enable the visualization of vessels by enhancing the signal of flowing blood and suppressing the signal from surrounding stationary tissue in a defined volume. The volume of blood moving is then approximated to the patent portion of the vessels. In a preliminary study, DAVIX was able to differentiate between SSc patients with DUs and those without and could predict the appearance of new DUs. Moreover, a significant negative correlation between nailfold capillaroscopy pattern and DAVIX was found [66].

Techniques to Assess Oxygenation

Spectroscopy and Multi- and Hyperspectral Imaging

Given the importance of oxygenation in the proposed hypoxia-fibrosis cycle [67], methods of measuring cutaneous vascular oxygenation offer great opportunity to understand more about the relationships between microvascular perfusion, oxygenation, and structure. Technologically this has been a difficult task but newer imaging and measurement techniques are now available to facilitate non-invasive oxygenation measurement and imaging. These tend to be optical (light based) techniques that use the microvascular haemoglobin's natural absorption of light and capitalize on the way that this alters between deoxygenation and oxygenation.

Spectroscopy is the single point measurement technique for collecting oxygenation data at a single point (analogous to perfusion measurement with LDF) and multispectral (or hyperspectral) imaging collects this data over an image (analogous to LDI). The techniques generally rely on illumination by 'broadband' or white (or IR) light. Certain wavelengths of light incident on the skin are then scattered and absorbed by the components in the skin (e.g. melanin and haemoglobin); other wavelengths are reflected back. The relative absorption of wavelengths provides information on the tissue components. In its simplest form this is a spectrum of absorption showing the relative amplitude of absorbed wavelengths (Fig. 4). In imaging, this tends to be a combination of images taken at different wavelengths and combined in a specific way to provide an image of e.g. oxygenation (Fig. 5). The term multispectral alludes to the collection of these discreet images taken at different wavelengths of light; this is possible using a camera with a set of wavelength filters, or a set of illumination wavelengths used and imaged, this is generally the whole field that is captured simultaneously. Hyperspectral refers to all wavelengths being captured and generally requires scanning by a spectrometer to provide all wavelengths at all pixels of an image; this information is dense but slow and not appropriate to record fast changes over an area (more useful for non-moving samples). Whilst there have been some studies using these techniques in the rheumatic diseases, they tend not to have comparisons to nailfold capillaroscopy. Teaw et al. used white light multispectral imaging and identified lower oxyhaemoglobin (non significant), higher deoxyheamoglobin ($p < 0.05$) and lower oxygen saturation measurements ($p < 0.05$) at baseline, in the hands of 13 patients with SSc as compared to a control group of 12. Following cold challenge, patients also experienced more of an decrease in oxyhaemoglobin, more of an increase in deoxyhemoglobin with a greater decline in oxygen saturation than the controls. No comparison to nailfold capillaroscopy was made [68]. Dinsdale et al. used white light single point spectroscopy to measure digital oxygenation and did compare this to nailfold capillaroscopy; whilst oxygenation was decreased in patients with SSc ($N = 82$) as compared to controls ($N = 24$), there was no significant correlation between oxygenation and capillary density ($r = 0.09$, $p = 0.26$) [14].

Two studies have been reported using near IR imaging systems. One small study reported lower oxygenation levels in the hands of 5 patients with SSc compared to in 5 controls (no nailfold measurements were made for comparison) [69]. A second study of 40 patients with SSc and 21 controls also reported decreased oxygenation levels at baseline and during brachial artery occlusion; semi-quantitative capillaroscopy was reported. Hand oxygenation was decreased in the patient group at baseline but no differences were found between oxygenation levels and the different capillaroscopy patterns [70].

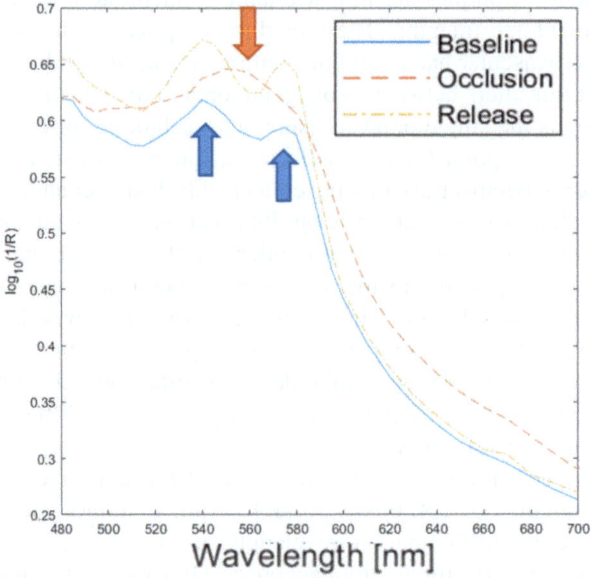

Fig. 4 A spectrum of absorption showing wavelength (x-axis, blue to red wavelengths) vs amplitude of reflected light (y-axis, relative log scale) returned from skin after illumination with white light. The individual lines show the differences that occur in a finger undergoing occlusion, with blue at baseline, dotted orange line during occlusion and yellow line immediately after occlusion (reactive hyperemia). The double peaks (blue arrows) represent presence of oxyhaemoglobin which dominates both at baseline and upon release of occlusion in a healthy control. The single peak in the orange curve (orange arrow) shows the dominance of the deoxyhaemoglobin during occlusion. (Image courtesy of Rosie Barnes)

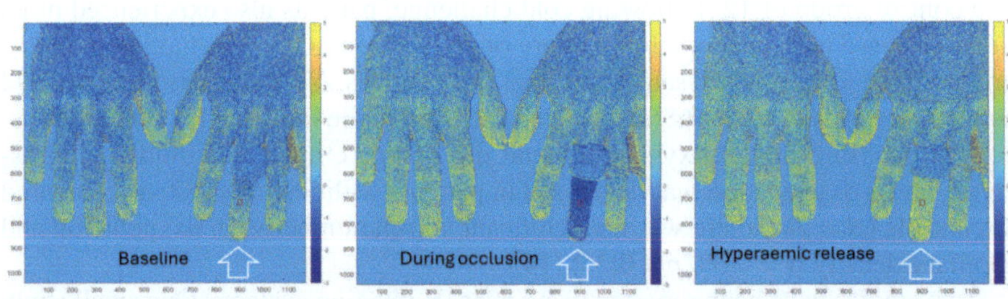

Fig. 5 An example of multispectral imaging of the hands before, during and immediately after middle finger occlusion (pressure cuff placed on left hand, highlighted by the white arrow). False coloured images (arbitrary oxygenation scale to the right with yellow being relatively high and dark blue being relatively low oxygenation, pixel numbers along the left and bottom edges). Note the middle finger shows decreased oxygenation under occlusion and increased oxygenation during hyperaemic release. (Images courtesy of Rosie Barnes)

Multispectral Photoacoustic Imaging

Multispectral photoacoustic imaging is a method combining the advantages of optical imaging and ultrasound. Laser pulses, with wavelengths tailored to preferential absorption of haemoglobin, induce ultrasonic waves that are detected by ultrasonic transducers. Since only the haemoglobin-rich regions of the tissue (i.e. the vessels) absorb the laser light, only the vessels emit the ultrasonic waves and thus the technique enables visualisation of 3D vascular networks within the tissue. Adding in the additional wavelengths relevant to oxy- and deoxy-haemoglobin absorption (i.e multispectral imaging as discussed above) facilitates oxygenation measurement within vessels. As with spectroscopy, due to the relatively new development of the technique there is a sparsity of studies applying these techniques in the rheumatic diseases. Liu et al., Daoudi et al. and Eisenbrey et al. [71–73] all carried out small studies with photoacoustic imaging of the fingers. Liu et al. used an early prototype to reconstruct cross-sections of the macrovascular structure in the fingers of 3 controls and 3 patients with SSc identifying reduced oxygenation in the patient group [71]. Daoudi et al. also identified decreased oxygenation in the fingers of 12 patients with SSc as compared to 9 controls [72]. Eisenbrey et al. used the oxygenation measures at the finger, combined with a cold challenge, to differentiate those with and without RP (with an area under the received operating curve of 0.91 post challenge) [73]. None of these studies included nailfold capillaroscopy. There have been two studies of photoacoustic imaging at the nailfold, but these have not included oxygenation measures [74, 75]. The use of imaging to measure oxygenation in capillaries is discussed further in chapter "Research Methods; Functional Measures of Nailfold Capillaroscopy Including Permeability, Perfusion and Oxygenation".

Conclusion

Microvascular abnormalities are a key issue in patients with rheumatic diseases. They are involved in the pathophysiology of SSc and they are also important in other rheumatic diseases including systemic lupus erythematosus, mixed connective tissue disease, inflammatory myopathies, among others. Nailfold capillaroscopy is currently the only validated method for the morphological assessment of microcirculation and the current gold standard for helping to differentiate between primary and secondary RP, as well as for the early diagnosis of SSc.

Combined analysis of the morphological aspects of the microcirculation observed in nailfold capillaroscopy with functional techniques including those measuring perfusion may complement traditional diagnostic methods for SSc spectrum disorders and RP, besides offering evaluation of different aspects of the microcirculation. Furthermore, combining methods might be useful to provide insights into disease pathophysiology, disease progression and treatment monitoring in clinical practice and in clinical trials [76]. It is important to note that most of the non-invasive techniques described in this chapter are safe, non-contact and with low risk for use in clinical practice; some laser-based techniques require user training and eye protection and some contrast agents (fluorescence optical imaging and MRI) may rarely induce anaphylaxis or other side effects. The choice of microvascular imaging will depend on many factors, including imaging rate, field of view, tissue penetration depth, and on the clinical application [3].

Most of the techniques described in this chapter are currently used mainly in clinical research and should be evaluated with further studies to validate their use in clinical practice. The cost of imaging should also be considered when considering clinical applicability. Design, availability and practicality, must also be addressed before any device can be applied [6].

Further perspectives include the use of multiple imaging strategies in a single platform to utilize their combined advantages. Possible future developments include strategies combining techniques, such as using LSCI, for example, to assess large areas of skin for the identification of potential areas of interest prior to a more in-depth investigation with a higher resolution technique, such as dynamic OCT. This may be a practical approach for increasing efficiency; that also aids in eliminating the inherent subjectivity in selection of assessment site [6]. Similarly, further validation of imaging modalities as outcome measures for treatment response is another area that warrants development and might be useful particularly for the assessment of new drugs and in clinical trials for the treatment of RP.

Lastly, the rapid development of automated processes and artificial intelligence might also bring exciting opportunities such as reducing the subjectivity present during manual image interpretation of some of these techniques and lowering the cost of interpreting results (although this will require large data sets of good quality images for training of algorithms and human oversight for quality assurance). Overall, the combination of non-invasive imaging techniques with nailfold capillaroscopy offers great promise for both research and clinical translation, for understanding pathogenesis, measuring severity and monitoring disease progression and treatment response.

References

1. Markousis-Mavrogenis G, Bournia VK, Sfikakis PP, et al. Raynaud phenomenon and microvasculopathy in systemic sclerosis: multi-modality imaging for diagnosis and evaluation. Curr Opin Rheumatol. 2023;35(6):324–33.
2. Murray AK, Moore TL, King TA, et al. Abnormal microvascular response is localized to the digits in patients with systemic sclerosis. Arthritis Rheum. 2006;54:1952–60.
3. Allen J, Howell K. Microvascular imaging: techniques and opportunities for clinical physiological measurements. Physiol Meas. 2014;35(7):R91–R141.
4. Herrick AL, Dinsdale G, Murray A. New perspectives in the imaging of Raynaud's phenomenon. Eur J Rheumatol. 2020;7(Suppl 3):S212–21.
5. Frech TM. Imaging techniques for assessment of vascular involvement in systemic sclerosis. Curr Opin Rheumatol. 2022;34(6):311–8.
6. Deegan AJ, Wang RK. Microvascular imaging of the skin. Phys Med Biol. 2019;64(7):07TR01.
7. Ruaro B, Bruni C, Wade B, et al. Laser speckle contrast analysis: functional evaluation of microvascular damage in connective tissue diseases. Is there evidence of correlations with organ involvement, such as pulmonary damage? Front Physiol. 2021;12:710298.

8. Ruaro B, Sulli A, Alessandri E, et al. Laser speckle contrast analysis: a new method to evaluate peripheral blood perfusion in systemic sclerosis patients. Ann Rheum Dis. 2014;73:1181–5.
9. Cutolo M, Ferrone C, Pizzorni C, et al. Peripheral blood perfusion correlates with microvascular abnormalities in systemic sclerosis: a laser-Doppler and nailfold videocapillaroscopy study. J Rheumatol. 2010;37:1174–80.
10. Rosato E, Rossi C, Molinaro I, et al. Laser Doppler perfusion imaging in systemic sclerosis impaired response to cold stimulation involves digits and hand dorsum. Rheumatology (Oxford). 2011;50(9):1654–8.
11. Ruaro B, Sulli A, Pizzorni C, et al. Correlations between skin blood perfusion values and nailfold capillaroscopy scores in systemic sclerosis patients. Microvasc Res. 2016;105:119–24.
12. Murray AK, Moore TL, Manning JB, et al. Noninvasive imaging techniques in the assessment of scleroderma spectrum disorders. Arthritis Rheum. 2009;61(8):1103–12.
13. Correa MJ, Andrade LE, Kayser C. Comparison of laser Doppler imaging, fingertip lacticemy test, and nailfold capillaroscopy for assessment of digital microcirculation in systemic sclerosis. Arthritis Res Ther. 2010;12(4):R157.
14. Dinsdale G, Wilkinson S, Wilkinson J, et al. State-of-the-art technologies provide new insights linking skin and blood vessel abnormalities in SSc-related disorders. Microvasc Res. 2020;130:104006.
15. Piotto DG, Correa MJ, Miotto e Silva VB, et al. Laser Doppler imaging for assessment of microcirculation in juvenile systemic sclerosis. Rheumatology (Oxford). 2014;53(1):72–5.
16. Ruaro B, Sulli A, Casabella A, et al. Peripheral blood perfusion in patients with systemic lupus erythematosus and in primary Raynaud's phenomenon. Eur J Rheumatol. 2021;8(1):7–11.
17. Szabo N, Csiki Z, Szanto A, et al. Functional and morphological evaluation of hand microcirculation with nailfold capillaroscopy and laser Doppler imaging in Raynaud's and Sjogren's syndrome and poly/dermatomyositis. Scand J Rheumatol. 2008;37(1):23–9.
18. Rosato E, Borghese F, Pisarri S, et al. Laser Doppler perfusion imaging is useful in the study of Raynaud's phenomenon and improves the capillaroscopic diagnosis. J Rheumatol. 2009;36(10):2257–63.
19. Ruaro B, Smith V, Sulli A, et al. Methods for the morphological and functional evaluation of microvascular damage in systemic sclerosis. Korean J Intern Med. 2015;30(1):1–5.
20. Pauling JD, Hackett N, Guida A, et al. Performance of laser-derived imaging for assessing digital perfusion in clinical trials of systemic sclerosis related digital vasculopathy: a systematic literature review. Semin Arthritis Rheum. 2020;50:1114–30.
21. Barbano B, Marra AM, Quarta S, et al. In systemic sclerosis skin perfusion of hands is reduced and may predict the occurrence of new digital ulcers. Microvasc Res. 2017;110:1–4.
22. Ring EF, Ammer K. Infrared thermal imaging in medicine. Physiol Meas. 2012;33:R33–46.
23. Lim R, Dinsdale G, Manning J, Heal C, Murray A, Herrick AL. Mobile phone thermography of the toes in patients with systemic sclerosis-a pilot study. Rheumatol Adv Pract. 2024;8:rkae068.
24. Dinsdale G, Nazeer S, Manning J, Murray A, Herrick AL. Mobile phone thermal imaging as an ambulatory assessment tool in Raynaud's phenomenon. Rheumatology. 2023;62:e311–2.
25. Miziołek B, Lis-Święty A, Kucharz E, Pieczyrak R, Polak K, Szczepanek M, Bergler-Czop B. Clinical assessment of patients with systemic sclerosis: is there a place for thermography? Arch Dermatol Res. 2023;315:387–93.
26. Herrick AL, Heal C, Wilkinson J, Dinsdale G, Manning J, Gunnarsson K, Jakobsson PJ, Murray A. Temperature response to cold challenge and mobile phone thermography as outcome measures for systemic sclerosis-related Raynaud's phenomenon. Scand J Rheumatol. 2021;50:479–84.
27. Wilkinson JD, Leggett SA, Marjanovic EJ, Moore TL, Allen J, Anderson ME, et al. A multicenter study of the validity and reliability of responses to hand cold challenge as measured by laser speckle contrast imaging and thermography: outcome measures for systemic sclerosis-related Raynaud's phenomenon. Arthritis Rheumatol. 2018;70:903–11.

28. Branco JHL, Branco RLL, Siqueira TC, de Souza LC, Dalago KMS, Andrade A. Clinical applicability of infrared thermography in rheumatic diseases: a systematic review. J Therm Biol. 2022 Feb;104:103172.
29. Pauling JD, Shipley JA, Harris ND, McHugh NJ. Use of infrared thermography as an endpoint in therapeutic trials of Raynaud's phenomenon and systemic sclerosis. Clin Exp Rheumatol. 2012;30:S103–15.
30. Herrick AL, Murray A. The role of capillaroscopy and thermography in the assessment and management of Raynaud's phenomenon. Autoimmun Rev. 2018;17:465–72.
31. Miziołek B, Lis-Święty A, Skrzypek-Salamon A, Brzezińska-Wcisło L. Correlation between the infrared thermogram and microvascular abnormalities of the nailfold in patients with systemic sclerosis. Postepy Dermatol Alergol. 2021;38:115–22.
32. Sebastiani M, Manfredi A, Colaci M, D'amico R, Malagoli V, Giuggioli D, Ferri C. Capillaroscopic skin ulcer risk index: a new prognostic tool for digital skin ulcer development in systemic sclerosis patients. Arthritis Rheum. 2009;61:688–94.
33. Hughes M, Wilkinson J, Moore T, Manning J, New P, Dinsdale G, Murray A, Herrick AL. Thermographic abnormalities are associated with future digital ulcers and death in patients with systemic sclerosis. J Rheumatol. 2016;43:1519–22.
34. Nolan E, Manning J, Heal C, Moore T, Herrick AL. Impact and associates of digital pitting in patients with systemic sclerosis: a pilot study. Scand J Rheumatol. 2020;49:239–43.
35. Scolnik M, Vasta B, Hart DJ, Shipley JA, McHugh NJ, Pauling JD. Symptoms of Raynaud's phenomenon (RP) in fibromyalgia syndrome are similar to those reported in primary RP despite differences in objective assessment of digital microvascular function and morphology. Rheumatol Int. 2016;36:1371–7.
36. Joyner MJ, Dietz NM, Shepherd JT. From Belfast to Mayo and beyond: the use and future of plethysmography to study blood flow in human limbs. J Appl Physiol. 2001;91:2431–41.
37. Cooke ED, Bowcock SA, Smith AT. Photoplethysmography of the distal pulp in the assessment of the vasospastic hand. Angiology. 1985;36(1):33–40.
38. Rosato E, Rossi C, Borghese F, Molinaro I, Pisarri S, Salsano F. The different photoplethysmographic patterns can help to distinguish patients with primary and sclerodermic Raynaud phenomenon. Am J Med Sci. 2010;340(6):457–61.
39. van Roon AM, Smit AJ, van Roon AM, Bootsma H, Mulder DJ. Digital ischaemia during cooling is independently related to nailfold capillaroscopic pattern in patients with Raynaud's phenomenon. Rheumatology. 2016;55:1083–90.
40. van Roon AM, van Roon AM, Stel AJ, Bootsma H, Smit AJ, Mulder DJ. Assessing recovery after cold challenge and thumb involvement can help to rule out systemic sclerosis in patients presenting with Raynaud's phenomenon. Scand J Rheumatol. 2020;49(2):137–40. https://doi.org/10.1080/03009742.2019.1643911. Epub 2019 Oct 22
41. Rosato E, Molinaro I, Rossi C, Pisarri S, Salsano F. The combination of laser Doppler perfusion imaging and photoplethysmography is useful in the characterization of scleroderma and primary Raynaud's phenomenon. Scand J Rheumatol. 2011;40:292–8.
42. Rosato E, Gigante A, Barbano B, Cianci R, Molinaro I, Pisarri S, Salsano F. In systemic sclerosis macrovascular damage of hands digital arteries correlates with microvascular damage. Microvasc Res. 2011;82:410–5.
43. Barth Z, Schwartz T, Flatø B, Aaløkken TM, Koller A, Lund MB, Sjaastad I, Sanner H. Association between nailfold capillary density and pulmonary and cardiac involvement in medium to longstanding juvenile dermatomyositis. Arthritis Care Res. 2019;71:492–7.
44. Ulrich M, Themstrup L, de Carvalho N, et al. Dynamic optical coherence tomography in dermatology. Dermatology. 2016;232:298–311.
45. Abignano G, Aydin SZ, Castillo-Gallego C, et al. Virtual skin biopsy by optical coherence tomography: the first quantitative imaging biomarker for scleroderma. Ann Rheum Dis. 2013;72:1845–51.
46. Themstrup L, Welzel J, Ciardo S, et al. Validation of dynamic optical coherence tomography for non-invasive, in vivo microcirculation imaging of the skin. Microvasc Res. 2016;107:97–105.

47. Ring HC, Themstrup L, Banzhaf CA, et al. Dynamic optical coherence tomography capillaroscopy: a new imaging tool in autoimmune connective tissue disease. JAMA Dermatol. 2016;152(10):1142–6.
48. Abignano G, Green L, Eng S, et al. Nailfold microvascular imaging by dynamic optical coherence tomography in systemic sclerosis: a case-controlled pilot study. J Invest Dermatol. 2022;142:1050–7.
49. Cutolo CA, Cere A, Toma P, et al. Peripheral and ocular microvascular alterations in systemic sclerosis: observations from capillaroscopic assessments, perfusion peripheral analysis, and optical coherence tomography angiography. Rheumatol Int. 2024;44(1):107–18.
50. Picasso R, Bica P, Pistoia F, Zaottini F, Sanguinetti S, Bovis F, Ponzano M, Pizzorni C, Paolino S, Sulli A, Gotelli E, Martinoli C, Cutolo M. High-resolution Doppler ultrasound in systemic sclerosis: analysis of digital arteries and nailfold microvasculature using 18-5 MHz and 33-9 MHz probes. Int J Rheum Dis. 2022;25:1288–94.
51. Schioppo T, Orenti A, Boracchi P, De Lucia O, Murgo A, Ingegnoli F. Evidence of macro- and micro-angiopathy in scleroderma: an integrated approach combining 22-MHz power Doppler ultrasonography and video-capillaroscopy. Microvasc Res. 2019;122:125–30.
52. Friedrich S, Lüders S, Klotsche J, Burmester GR, Riemekasten G, Ohrndorf S. The first composite score predicting Digital Ulcers in systemic sclerosis patients using Clinical data, Imaging and Patient history-CIP-DUS. Arthritis Res Ther. 2020;22:144.
53. D'Alessandro R, Garcia Gonzalez E, Falsetti P, Conticini E, d'Alessandro M, Selvi E, et al. Peripheral macrovascular involvement in systemic sclerosis: a cohort study by color and spectral Doppler ultrasonography. Life. 2023;13:487.
54. Colalillo A, Vaiarello V, Pellicano C, Leodori G, Gigante A, Rosato E. Color Doppler Ultrasonography of digital arteries and digital ulcers development in systemic sclerosis. Microvasc Res. 2021;138:104210.
55. Bieber A, Dolnikov K, Chizik V, Novofastovsky I, Fawaz A, Balbir-Gurman A, Mader R. Microangiopathy and forearm arterial blood flow in systemic sclerosis: a controlled study. Clin Rheumatol. 2020;39:2671–6.
56. Jonak C, Skvara H, Kunstfeld R, et al. Intradermal indocyanine green for in vivo fluorescence laser scanning microscopy of human skin: a pilot study. PLoS One. 2011;6:e23972.
57. Werner SG, Langer HE, Ohrndorf S, et al. Inflammation assessment in patients with arthritis using a novel in vivo fluorescence optical imaging technology. Ann Rheum Dis. 2012;71(4):504–10.
58. Kang Y, Lee J, An Y, et al. Segmental analysis of indocyanine green pharmacokinetics for the reliable diagnosis of functional vascular insufficiency. J Biomed Opt. 2011;16(3):030504.
59. Pfeil A, Drummer KF, Oelzner P, et al. Fluorescence optical imaging as a novel technique for the visualisation of inflammation in patients with systemic sclerosis with Raynaud's phenomenon: a pilot study. Ann Rheum Dis. 2014;73(6):1279–80.
60. Pfeil A, Drummer KF, Böttcher J, et al. The Application of Fluorescence Optical Imaging in Systemic Sclerosis. Biomed Res Int. 2015;2015:658710.
61. Friedrich S, Lüders S, Werner SG, et al. Disturbed microcirculation in the hands of patients with systemic sclerosis detected by fluorescence optical imaging: a pilot study. Arthritis Res Ther. 2017;19(1):87.
62. Friedrich S, Lüders S, Glimm AM, et al. Association between baseline clinical and imaging findings and the development of digital ulcers in patients with systemic sclerosis. Arthritis Res Ther. 2019;21(1):96.
63. Hasegawa M, Nagai Y, Tamura A, et al. Arteriographic evaluation of vascular changes of the extremities in patients with systemic sclerosis. Br J Dermatol. 2006;155(6):1159–64.
64. Janevski B. Arteries of the hand in patients with scleroderma. Diagn Imaging Clin Med. 1986;55(4-5):262–5.
65. Allanore Y, Seror R, Chevrot A, et al. Hand vascular involvement assessed by magnetic resonance angiography in systemic sclerosis. Arthritis Rheum. 2007;56:2747–54.

66. Hughes M, Di Donato S, Gjeloshi K, et al. MRI Digital Artery Volume Index (DAVIX) as a surrogate outcome measure of digital ulcer disease in patients with systemic sclerosis: a prospective cohort study. Lancet Rheumatol. 2023;5(10):e611–21.
67. Ren H, Liu L, Xiao Y, Shi Y, Zeng Z, Ding Y, Zou P, Xiao R. Further insight into systemic sclerosis from the vasculopathy perspective. Biomed Pharmacother. 2023;166:115282.
68. Teaw S, Gupta A, Williams A, Wilson FP, Sumpio BJ, Sumpio BE, Hinchcliff M. Hyperspectral imaging in systemic sclerosis-associated Raynaud phenomenon. Arthritis Res Ther. 2023;25:10.
69. Jalil B, Hartwig V, Salvetti O, Potì L, Gargani L, Barskova T, Matucci Cerinic M, L'Abbate A. Assessment of hand superficial oxygenation during ischemia/reperfusion in healthy subjects versus systemic sclerosis patients by 2D near infrared spectroscopic imaging. Comput Methods Prog Biomed. 2018;155:101–8.
70. Gargani L, Bruni C, Barskova T, Hartwig V, Marinelli M, Trivella MG, Matucci-Cerinic M, L'Abbate A. Near-infrared spectroscopic imaging of the whole hand: a new tool to assess tissue perfusion and peripheral microcirculation in scleroderma. Semin Arthritis Rheum. 2019;48:867–73.
71. Liu Y, Zhang L, Li S, Han X, Yuan Z. Imaging molecular signatures for clinical detection of scleroderma in the hand by multispectral photoacoustic elastic tomography. J Biophotonics. 2018;11:e201700267.
72. Daoudi K, Kersten BE, van den Ende CHM, van den Hoogen FHJ, Vonk MC, de Korte CL. Photoacoustic and high-frequency ultrasound imaging of systemic sclerosis patients. Arthritis Res Ther. 2021;23:22.
73. Eisenbrey JR, Stanczak M, Forsberg F, Mendoza-Ballesteros FA, Lyshchik A. Photoacoustic oxygenation quantification in patients with Raynaud's: first-in-human results. Ultrasound Med Biol. 2018;44:2081–8.
74. Aguirre J, Hindelang B, Berezhnoi A, Darsow U, Lauffer F, Eyerich K, Biedermann T, Ntziachristos V. Assessing nailfold microvascular structure with ultra-wideband raster-scan optoacoustic mesoscopy. Photoacoustics. 2018;10:31–7.
75. Nitkunanantharajah S, Haedicke K, Moore TB, Manning JB, Dinsdale G, Berks M, Taylor C, et al. Three-dimensional optoacoustic imaging of nailfold capillaries in systemic sclerosis and its potential for disease differentiation using deep learning. Sci Rep. 2020;10:16444.
76. Ruaro B, Nallino MG, Casabella A, et al. Monitoring the microcirculation in the diagnosis and follow-up of systemic sclerosis patients: focus on pulmonary and peripheral vascular manifestations. Microcirculation. 2020;27(8):e1264.

Practical Approaches to Nailfold Capillaroscopy—Case Studies

Michael Hughes, Alberto Sulli, and Ivan Foeldvari

Key Points

- In a patient presenting with Raynaud's phenomenon (RP), nailfold capillaroscopy (NFC) combined with autoantibody testing can help to stratify the risk of progression to definitive connective tissue disease (CTD)/systemic sclerosis (SSc).
- In general, nailfold capillaroscopy should be repeated at an interval of 6–12 months in patients who are at 'risk'.
- Nailfold capillaroscopy allows visualisation of the microvascular component of CTDs, providing novel insights into disease pathogenesis, including to help rationalise the therapeutic strategy.
- Thermography provides complementary functional vascular assessment to NFC in patients presenting with RP.
- In patients with RP, patient education and easy access to urgent digital ulcer care is essential.

M. Hughes (✉)
Division of Musculoskeletal and Dermatological Sciences, School of Biological Sciences, Centre for Musculoskeletal Research, The University of Manchester, Manchester Academic Health Science Centre, Manchester, UK

Department of Rheumatology, Northern Care Alliance NHS Foundation Trust, Salford Care Organisation, Salford, UK

NIHR Manchester Biomedical Research Centre, Manchester University NHS Foundation Trust, Manchester, UK
e-mail: Michael.hughes-6@manchester.ac.uk

A. Sulli
Laboratory of Experimental Rheumatology and Academic Division of Clinical Rheumatology, Department of Internal Medicine, University of Genova, Genoa, Italy

IRCCS Ospedale Policlinico San Martino, Genoa, Italy
e-mail: albertosulli@unige.it

I. Foeldvari
Hamburger Zentrum für Kinder- und Jugendrheumatologie, Hamburg, Germany
e-mail: foeldvari@t-online.de

A. L. Herrick et al. (eds.), *Nailfold Capillaroscopy in Rheumatological Diseases*,
https://doi.org/10.1007/978-3-032-03970-5_13

- In patients presenting with significant digital ischaemia, a multi-disciplinary approach to management is essential. Proximal (macrovascular) disease should be excluded.
- There is a range of potent vasodilating/vasoactive therapies available for the management of RP. Many of these are also used for the treatment of broader vasculopathic sequelae in SSc (e.g., for digital ulcers and pulmonary artery hypertension).

This chapter presents 5 cases which together exemplify many of the points made in previous chapters. The cases demonstrate a practical approach to management, highlighting the role of nailfold capillaroscopy (NFC). Although the main role of NFC in both adult and paediatric clinical practice is in diagnosis, NFC is also useful in predicting risk, not only the risk of developing a systemic sclerosis (SSc)-spectrum disorder but also (as in Case 5) the risk of disease progression.

Case 1: Systemic sclerosis (SSc)-CTD Overlap with SSc-Associated Vasculopathy

A 42-year-old female patient with established systemic lupus erythematosus (SLE) with past lupus nephritis presented with acute bilateral digital (finger) ischaemia without provocation (Fig. 1). The lesions were exquisitely painful and associated with significant sleep disturbance. The patient had longstanding Raynaud's

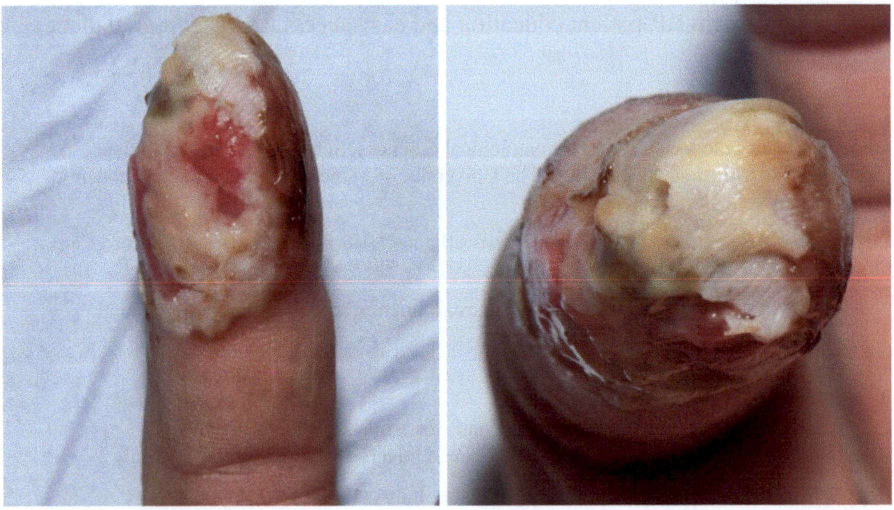

Fig. 1 Digital ischaemia of the fingers with significant slough and superficial soft tissue infection. There was a clear (horizontal) line of demarcation which is suggestive of proximal (macrovascular) vessel involvement

phenomenon (RP) affecting the hands and feet, and without a history of previous digital ulcers and/or chilblains.

Their current treatment consisted of methotrexate (MTX) (oral, 20 mg weekly), hydroxychloroquine (200 mg daily), low-dose prednisolone (5 mg daily), oral calcium/vitamin D supplementation, and weekly bisphosphonate (risedronate). Existing nifedipine (modified release) was optimised to 40 mg twice daily immediately prior to hospitalisation. The patient had previously tried sildenafil, but this was not tolerated due to systemic vasodilatory side effects. Historically, an inflammatory arthritis had been active but was presently quiescent. No other major internal organ involvement was known from their SLE. There was no history of thromboembolic disease or pregnancy morbidity/mortality. The patient was a lifelong non-smoker.

Examination of the hands revealed digital ischaemia of the left middle and right index fingers (Fig. 1). There were obvious signs of superficial soft tissue infection with purulent material and discharge. The other fingers demonstrated no signs of persistent digital ischaemia including digital pitting scars or ulcers. The peripheral pulses were symmetrical and strong including at the level of the wrists. There was obvious evidence of nailfold vasculopathy (with macroscopically dilated vessels and haemorrhages) to visual inspection. Systemic examination was other unremarkable including no musculocutaneous signs of active SLE. There was no peripheral/central nervous system deficit and proximal muscle strength was normal.

Urine dipstick examination showed no significant active renal sediment (mild proteinuria only).

Investigations were in keeping with known SLE. BioPlex CTD screen was positive including anti-Sm, anti-chromatin, and weakly positive anti-dsDNA antibodies. Extractable nuclear antibody (ENA) positivity was observed to anti-SSA and SS-B antibodies. There was no evidence of complement (C3 or C4) consumption. Full blood count demonstrated mild lymphopenia and neutrophilia. C-reactive protein (CRP) was mildly raised (<20 mg/L) and erythrocyte sedimentation rate (ESR) was very high at >100 mm/h. Renal function was stable for the patient. ANCA was negative. There was no evidence of antiphospholipid syndrome on testing (negative lupus anticoagulant, and negative IgG and IgM anticardiolipin and anti-beta-2-glycoprotein-1 antibodies). Chest radiograph was unremarkable. Hand radiographs revealed soft tissue swelling of the affected ischaemic digits without features of established osteomyelitis. Promptly arranged arterial Doppler ultrasound upper limb examinations showed no significant proximal (large) vessel disease.

'Bedside' nailfold capillaroscopy (Fig. 2) was performed (using a Dino-Lite microscope) which revealed significantly enlarged capillaries, reduced capillary density, and multiple large microhaemorrhages.

The patient was urgently hospitalised and treated with intravenous iloprost (5 days initially, and with several further days completed). Meticulous attention was made to provision of appropriate dressings, optimisation of analgesia (including opioid-based), and treatment of superadded infection with intravenous antibiotic therapy. Background immunosuppression with MTX was discontinued (due to the presence of significant infection). There was no strong evidence to support intensification/escalation of immunosuppression (e.g. for active SLE and/or vasculitis). To

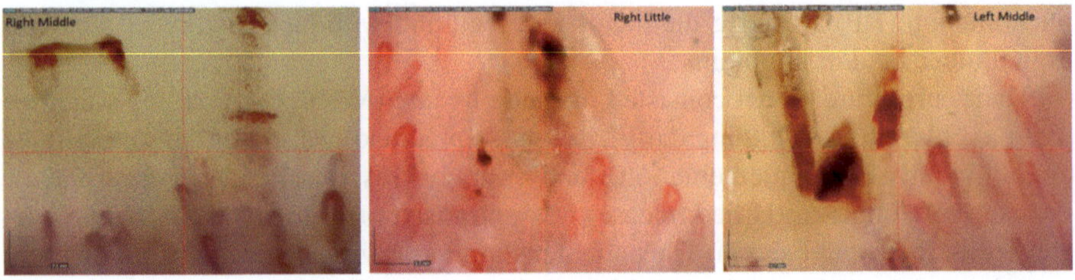

Fig. 2 Nailfold capillaroscopy showing evidence of capillary enlargement, reduced density, and large microhaemorrhages throughout the fingers. (Copyright. Salford Care Organisation, Northern Care Alliance NHS Foundation Trust)

target potentially broad-ranging vascular disease effector mechanisms, low-dose aspirin (75 mg daily) and statin (atorvastatin 40 mg) therapies, were introduced.

The patient subsequently made excellent progress with very minimal residual tissue loss, and with maintenance of their hand function and quality of life. CRP normalised, as did ESR (to the usual level for the patient) after treatment of infection (and this would lend further weight to the vasculopathy being 'non-inflammatory'). After one-year, there were *new* concerns of lupus nephritis activity (e.g., significant proteinuria) and she has been commenced on mycophenolate mofetil (MMF) (1g BD), discontinuing MTX. Candesartan was introduced and uptitrated from a renal perspective (for blood pressure and proteinuria control). The patient has received a further course of iloprost after 1 year (on a semi-elective basis) for their RP and without any further episodes of digital ischaemia.

Discussion Points

1. What was the role of NFC in the management of this patient?

   NFC enabled the timely *early* recognition of significant SSc-CTD overlap vasculopathy. This provided evidence for targeting 'non-inflammatory' vascular disease effector mechanisms, including introduction of anti-platelet and statin therapy (the latter has pleiotropic effects on the vasculature) [1, 2]. This also avoided unnecessary escalation and/or intensification of their existing immunosuppression, especially important in the context of infected digital lesions.
2. What are the therapeutic options longer-term for digital vasculopathy?

   The patient receives treatment now with maximum dose calcium-channel blocker and angiotensin receptor blocker therapies. They have previously been intolerant of sildenafil, but this would not preclude careful rechallenging, including with another phosphodiesterase-type 5 inhibitor (e.g., tadalafil) [3]. If systemic vasodilatory side effects remain an issue, other treatment options could include (but are not limited to) selective serotonin reuptake inhibitors (e.g., fluoxetine) for Raynaud's phenomenon, avoiding systemic vasodilation. If the patient develops recurrent digital ulceration, then an endothelin receptor antagonist (i.e., bosentan) would strongly be considered [4].

3. The role of the multi-disciplinary team

   This was critical. Prompt recognition of digital ischaemia (by the patient and their treating clinicians) facilitated prompt hospitalisation and introduction of digit-saving treatment. Patients require timely access to specialist (including dedicated digital ulcer) services [5]. Careful, 'non-surgical' 'sharp' (e.g., using a scalpel) and 'autolytic' (by using dressings to enhance naturally occurring lysis) debridement is crucial to promote healing and prevent further complications [6]. Currently, there is no agreed general standard of care for digital ulcer debridement (and with substantial international variation in use). However, significant ongoing international collaborative work is investigating the safety and efficacy of digital ulcer debridement [7]. Hand therapy input is essential in this setting to optimise function and promotes improved digital perfusion.
4. The importance of large vessel disease

   This was excluded *early* in her presentation. The peripheral pulses should be examined as part of the initial assessment of digital ischaemia, and these should be strong and symmetrical [8]. Prompt recognition of proximal (macrovascular) disease is essential because this could be amenable to intervention (e.g., revascularisation procedures).
5. What is the likely longer-term outcome for the patient?

   By recognition of the SSc-vasculopathic component to her CTD as demonstrated by NFC, 'vascular' treatments could be optimised, including targeting different disease effector mechanisms.

Case 2: The Role of Capillaroscopy in Predicting 'Risk' of Developing SSc

A 59-year-old male patient was referred with late-onset RP (duration of 1–2 years). He reported white colour change only which mainly affected his right index finger. There was no history of digital ulcers. He described episodic 'tingling' in the feet (which was not necessarily confined temporally to attacks of RP), and previous nerve conduction studies were normal.

He had noticed that his fingers had become slightly larger in appearance, but not puffy in his opinion, over the past several years. He reported mild acid reflux symptoms and previous endoscopy had demonstrated a small hiatus hernia. Subjectively, he felt only occasionally short of breath including ascending the stairs at home. Chest radiograph, transthoracic echocardiogram and advanced lung function showed no cause of concern. He reported non-inflammatory small joint symptoms in keeping with osteoarthritis. His medical history consisted of (treated) hypothyroidism, 'white coat' hypertension, and obstructive sleep apnoea (with use of a continuous positive airway pressure machine at home). There were no relevant occupational exposures or family history. The patient was a lifelong non-smoker. His prescribed medication consisted of amlodipine (5 mg daily) and low-dose proton pump inhibitor (omeprazole 20 mg daily).

On examination, there were osteoarthritis features of the hands and with no evidence of active peripheral joint synovitis. There was no definitive puffiness to the fingers or obvious sclerodermatous skin changes, specifically no sclerodactyly. Nor were there any other cutaneous stigmata of SSc including digital pitting scars or ulcers. Proximal muscle strength was normal and systemic examination was normal.

Investigations showed weakly positive ANA 1:300 (anticentromere pattern). Anticentromere antibodies were not elevated (0.9, range 0.0–0.9). Myositis-associated and anti-RNA polymerase antibodies were negative. Radiographs of the hands and feet showed degenerative changes only and chest radiograph disclosed no interstitial lung disease. Nailfold capillaroscopy (Fig. 3) revealed mostly normal capillaries, with only a few being slightly widened, with no microhaemorrhages seen, and capillary density was within the normal range. Thermographic assessment (Fig. 4) showed no significant temperature gradients along the fingers at baseline room temperature of 23 °C and with normal rewarming after cold challenge testing.

The patient was appropriately counselled concerning his late-onset RP. His Raynaud's symptoms were only mild, and he elected to follow a non-pharmacological approach to management. He was provided with written information about RP and general/lifestyle adaptations, including being directed to patient organisations for further information. The concept of 'risk' was discussed with the patient including possible progression to SSc. He was counselled to seek advice if his Raynaud's worsened, including the need for urgent medical attention if he developed digital ulcers. Repeat nerve conduction studies were recommended in view of the patient's neurosensory symptoms. The patient will be monitored closely in rheumatology (at least for a few years) including to repeat the nailfold capillaroscopy (e.g., on a 6–12 monthly basis) to see if whether any capillaroscopic abnormalities develop.

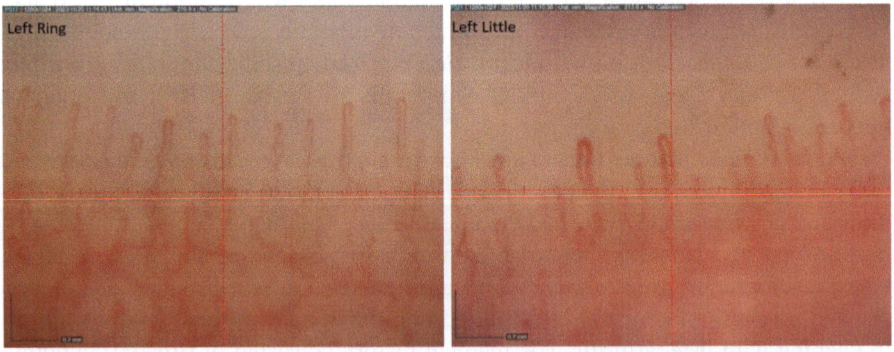

Fig. 3 Nailfold capillaroscopy. This was quite reassuring, with overall normal capillary size (with slight widening of a small number of capillaries), preserved density, and no haemorrhages seen. (Copyright. Salford Care Organisation, Northern Care Alliance NHS Foundation Trust)

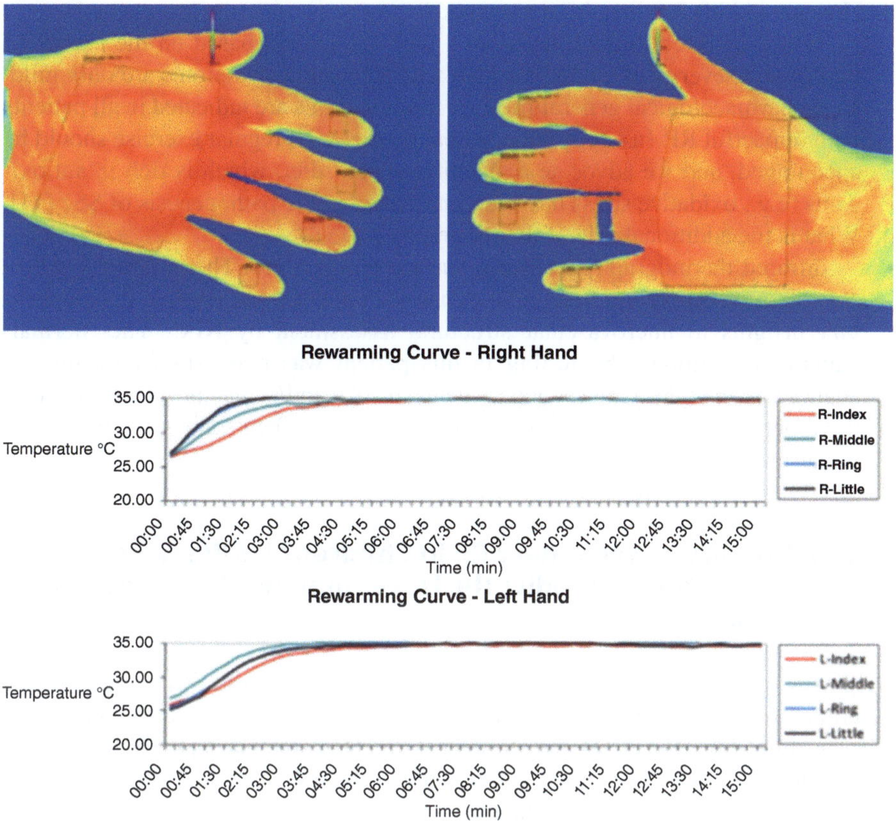

Fig. 4 Thermography. Thermographic assessment showed no significant temperature gradients (between the fingers and dorsum of the hand) at baseline room temperature of 23 °C (upper panel). There was good rewarming observed after cold challenge testing (lower panel). (Copyright. Salford Care Organisation, Northern Care Alliance NHS Foundation Trust)

Discussion Points

1. What is the risk of progression to definitive SSc?

   He presents with late-onset RP and therefore this requires further investigation and monitoring. The ANA was only weakly positive (with a centromere pattern) and anticentromere antibodies were not elevated. Nailfold capillaroscopy was very helpful here with no significant (diagnostic) abnormalities seen at this point but this should be monitored for progression over time. He had no puffy fingers. Practical insights can be gained from the published studies concerning the VEDOSS cohort including risk of progression in patients with RP [9].
2. How long should he be followed up for?

   There is no definitive answer to this. However, it would be reasonable to monitor the patient for at least at least 3–5 years. We would repeat the capillaroscopy every 6–12 months in the first instance (12 monthly if things remain stable).

3. How should his Raynaud's be managed?

   This is directed through discussion with the patient based on the perceived impact and severity of symptoms [10]. His Raynaud's symptoms are only mild. Non-pharmacological general/lifestyle modifications are indicated in all patients with impactful RP. In our opinion, a healthy diet with regular exercise should be encouraged, and we advocate a 'Mediterranean' diet, which is rich in antioxidants (e.g., oxidative stress has been implicated in the pathogenesis of SSc [11].
4. What is the additional role of thermography?

   Infrared thermography measures surface temperature. Thermography protocols often incorporate a functional dynamic challenge and provide *complementary* insights to microvascular structural assessment by NFC. The 'normal' pattern of thermography testing in this patient was reassuring, reducing the chances of an underlying secondary cause for RP and/or risk progression than if thermography had shown significant temperature gradients along the fingers, or impairment of rewarming.

Case 3: Primary or Secondary RP in Children? Do We Have Prognostic Factors to Predict the Development of a Connective Tissue Disease

A 13-year-old, Caucasian, non-consanguine girl presented with white and blue discoloration of all her fingers in the cold. No ulcerations occurred and she was otherwise healthy. She had a regular menstruation. Her stamina was 100% and she participated in all kinds of sports without any problems. She had a normal psychosocial development. She had no diagnosis of any chronic diseases. There was positive family history of primary RP in her mother, but not any connective tissue disease or autoimmune disease in close relatives (siblings, parents or grandparents).

Physical examination revealed palmar and plantar erythema, besides that, no other significant findings. She was Tanner (a scale of physical development) stage 4.

Blood tests showed a normal blood count, biochemistry, ESR and CRP. Urine test was normal. ANA, ENA were negative.

Nailfold capillaroscopy (Fig. 5) showed normal findings, with 8 capillaries/mm and no abnormal capillaries, no giants or avascular areas.

Discussion Points

1. Can we differentiate between primary and secondary RP in children?
   A. With Nailfold Capillaroscopy?
      - Primary RP has a normal capillaroscopy pattern [12]. The normal pattern in children can be different from the "adult normal pattern", as the capillary number/mm changes in healthy children during growth as shown by

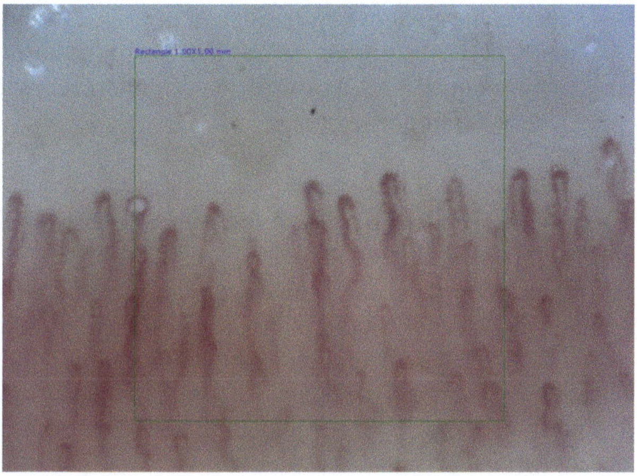

Fig. 5 Nailfold capillaroscopy, showing no abnormalities Capillaroscopy conducted by Özcan Zeynep, study nurse, Hamburger Zentrum für Kinder- und Jugendrheumatologie. This case clearly presents a primary RP.

Terreri et al. [13] and Piotto [14] and the capillary length and the capillary width too [14]. Piotto et al. finds:

- **Avascular area** is defined when ≥2 capillaries are missing in a distal row. This occurs in 10% of healthy children.
- **Enlarged capillaries** are defined as >2 times the normal diameter (20–50 um loops), these are of concern as they associate with SSc, but may be present in up to 11% healthy children.
- **Giant capillaries**, defined as enlarged >4 times the normal diameter or ≥ 50 μm apical diameter are always considered pathologic.

Farenhorst at al [15] compared primary and secondary RP patients and showed that significantly more patients have lower number of capillaries, and have capillary loss, defined <6/mm in the secondary RP group.

B. By ANA positivity?
   - In the study from Farenhorst at al [15] it was shown that ANA or ENA positivity were stronger predictors of development of a connective tissue disease than the capillaroscopic findings.
   - Torrente-Segarra [16] showed that ANA negative patients more frequently showed "normal" NFC pattern compared to ANA positive patients (71% *vs*. 48%, respectively; p = NS). None of ANA negative patients showed "scleroderma pattern" on NFC.

2. How many patients develop a connective tissue disease?
   - Studies in children have shown that patients showing no pathologic nailfold capillaroscopy findings, have a very low risk to develop a connective tissue disease [17, 18]. In these studies, ANA positivity and pathologic nailfold capillaroscopy pattern were the predictors to develop an CTD, which developed in approximately 10% of the patients over 2 to 3 years.
3. Recommendation for follow of patients with RP in children.
   - Following on from a Consensus Meeting held in Hamburg, a proposal for the follow up of patients with RP was published [19]. It is recommended that patients with ANA positivity and nailfold capillaroscopy changes should have

the highest follow up frequency at every 3 months, followed by those with either ANA positivity or capillaroscopy changes at every 6 months. Patients with neither ANA positivity nor capillaroscopy changes should be followed every 12 months.

Case 4: Nailfold Capillaroscopy in Juvenile SSc

At the age of 9 years, a female, Caucasian patient started to have difficulties closing her fingers. A blue discoloration was observed at cold temperature. Later on, she developed fingertip ulceration of the index and middle finger of both hands. A year later she started to get problems with breathing, when she was running. At that time, she presented to pediatric rheumatology, where the diagnosis of the limited cutaneous subtype of juvenile SSc was made.

On physical exam her modified Rodnan skin score (mRSS) was 6, she had sclerodactyly, on her index and middle fingertips she had signs of healed ulceration. She had palmar- and plantar erythema. Her mouth opening was decreased, it was only 3 cm. On musculoskeletal examination her shoulder abduction was decreased, it was 80°, her elbows were in slight flexion contracture, both wrists had only 30° palmar and dorsiflexion, she had around 3 cm palm- finger distance; her hip internal rotation was decreased to 15° on both sides and both knees had slight flexion contractures.

Her antibody profile showed anticentromere antibody positivity. Anti-Scl-70 was negative.

On chest high resolution computerized tomography (HRCT) she had already significant features of interstitial lung disease. Her pulmonary function test revealed a decreased FVC of 65% and DLCO of 60%.

NFC (Fig. 6) revealed decreased number of capillaries 4/mm with giants, typical for SSc.

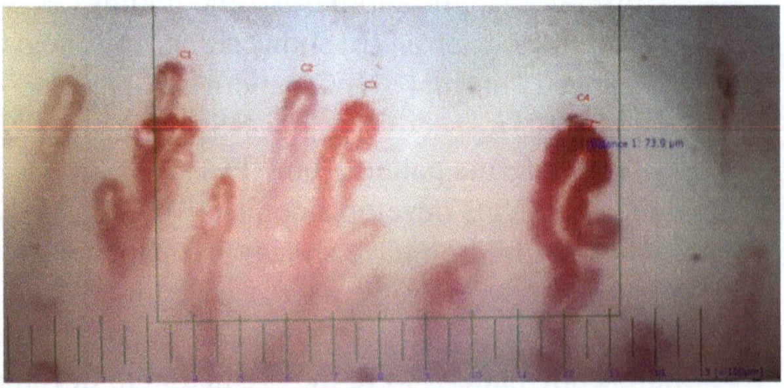

Fig. 6 Capillaroscopy showing reduced capillary density and a giant capillary. Capillaroscopy conducted by Özcan Zeynep, study nurse, Hamburger Zentrum für Kinder- und Jugendrheumatologie

Discussion Points

A. Classification of juvenile SSc and use of nailfold capillaroscopy
   - The applied classification for juvenile SSc is the adult classification from 2013. There is an added definition, that the first non-Raynaud symptom should occur under the age of 16. It is used for inclusion for the juvenile scleroderma inception cohort [20]. One item of this classification is abnormal nail fold capillaries with weight of 2 points.
   - The proposed juvenile classification [21], which requires "Skin thickening of the fingers of both hands extending proximal to the metacarpophalangeal joints", already scores 9 points, which is sufficient to fulfill the adult criteria.

B. Does the presence of scleroderma pattern predict severity of juvenile SSc?
   - We do not currently have sufficient pediatric data regarding the prognostic value of the nailfold changes for internal organ involvement, but in a presented poster at the ACR 2024 by Foeldvari et al. [22] from the juvenile scleroderma inception cohort (www.juvenile-scleroderma.com), patients with nailfold capillaroscopy changes had more severe organ involvement compared with patients with no nailfold changes.

C. Is there a juvenile scleroderma "nailfold pattern"?
   - In the EULAR Study Group on Microcirculation in Rheumatic Diseases publication by Melsens [12], using the SCTC/EULAR consensus on standardized reporting of capillaroscopy and evaluating children from several continents, patients with juvenile SSc, indeed had scleroderma patterns like adults. In line with this they differed significantly from healthy controls in relation number of capillaries, capillary density, number of capillaries with abnormal shapes and number of hemorrhages.

D. How often should nailfold capillaroscopy be conducted?

In the juvenile scleroderma inception cohort (www.juvenile-scleroderma.com) it is suggested to assess every patient every 6 months with nailfold capillaroscopy to gain more insight into their disease.

Case 5: Progression of Internal Organ Involvement Associated with the Severity of Nailfold Capillary Microangiopathy

This is a 52-year-old female patient, working as a painter, with a recent history of RP (one year) and arthralgia of both hands. There were no other symptoms.

In her past medical history, she reported appendectomy, saphenectomy and left ankle fracture due to accidental fall.

Physical examination demonstrated the presence of RP (with mild white and cyanotic changes during cold exposure) (Fig. 7), slightly puffy fingers, absence of digital ulcers/telangiectasias, absence of sclerodactyly/skin involvement. The mRSS was 0. No other clinically relevant findings were present.

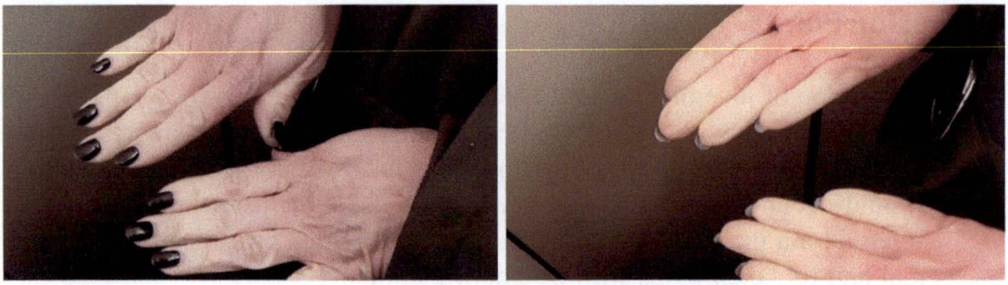

Fig. 7 Raynaud's phenomenon showing 'white/pallor' phase

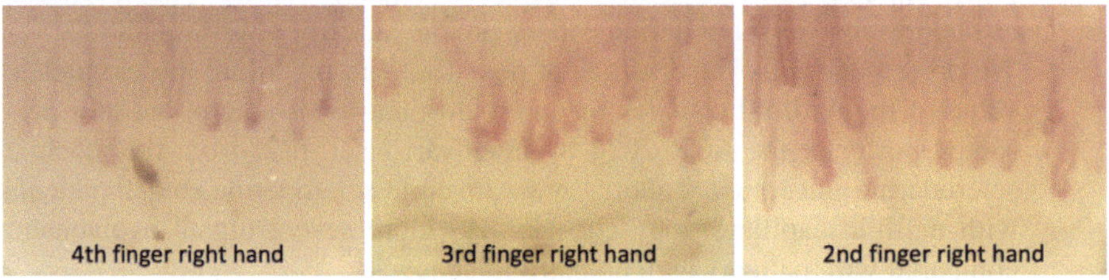

Fig. 8 Baseline nailfold videocapillaroscopy showing the "Early" scleroderma-pattern (×200). The "Early" pattern of microangiopathy is characterized by the presence of giant capillaries (homogeneously enlarged capillaries with a normal morphology and a limb diameter > 50 µm), possible microhaemorrhages (brown dark masses) and normal capillary density (>7–8 capillaries/mm)

All the following laboratory findings were normal or negative: haematology, biochemistry, urinalysis, erythrocyte sedimentation rate, C-reactive protein, complement, immunoglobulins, thyroid function, cryoglobulins, markers for HCV and HBV, anti-phospholipid antibodies. Antinuclear antibodies (ANA) were positive (titre1:640, IIF pattern nucleolar). The ENA were negative including anti-topoisomerase antibodies. Specific scleroderma-associated autoantibodies had not been searched for at that time.

NFC demonstrated an "Early" scleroderma-pattern of microangiopathy (Fig. 8) [23–26].

Screening for internal organ involvement did not demonstrate other clinical manifestations:

Hand X-rays: normal,
Chest X-ray: normal,
Spirometry + DLCO: normal, FVC 100%, DLCO 94%,
Esophageal manometry: normal esophageal motility,
Renal Doppler-echography: normal renal artery resistive indexes (0,65 bilaterally),
Echocardiogram: no pathological findings. Estimated pulmonary artery pressure 25 mmHg.

Although the ACR/EULAR 2013 criteria for SSc were not fulfilled, she fulfilled the LeRoy & Medsger 2001 criteria for early SSc [27, 28]. Also, VEDOSS criteria for possible progression to definite SSc were in this case fulfilled (RP, positive capillaroscopy, puffy fingers) [9, 29].

A diagnosis of early SSc was made, and treatment with etoricoxib, aspirin and aminaphtone started. Arthralgias disappeared after two cycles of etoricoxib for 10 days.

Six months later the patient returned for the follow-up visit. The patient had stopped all treatments, without change in her clinical condition:

RP was still present, a little bit more evident,
Slight puffy fingers,
Absence of digital ulcers/telangectasias,
Absence of sclerodactyly/skin involvement (mRSS = 0),
No symptoms of internal organ involvement.

However, the NFC (×200) demonstrated a progression of the microvascular damage to the "Active" scleroderma-pattern (Fig. 9) [23–26].

At this point, three important clinical aspects were taken into consideration: (1) The nucleolar pattern of ANA is associated with a more rapidly progressive microangiopathy [24, 30]; (2) The quick progression from the "Early" to the "Active" pattern of microangiopathy is a risk factor for a rapid progression to the "Late" pattern, which correlates with a more advanced organ involvement [31–34]; (3). NFC is a recognized tool to predict future severe organ involvement in SSc [35, 36].

Following these considerations, we decided to start treatment with mycophenolate 1g BD and aspirin.

The patient was lost to follow-up for 18 months, then she returned for a further visit. She reported her decision not to start the suggested treatment. Her clinical condition had changed:

RP was present with classical triphasic colour changes which were witnessed during the visit, the fingers were very puffy, and she was complaining of disabling arthralgias at hands and shoulders.

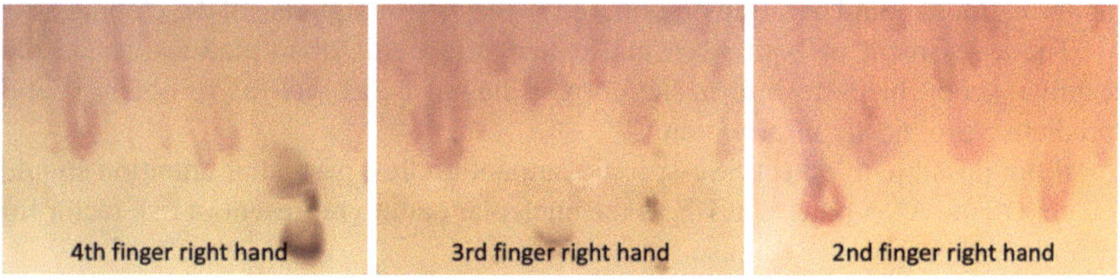

Fig. 9 Nailfold videocapillaroscopy 6 months later, showing the "Active" scleroderma-pattern (×200). The "Active" scleroderma-pattern of microangiopathy presents with lowered capillary density (<7 capillaries/mm), frequent giant capillaries and microhaemorrhages

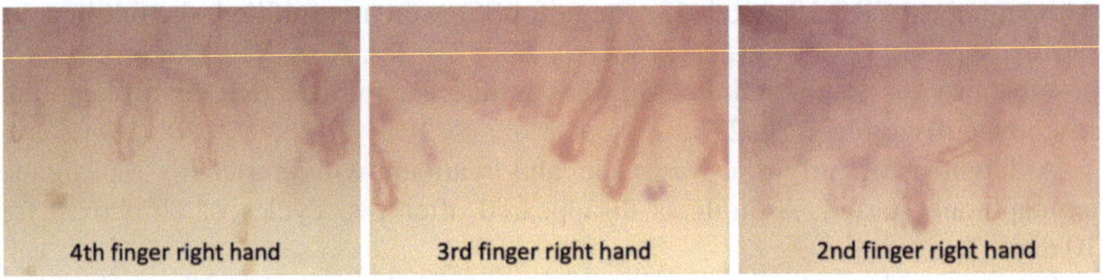

Fig. 10 Nailfold videocapillaroscopy 18 months later (3 years after RP onset), showing the "Late" scleroderma-pattern (×200). The "Late" scleroderma-pattern of microangiopathy is characterized by loss of capillaries combined with abnormal shaped capillaries (representing neoangiogenesis), while giant capillaries are not present

Sclerodactyly and diffuse skin involvement were present, with a mRSS of 19. She was also complaining of mild dysphagia.

NFC demonstrated a "Late" pattern of microangiopathy (Fig. 10) [35, 36].

Together with the severity of nailfold capillary abnormalities, internal organ involvement was also found to have developed:

High resolution computed tomography scan of thorax: interstitial lung disease,
Spirometry + DLCO: FVC 86%, DLCO 83%, still normal but function decreased,
Esophageal manometry: esophageal dysmotility,
Renal Doppler-echography: normal/borderline renal artery resistive indexes (0.69 bilaterally),
Echocardiogram: Estimated PAPs 36 mmHg (increased since last visit),
ANA positive (title 1:640) with the nucleolar IIF pattern, and among SSc-specific autoantibodies, anti-fibrillarin were detected positive.

Discussion

This clinical case describes the "natural" evolution of SSc in a patient with RP at initial clinical presentation.

Patients with RP, positive antinuclear antibodies and specific nailfold capillary abnormalities should be strictly monitored as they are at high risk of developing SSc.

The assessment of both ANA and extent of specific abnormalities at nailfold capillaroscopy helps to inform the correct diagnosis, as well as to obtain useful predictive/prognostic information.

If not possible to detect SSc-specific autoantibodies, particular attention should be paid to the ANA pattern at IIF, as the nucleolar pattern represents a risk factor for a faster and progressive disease.

SSc patients whose nailfold microangiopathy rapidly progresses over a few months are at high risk of developing severe organ involvement.

References

1. Hughes M, Allanore Y, Chung L, Pauling JD, Denton CP, Matucci-Cerrinic M, et al. Raynaud's phenomenon and digital ulcers in systemic sclerosis. Nat Rev Rheumatol. 2020;4(4):208–21.
2. Abou-Raya A, Abou-Raya S, Helmii M. Statins: potentially useful in therapy of systemic sclerosis-related Raynaud's phenomenon and digital ulcers. J Rheumatol. 2008 Sep;35(9):1801–8.
3. Hughes M, Ong VH, Anderson ME, Hall F, Moinzadeh P, Griffiths B, et al. Consensus best practice pathway of the UK scleroderma study group: digital vasculopathy in systemic sclerosis. Rheumatology (Oxford). 2015;54(11):2015–24.
4. Matucci-Cerinic M, Denton CP, Furst DE, Mayes MD, Hsu VM, Carpentier P, et al. Bosentan treatment of digital ulcers related to systemic sclerosis: results from the RAPIDS-2 randomised, double-blind, placebo-controlled trial. Ann Rheum Dis. 2011 Jan;70(1):32–8.
5. Ngcozana T, Ong VH, Denton CP. Improving access to digital ulcer care through nurse-led clinic: a service evaluation. Musculoskeletal Care. 2020 Mar;18(1):92–7.
6. Hughes M, Alcacer-Pitarch B, Gheorghiu AM, Praino E, Sandler RD, Tavor Y, et al. Digital ulcer debridement in systemic sclerosis: a systematic literature review. Clin Rheumatol. 2020;39(3):805–11.
7. Hughes M, Alcacer-Pitarch B, Allanore Y, Baron M, Boin F, Bruni C, et al. Digital ulcers: should debridement be a standard of care in systemic sclerosis? Lancet Rheumatol. 2020;2(5):e302–7.
8. Sharp CA, Akram Q, Hughes M, Muir L, Herrick AL. Differential diagnosis of critical digital ischemia in systemic sclerosis: report of five cases and review of the literature. Semin Arthritis Rheum. 2016;46(2):209–16.
9. Bellando-Randone S, Del Galdo F, Lepri G, Minier T, Huscher D, Furst DE, et al. Progression of patients with Raynaud's phenomenon to systemic sclerosis: a five-year analysis of the European scleroderma trial and research group multicentre, longitudinal registry study for very early diagnosis of systemic sclerosis (VEDOSS). Lancet Rheumatol. 2021;3(12):e834–43.
10. Pauling JD, Hughes M, Pope JE. Raynaud's phenomenon—an update on diagnosis, classification and management. Clin Rheumatol. 2019;38(12):3317–30.
11. Doridot L, Jeljeli M, Chêne C, Batteux F. Implication of oxidative stress in the pathogenesis of systemic sclerosis via inflammation, autoimmunity and fibrosis. Redox Biol. 2019;25:101122.
12. Melsens K, Cutolo M, Schonenberg-Meinema D, Foeldvari I, Leone MC, Mostmans Y, et al. Standardized nailfold capillaroscopy in children with rheumatic diseases: a worldwide study. Rheumatology. 2023;62(4):1605–15.
13. Terreri MTRA, Andrade LEC, Puccinelli ML, Hilário MOE, Goldenberg J. Nail fold capillaroscopy: normal findings in children and adolescents. Semin Arthritis Rheum. 1999;29(1):36–42.
14. Piotto DP, Sekiyama J, Kayser C, Yamada M, Len CA, Terreri MT. Nailfold videocapillaroscopy in healthy children and adolescents: description of normal patterns. Clin Exp Rheumatol. 2016;34(Suppl 100):193–9.
15. Farenhorst CA, Roon AM, Gessel AI, Stel AJ, Bootsma H, Armbrust W, et al. Capillary microscopy is a potential screening method for connective tissue disease in children with Raynaud's phenomenon. Pediatr Rheumatol. 2022;20(1):11.
16. Torrente-Segarra V, Hernández-Baldizón S, Mosquera JM, Antón J. The importance of nailfold capillaroscopy in children with rheumatic diseases. Clin Exp Rheumatol. 2021;39(Suppl 128):35.
17. Falcini F, Rigante D, Candelli M, Martini G, Corona F, Petaccia A, et al. Anti-nuclear antibodies as predictor of outcome in a multi-center cohort of Italian children and adolescents with Raynaud's phenomenon. Clin Rheumatol. 2015;34(1):167–9.
18. Nigrovic PA, Fuhlbrigge RC, Sundel RP. Raynaud's phenomenon in children: a retrospective review of 123 patients. Pediatrics. 2003 Apr;111(4 Pt 1):715–21.
19. Pain CE, Constantin T, Toplak N, Moll M, Iking-Konert C, Piotto DP, et al. Raynaud's syndrome in children: systematic review and development of recommendations for assessment and monitoring. Clin Exp Rheumatol. 2016;34(Suppl 100):200–6.

20. Foeldvari I, Klotsche J, Kasapcopur O, Adrovic A, Terreri MT, Sakamoto AP, et al. Differences sustained between diffuse and limited forms of juvenile systemic sclerosis in an expanded international cohort. Arthritis Care Res. 2022;74(10):1575–84.
21. Zulian F, Woo P, Athreya BH, Laxer RM, Medsger TAJ, Lehman TJA, et al. The Pediatric rheumatology European society/American College of Rheumatology/European league against rheumatism provisional classification criteria for juvenile systemic sclerosis. Arthritis Rheum. 2007;57(2):203–12.
22. Foeldvari I, Klotsche J, Torok K, Kasapcopur O, Adrovic A, Feldman B, et al. POS0758 presence of nailfold capillary changes correlates with more severe organ involvement in juvenile systemic scleroderma. Results of the juvenile scleroderma inception cohort. Ann Rheum Dis. 2024;83:1165–6.
23. Cutolo M, Sulli A, Pizzorni C, Accardo S. Nailfold videocapillaroscopy assessment of microvascular damage in systemic sclerosis. J Rheumatol. 2000;27(1):155–60.
24. Cutolo M, Pizzorni C, Tuccio M, Burroni A, Craviotto C, Basso M, et al. Nailfold videocapillaroscopic patterns and serum autoantibodies in systemic sclerosis. Rheumatology (Oxford). 2004;43(6):719–26.
25. Smith V, Ickinger C, Hysa E, Snow M, Frech T, Sulli A, et al. Nailfold capillaroscopy. Best Pract Res Clin Rheumatol. 2023;37(1):101849.
26. Smith V, Herrick AL, Ingegnoli F, Damjanov N, De Angelis R, Denton CP, et al. Standardisation of nailfold capillaroscopy for the assessment of patients with Raynaud's phenomenon and systemic sclerosis. Autoimmun Rev. 2020;19(3):102458.
27. van den Hoogen F, Khanna D, Fransen J, Johnson SR, Baron M, Tyndall A, et al. 2013 classification criteria for systemic sclerosis: an American College of Rheumatology/European league against rheumatism collaborative initiative. Arthritis Rheum. 2013;65(11):2737–47.
28. LeRoy EC, Medsger TA. Criteria for the classification of early systemic sclerosis. J Rheumatol. 2001;28(7):1573–6.
29. Minier T, Guiducci S, Bellando-Randone S, Bruni C, Lepri G, Czirják L, et al. Preliminary analysis of the very early diagnosis of systemic sclerosis (VEDOSS) EUSTAR multicentre study: evidence for puffy fingers as a pivotal sign for suspicion of systemic sclerosis. Ann Rheum Dis. 2014;73(12):2087–93.
30. Sulli A, Ruaro B, Smith V, Pizzorni C, Zampogna G, Gallo M, et al. Progression of nailfold microvascular damage and antinuclear antibody pattern in systemic sclerosis. J Rheumatol. 2013;40(5):634–9.
31. Sulli A, Pizzorni C, Smith V, Zampogna G, Ravera F, Cutolo M. Timing of transition between capillaroscopic patterns in systemic sclerosis. Arthritis Rheum. 2012;64(3):821–5.
32. Sulli A, Paolino S, Pizzorni C, Ferrari G, Pacini G, Pesce G, et al. Progression of nailfold capillaroscopic patterns and correlation with organ involvement in systemic sclerosis: a 12 year study. Rheumatology (Oxford). 2020;59(5):1051–8.
33. Marino Claverie L, Knobel E, Takashima L, Techera L, Oliver M, Gonzalez P, et al. Organ involvement in Argentinian systemic sclerosis patients with "late" pattern as compared to patients with "early/active" pattern by nailfold capillaroscopy. Clin Rheumatol. 2013;32(6):839–43.
34. Ingegnoli F, Ardoino I, Boracchi P, Cutolo M. Nailfold capillaroscopy in systemic sclerosis: data from the EULAR scleroderma trials and research (EUSTAR) database. Microvasc Res. 2013;89:122–8.
35. Smith V, Riccieri V, Pizzorni C, Decuman S, Deschepper E, Bonroy C, et al. Nailfold capillaroscopy for prediction of novel future severe organ involvement in systemic sclerosis. J Rheumatol. 2013;40(12):2023–8.
36. Paxton D, Pauling JD. Does nailfold capillaroscopy help predict future outcomes in systemic sclerosis? A systematic literature review. Semin Arthritis Rheum. 2018;48(3):482–94.

MIX
Papier aus verantwortungsvollen Quellen
Paper from responsible sources
FSC® C105338

If you have any concerns about our products,
you can contact us on
ProductSafety@springernature.com

In case Publisher is established outside the EU,
the EU authorized representative is:
Springer Nature Customer Service Center GmbH
Europaplatz 3, 69115 Heidelberg, Germany

Printed by Libri Plureos GmbH
in Hamburg, Germany